EDUCATING THE BODY

A History of Physical Education in Canada

Educating the Body

A History of Physical Education in Canada

M. ANN HALL, BRUCE KIDD,
AND PATRICIA VERTINSKY

UNIVERSITY OF TORONTO PRESS
Toronto Buffalo London

© University of Toronto Press 2024
Toronto Buffalo London
utorontopress.com

ISBN 978-1-4875-0856-2 (cloth) ISBN 978-1-4875-3851-4 (EPUB)
ISBN 978-1-4875-2594-1 (paper) ISBN 978-1-4875-3850-7 (PDF)

Library and Archives Canada Cataloguing in Publication

Title: Educating the body : a history of physical education in Canada /
M. Ann Hall, Bruce Kidd, and Patricia Vertinsky.
Names: Hall, M. Ann (Margaret Ann), 1942– author. | Kidd, Bruce, author. |
Vertinsky, Patricia Anne, 1942– author.
Description: Includes bibliographical references and index.
Identifiers: Canadiana (print) 2023046792X | Canadiana (ebook) 20230467954 |
ISBN 9781487508562 (cloth) | ISBN 9781487525941 (paper) |
ISBN 9781487538507 (PDF) | ISBN 9781487538514 (EPUB)
Subjects: LCSH: Physical education and training – Canada – History.
Classification: LCC GV225.A1 H35 2024 | DDC 796.071071 – dc23

Cover design: Brad Norr Design
Cover images: (top left, middle) *Syllabus of Physical Exercises for Schools*, published by the Executive Council, Strathcona Trust, 1911, 40; (bottom) City of Vancouver Archives, 1184-2355, photograph by Jack Lindsay; (back) City of Vancouver Archives, Sp P46.4

We wish to acknowledge the land on which the University of Toronto Press operates. This land is the traditional territory of the Wendat, the Anishnaabeg, the Haudenosaunee, the Métis, and the Mississaugas of the Credit First Nation.

This book has been published with the help of a grant from the Federation for the Humanities and Social Sciences, through the Awards to Scholarly Publications Program, using funds provided by the Social Sciences and Humanities Research Council of Canada.

University of Toronto Press acknowledges the financial support of the Government of Canada, the Canada Council for the Arts, and the Ontario Arts Council, an agency of the Government of Ontario, for its publishing activities.

 Canada Council   Conseil des Arts
for the Arts   du Canada

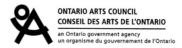

ONTARIO ARTS COUNCIL
CONSEIL DES ARTS DE L'ONTARIO
an Ontario government agency
un organisme du gouvernement de l'Ontario

Funded by the   Financé par le
Government   gouvernement
of Canada   du Canada

*We dedicate this book to the memory of two outstanding
Canadian physical educators:*

Dr. Doris Plewes (1898–1994)
Teacher, volunteer, physical fitness advocate, bureaucrat, visionary

Dr. Stewart Davidson (1921–2002)
*University professor and administrator, national
and international leader, historian*

Contents

List of Illustrations   xi

Acknowledgments   xv

INTRODUCTION   3

1 RYERSON AND HIS VISION   15

    Ryerson and His Times   16
    Creating the Educational State   19
    Developing Physical Education   20
    Ryerson, Industrial Schools, and Physical Education   24
    Physical Education after Ryerson   28
    Expanding Physical Education in the Schools   36
    Indigenous Schooling in the Late Nineteenth Century   38
    Calisthenics, Drill, and Recreation in Indigenous Schools   41

2 TOWARDS A PAN-CANADIAN CURRICULUM   45

    Canadian Imperialism and Lord Strathcona   47
    Indigenous Schooling and Physical Education   52
    Cadet Movement and Militarism   55
    Challenging the Military Drill Approach   58
    Early Youth Movements and Physical Education   65

3 THE MARGARET EATON SCHOOL: FORTY YEARS OF WOMEN'S PHYSICAL EDUCATION — 75

- The Female Tradition in Physical Education — 77
- The New Kinesthetic of Modernism — 78
- Emma Scott Raff: Elegance and Expression — 82
- Mary Hamilton: Beauty and Fitness — 86
- Florence Somers: Femininity and Charm — 94
- The Margaret Eaton School in Retrospect — 98

4 FIT FOR LIVING — 100

- Creating a National Association for Physical Education — 101
- School Physical Education across the Provinces — 103
- Physical Education in the Indian Residential Schools — 108
- Dominion–Provincial Physical Training Programs — 112
- Wartime National Physical Fitness Act — 117
- Youth Movements in the Depression and Wartime — 120

5 SETTING A HEROIC AGENDA – REALIZING THE POSSIBILITIES — 126

- Promoting Fitness for the Masses — 127
- Sad State of Physical Education in Canadian Schools — 133
- Contested Terrain of Movement Education — 137
- Physical Education in the Indian Residential and Day Schools — 148

6 CHANGING TIMES AND NEW INITIATIVES — 157

- Changing Context — 157
- Making Physical Education Relevant — 160
- Max Fourestier and the Vanves Experiment — 163
- Children and Physical Activity — 166
- ParticipACTION — 168
- Quality Daily Physical Education — 171
- Establishing Dance within Physical Education — 173
- Sport in Schools — 174
- Physical Education and Sport in the Universities — 179
- The Rise of Kinesiology — 182

7 SEEKING OPTIMISM IN A CONTESTED FIELD — 188

Physical and Health Education Curricula across Canada: A Snapshot — 189
Physically Educated versus Physically Literate — 193
Training Physical Education Teachers — 198
Physical Education versus Kinesiology in Higher Education — 200
Equity, Diversity, Inclusion, and Social Justice — 202
Disability Inclusion through Adaptive Physical Activity — 209
Promoting Sport and Physical Activity for All — 213

AFTERWORD: PHYSICAL EDUCATION FOR THE FUTURE — 217

Rediscovering the Benefits of the Outdoors — 219
Physical and Health Education Using Digital Technologies — 221
Ongoing Struggle over Health and Physical Education
    Curriculum Development — 223
Higher Education Training in Physical and Health Education — 226
Meaningful Physical Education: A New Approach? — 228
Indigeneity and EDI Initiatives: Still a Long Way to Go — 229

Appendix: R. Tait McKenzie Honour Award Winners — 235
Notes — 245
Bibliography — 267
Index — 287

Illustrations

Figures

I.1	Kahnawake Lacrosse Club, Montreal, Quebec, 1867	9
1.1	Rev. Egerton Ryerson, D.D., L.L.D., 1886	18
1.2	An example of Ryerson's gymnastic exercises	22
1.3	Frederick S. Barnjum, 1863	30
1.4	Competition for the Wickstead Medals, McGill University, 1886–7	32
1.5	Frederick Barnjum's women's gymnastic group, Montreal, Quebec, 1870	32
1.6	Shingwauk Home for Boys, Sault Ste. Marie, Ontario, 1886	40
1.7	Annual sports day at the Battleford Indian Industrial School, Saskatchewan, 1895	43
2.1	Sir Donald Smith, Lord Strathcona, 1895	48
2.2	*Syllabus of Physical Exercises for Schools*, 1911	51
2.3	Cadet Corps, St. Paul's Industrial School (near Winnipeg), 1900	58
2.4	Band of St. Paul's Industrial School, 1900	59
2.5	Girls' Calisthenic Club, St. Paul's Industrial School, 1900	59
2.6	Arthur S. Lamb, 1926	61
2.7	Ethel Mary Cartwright, 1927	63
2.8	Exercise lawn drill at Mount Allison Ladies College, Sackville, New Brunswick, 1918	65
2.9	John Howard Crocker, L.L.D., University of Western Ontario, 1950	67

2.10	Mary Beaton instructs swimmers at the McGill Street YWCA, Toronto, 1910	69
3.1	Genevieve Stebbins, principal of the New York School of Expression, 1892	81
3.2	Emma Scott Raff and Margaret Wilson Beattie Eaton	83
3.3	Margaret Eaton School of Literature and Expression, c. 1908	85
3.4	Mary Ross Barker	87
3.5	Mary Hamilton, c. 1925	89
3.6	Counsellors at Camp Tanamakoon with Mary Hamilton, 1946	91
3.7	Mary Hamilton and a counsellor at Camp Tanamakoon	92
3.8	Florence A. Somers	95
4.1	Ethel Mary Cartwright, 1942	105
4.2	Cécile G. Grenier, 1939	107
4.3	Specialists in Physical Education, Ontario College of Education, 1930–1	109
4.4	Pelican Lake Indian Residential School, c. 1927	110
4.5	Girls' physical training class at Pelican Lake Indian Residential School, 1941	111
4.6	Women in a Pro-Rec fitness display in Stanley Park, Vancouver, 1940	114
4.7	Pro-Rec members putting on a display at the University of British Columbia, c. 1940	115
4.8	Poster announcing a camp for girl athletes at the Ontario Athletic Commission Camp, c. 1938	116
4.9	Ian Eisenhardt cartoon in the *Montreal Herald*, 1944	119
4.10	Kathlyn Hall as a Girl Guide, 1930	121
5.1	Dr. Doris W. Plewes, 1948	131
5.2	Lloyd Percival teaching young boys the sprint start, 1966	131
5.3	First Ontario Athletic Leadership Camp for boys, Lake Couchiching, Ontario, 1948	136
5.4	Ontario Athletic Leadership Camp for girls, Lake Couchiching, Ontario, 1958	137
5.5	Rudolf Laban with dancers of the Berlin State Opera, 1934	139
5.6	Movement education in elementary school	143
5.7	Creative dance in elementary school	149
5.8	Ian Eisenhardt, 1950	150
5.9	Skating on Round Lake at Celia Jeffrey Indian Residential School, Kenora, Ontario, c. 1951	151

5.10	Tobogganing at Birtle Indian Residential School, Manitoba, c. 1950	152
5.11	Boys playing hockey at Pelican Lake Indian Residential School, c. 1951	155
6.1	Donald Macintosh	161
6.2	Children from the Gambetta School Kindergarten in Vanves, France, 1959	164
6.3	Professor Donald Bailey, Physical Education, University of Saskatchewan, measuring vertical jumps, 1960	167
6.4	ParticipACTION poster from the early years of the fitness campaign, 1973–9	169
6.5	Useful Canadian resource on quality daily physical activities	172
6.6	Founding members of the Canadian Association for the Advancement of Women and Sport, 1981	177
6.7	Canadian university women athletes in action	181
6.8	Students in the Bachelor of Kinesiology program, Faculty of Kinesiology, Sport, and Recreation, University of Alberta	186
7.1	Recommended time allocations for physical education instruction by province, 2014	191
7.2	Physical literacy for life, a model for physical education promoted by PHE Canada	195
7.3	Earle F. Zeigler, early portrait	203
7.4	Earle F. Zeigler, later portrait	204
7.5	First Nations youth participating in a traditional lacrosse game in Montreal, Quebec, 2017	206
7.6	Ice Hockey in Gjoa Haven, an Inuit hamlet in Nunavut	208
7.7	Children experiencing disability playing with basketballs	212

Tables

1.1	Growth of the Ontario School System, 1847–76	37
1.2	Growth of physical education in Ontario, 1871–1901	38
2.1	Influence of the Strathcona Trust in Ontario, 1911–31	52

Acknowledgments

As authors, both individually and collectively, we have a long association with physical education – together it adds up to over 150 years and counting. It would be impossible to thank the many students and colleagues who have helped shaped our view of this field, and who like us have witnessed its ongoing changes and challenges. Many of these colleagues have long since passed away. However, for this particular project, we would like to mention several individuals who were more than generous with their time and expertise. They are Peter Donnelly, Janice Forsyth, Donna Goodwin, Joannie Halas, Douglas Gleddie, Michael Heine, Michelle Kilborn, Anna Lathrop, Jenna Lorusso, and Stephen McGinley.

Finding photographs for this project was challenging, but the task was made so much easier by the many archivists and librarians who responded to our requests. We are particularly grateful to the archives, universities, organizations, and individuals who provided these images free of charge. We would especially like to thank Marnee Gamble, Special Media Archivist at the University of Toronto Archives for her assistance.

We were probably able to complete this project faster than normally because for over two years, we could not go anywhere due to COVID. No doubt our spouses and partners were subjected to more discussion about this research than they wished to hear. In this regard, we thank Jane Haslett for her careful reading of our initial drafts, which became more coherent because of her input.

Finally, we thank all those at the University of Toronto Press (UTP) who helped with the production of *Educating the Body*. We are especially grateful to our editor Len Husband for recognizing the value of this project, and encouraging us throughout the writing process. We also appreciated the comments and suggestions made by several anonymous reviewers of the first draft of the manuscript, all of which improved the book. James Leahy did a masterful job of copy-editing, improving our writing immeasurably, and the production process was smoothly coordinated by Janice Evans. A book like this one requires a comprehensive index, and we thank Judy Dunlop of Judy Dunlop Information Services for her masterly job. If we have forgotten anyone else, especially at UTP, who helped bring this book to an audience, we thank you too.

EDUCATING THE BODY

A History of Physical Education in Canada

Introduction

Humans have always sought to instruct their young in what they believed to be the healthy and socially appropriate use and display of their bodies, as well as the practices of valued games and dances. We can call it physical education. It is indispensable for growth, development, and culture. In the territory now known as Canada, virtually every group that has lived here, beginning with the Indigenous peoples who arrived millennia ago, has provided for and engaged in such instruction. This also includes the French fur traders, fishers, farmers, and loggers who settled the St. Lawrence basin in the seventeenth century; the British militias, merchants, and settlers who won military, economic, and political control in the eighteenth century; and the successive diasporas of nineteenth-, twentieth-, and twenty-first-century immigrants. But the ways in which different peoples have fashioned and carried out this instruction have differed significantly from group to group, time to time, and place to place.

This book sets out a history of physical education in Canada, with a focus on the major advocates, innovators, and institutions that have steered and conducted it, and the conditions that have shaped their efforts. We consider the primary intents, methods, and institutions of different groups, as well as the differences between them. We also examine the ways in which the young have taken up, revised, or resisted these different precepts and practices. It is a remarkable story of vision, innovation, persistence, and achievement.

In recent times, the most widely recognized form of physical education has been conducted in the state schools, which is a central theme of this book. In fact, the Euro-Canadian beginnings of physical education began with efforts to create state-supported schooling in pre-Confederation Canada. We also examine the purposes and activities of the playgrounds, public recreation programs, summer camps, youth groups, and, to a lesser extent, the various ethnic, political, and religious organizations, community clubs, and private entrepreneurs who conducted forms of physical education. Of course, groups within society have also instructed their young in other forms of physical exertion. Labour and military historians have examined the embodied knowledge, skills, and habits required by productive activity, the workplace, and military service. Before the modern era, training for production, including warfare, was the most prevalent form of physical instruction. But while such regimes trained the body in significant ways, often requiring great skill, courage, and tremendous amounts of physical energy, such activities are beyond the scope of this book.

The history of physical education cannot be told in isolation from the economic, political, and social circumstances in which it took place, and especially the character and ideology of the groups who championed it. This also applies to the institutions and resources they possessed to make it available. Most physical education has been imagined, argued for, developed, carried out, or, on the other hand, neglected, with an explicit social purpose. While individual lessons are planned and delivered with the acquisition of discrete knowledge, physical skills, and strengths as immediate outcomes – think instruction in sports, dance, or fitness – most forms of the enterprise have been linked to larger objectives such as social stability, public health, gender relations, and cultural identity. Given the central role of the Canadian state in the development and conduct of physical education, and the largely white, male Euro-Canadian groups who led the country, the narratives of national defence, health, and "nation-building" play a major role in our story.

We recognize that Canada is not a homogeneous country, and although we have tried to describe and analyse developments in all parts of the country, we were not as successful as we would have liked. There is far more information available from Ontario than from any other jurisdiction. Canada is a classed, gendered, and racialized society, and we pay attention to these realities throughout. The way the state included children of different classes, genders, and social backgrounds in physical education differed significantly, as our discussion of physical education for girls and young women, as well as children and youth in the Indigenous residential schools, will disturbingly show. On the other hand, outside the state schools, many youth groups developed powerfully affirming programs for the children and youth under their care. Some subordinate groups taught physical education as a means of strengthening adherence to other ideas, even opposition to the dominant order. For example, long before the Quiet Revolution, the Catholic youth movement's vast sports programs in Quebec sought to inculcate francophone youth in distinctly Quebecois – not Canadian – allegiances. During the 1920s and 1930s, the Workers'

Sports Association of Canada sought to socialize and strengthen young men and women for activism against the capitalist state. In Black churches, and immigrant clubs and summer camps, physical education and sports were conducted to inculcate pride in their cultures of origin, and in women's clubs, an assertive feminism. These efforts were carried out in parallel with school-based physical education. We cannot fully understand how physical education has been planned, rolled out, and experienced without some understanding of the ideologies, political economy, and social structure of Canada.

The history of physical education is also inseparable from the changing scholarship about Canada, the Canadian state, public education, health, physical activity, sport, and the body. It is also tied to the changing nature of the major institutions that stimulate this scholarship, especially the universities, which grant degrees in physical education and encourage their faculty and students to conduct relevant research. Three developments in particular have shaped our analysis. In the first place, the significant growth of critical, social scientific research about physical education and sport during the last fifty years, written from an evolving series of perspectives, has given us a wealth of material to draw upon. In keeping with wider trends in the social sciences, scholars have adapted and in turn integrated social history, materialist, feminist, post-structuralist, queer studies, and other theoretical approaches to examine the changing nature of physical education. Most recently, the focus has been on the impact of different practices upon different abilities, genders, sexualities, racialized people, and the way these are incorporated into the "body," a concept with its own elaborate vocabulary and analysis.

These trends in scholarship have in turn been shaped by a second, simultaneous shift in North American universities. The preparation of teachers, coaches, and fitness leaders that preoccupied the early decades of university physical education has been replaced by a new ambition known as kinesiology.[1] In some institutions, kinesiology connotes a broad, multi-disciplinary effort to study and teach about all aspects of human movement, drawing upon the major disciplines from the humanities and social sciences to the biological and physical sciences. In such degree programs, kinesiology has become a comprehensive liberal arts program focused on the human body. In other universities, kinesiology has come to mean a new health profession, employing the movement sciences to enhance various forms of rehabilitation. The displacement of university-based physical education by kinesiology is both subject and context for our story.

The third change that informs this book is the rethinking of the nature of Canada and the Canadian state that has taken place in recent years. The revision of received wisdom is an ongoing dynamic of research, scholarship, and debate, as unexpected events and changing circumstances pose new questions. Scholars must also develop new ways of seeing, pursue new approaches to investigation and explanation, and generate and wrestle with new evidence. This process has been accelerated by the publication in 2015 of the *Final Report of the Truth and Reconciliation Commission of Canada*.[2] The major findings of the Truth and Reconciliation Commission (TRC) about the residential schools were already known to Indigenous communities, and scholars have written extensively about them.[3] They built upon the oral histories of Indigenous peoples, the work of earlier scholars, court documents, and other public inquiries such as the 1996 Royal Commission on Aboriginal Peoples in Canada. But the TRC caused a sea change in scholarly and public understanding. As the Canadian Historical Association observed, the "TRC became a vehicle for a wider, more critical discussion of the past *and* the present of Canadian colonialism, and the multiple ways it has cost Indigenous people and shaped Canada. The TRC was in no small way a reckoning with Canadian history."[4]

The TRC was a mammoth undertaking. It was established in 2008 as part of the Indian Residential Schools Settlement Agreement between the federal government and the approximately 8,000 Indigenous children and youth who had attended residential schools operating in Canada between 1883 and 1996. Led by commissioners Murray Sinclair, Wilton Littlechild, and Marie Wilson, the TRC conducted extensive research, public engagement, and advocacy. The commissioners and research staff pored over the records left in various archives by Canadian governments and the churches that ran the schools, repeatedly going to court to compel Canada to produce them. They interviewed more than 6,000 people, most of whom were survivors of the schools, to produce an oral history archive.

The TRC commissioners argue that if the constitutional and treaty rights of First Nations, Inuit, and Métis, as the original, self-determining people of the land known as Canada, are to be recognized and respected, a new dialogue between settlers and Indigenous peoples is urgently needed. They call such dialogue "reconciliation." For mutual healing, reconciliation requires "public truth sharing, apology, and commemoration that acknowledge and redress past harms."[5] Truth-telling also requires that the full history of residential schools – why they were established, how they were conducted, and their impact upon Indigenous children and communities – should be known to all, so that it can never be forgotten. Several of the TRC's ninety-six recommendations or "calls to action" speak to the practice of researching, writing, and teaching this history. For example, the commissioners called upon governments to "provide the necessary funding to post-secondary institutions to educate teachers on how to integrate Indigenous knowledge and teaching methods into classrooms."[6] They also recommended commemorative projects on the theme of reconciliation, including a national heritage plan for commemorating residential schooling, a statutory holiday, and monuments to residential schools in capital cities. On 30 September 2021, the first National Day for Truth and Reconciliation honoured the lost children and survivors of residential schools, their families, and communities.

Not surprisingly, because Sinclair and Littlechild began their careers as physical educators, and Littlechild is a distinguished sports leader, five calls to action addressed physical activity and sport. In brief, the commissioners recommended public education that tells the national story of Indigenous athletes in history; long-term Indigenous athlete development and growth; continuous support for the North American Indigenous Games; mainstream physical activity and sport policies, programs, and competitions that include Indigenous peoples and also reflect their diverse cultures and traditional sporting activities; and full consultation when international games are located on Indigenous territories.[7]

The TRC challenges us to rethink the history of Canada and the relationship between settler Canadians and Indigenous peoples, as well as the creation and extension of the Canadian state. It illuminates the erasures in historical memory that have taken place about the role of Indigenous people in the development of Canadian society. It sheds harsh light upon settler governments' failure to honour the various treaties they signed with the Indigenous peoples, and the brutal forced removals, deliberate neglect, incarcerations, and cultural genocide practised by successive governments as a way of opening and securing the northern land mass for European settlement and capitalist development. It challenges every one of us to understand the story of Canada in terms of the dynamic interaction between Indigenous peoples and the various forms of "colonialism" practised and enjoyed by those of us who arrived over the last 500 years.[8] With the revelations in 2021 of the remains of over 200 Indigenous children at the former Kamloops Indian Residential School and at other sites, the grim realization of the true nature and trajectory of Canadian history has only intensified. This reckoning has led cities, universities, schools, and sports organizations to reconsider their role in Canadian history, and in some cases, change the names of institutions, streets, teams, and awards, or remove statues, including those of John A. Macdonald, Canada's first prime minister.

As historians of physical education, it is incumbent upon us to keep in play the disturbing dynamics between Euro-Canadian and Indigenous schooling, and the very different consequences for both groups. While settler physical education was planned and delivered to build up the Euro-Canadian nation, it was simultaneously promoted and taught in the residential schools to break down and suppress traditional Indigenous knowledge and practices, and to assimilate Indigenous children to Euro-Canadian ways. As the TRC recommends: "All Canadian children and youth deserve to know Canada's honest history, including what happened in the residential schools."[9]

At the time of first European contact, physical activity was integral to Indigenous peoples across North America. They ran, swam, paddled, constructed dwellings and watercraft, transported packs and children, hunted, fished, and much else. These were survival skills. The semi-nomadic Indigenous cultures required frequent travel in search of food and shelter, aerobic fitness to venture and communicate across long distances, speed and dexterity to chase down game, strength and balance to move heavy loads from camp to camp, and courage, pain endurance, and stamina for moments of crisis, including harsh weather, childbirth, encounters with large game, and warfare. Since so many of these skills and strengths were necessary for travel, hunting, and fishing, they reinforced the Indigenous peoples' close connection to the land and gave them a comprehensive source of practical, embodied, and spiritual knowledge about the natural environment. Indigenous peoples also engaged in a rich variety of competitions, games, and dances. They tested each other in all manner of life skills through indoor and outdoor games. Their ball games, like the Haudenosaunee *tewaarathon*, could engage hundreds of players, both men and women, and thousands of spectators, and often served as occasions for spiritual ceremonies and diplomacy. All these skills and games were taught to the young.

In their first encounters with Indigenous peoples, Europeans admired these practices and sang their praises to their patrons and readers back home. They commended them for ensuring that all members of their communities became proficient in such skills and recommended that European societies emulate them. One French explorer noted that the Indigenous peoples he met were "very robust; men, women and even children are extremely vigorous ... they escape maladies which beset most of our Europeans for want of exercise."[10] George W. Beers, the father of modern lacrosse, speculated about the "unparalleled union of strength, agility and wind" developed by and necessary for the original Indigenous game. The sport, he argued, "brought out the very finest physical attributes of the finest made men in the world," given that "all the education of an Indian from cradle to manhood tended to physical development."[11]

Yet in the course of contact, much of this remarkable culture of physical activity was undermined, even lost. Most Indigenous communities, even those with no direct contact, were decimated by influenza, smallpox, measles, and other diseases brought by the Europeans to which they had no immunity. Others fell to European violence and Indigenous conflicts inflamed by European trading rivalries and guns. Such devastating losses, migration and integration with other groups, and continual interaction with European cultures, significantly altered traditional beliefs and living

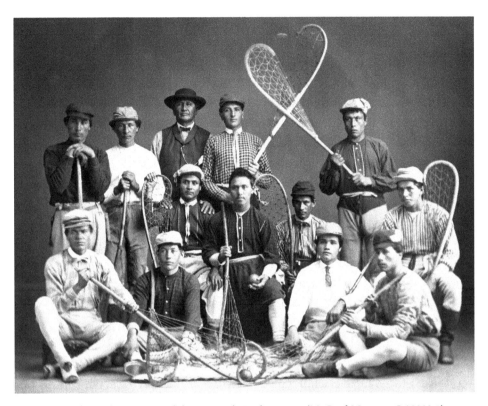

Figure I.1. Kahnawake Lacrosse Club, Montreal, Quebec, 1867 (McCord Museum, I-29099.1)

patterns. Some Indigenous games were appropriated and turned into Euro-Canadian sports. *Tewaarathon*, for example, was refashioned into lacrosse, while Indigenous players were banned from participation.[12] By the late nineteenth century, when the new state of Canada forced the removal of Indigenous people onto small, remote reserves, and then sought to assimilate their children in residential schools, much traditional knowledge was completely abandoned or forgotten.

Very little of the extraordinary Indigenous tradition of physical activity, with its remarkable record of instruction and inclusion, including the full participation of girls and women, was incorporated into what became Canadian physical education. It has been poorer for this failure. By the time we start our story with the development of school-based programs in the mid-nineteenth century, the educational leaders of the emerging Canadian state looked only to Europe and the United States for inspiration. It was not only that Indigenous peoples were no longer needed for exploration, trade, and military defence, the European entrepreneurs and settlers flooding into Canada wanted their land for logging, mining, farming, cities, and towns, and to that end, wanted them gone. They wanted no part of the imperial government's recognition of Indigenous rights and the promise of protection in the Royal Proclamation of 1763, the Niagara Treaty of 1764, and other treaties and agreements. As historian Allan Greer has argued, settlers were passionate about the Enlightenment ideals of individual rights to the possession of property, and therefore looked down upon Indigenous peoples for their fiercely prized sense of collective ownership. The logical outcomes of this ideology were the reserve system created by Canadian governments; the systemic neglect of the treaty undertakings they made; the Indian Act that infiltrated every aspect of Indigenous peoples' lives; and the residential schools that seized them from reserves to assimilate them.[13] We tell this part of the difficult story in our account of physical education in the residential schools.

We were led to write this book by our shared concern for the marginalization of physical education in many Canadian schools and universities in recent years, and the relative decline in historical scholarship about the field. After several worrying conversations at conferences, we decided to write an up-to-date history ourselves. Our understanding of physical education has been shaped by engaged experience as well as critical scholarship. The three of us are white, privileged, cisgender academics who attended state schools (two of us in Ontario, the third in the United Kingdom) in the period immediately following the Second World War, when physical education was a taken-for-granted essential component of every child's education. We also took part in community sport and physical activity, and one of us was talented enough to become an Olympic athlete. We played leadership roles in the schools we attended, the youth groups we joined, and the universities where we have worked. We have all have taught physical education and coached sports at some point in our lives. In many ways we are both "products" and exemplars of physical education.

In addition to these shared experiences, each of us brings distinct strengths to this analysis. During her long career at the University of Alberta as a sport sociologist and historian, Ann Hall has written extensively on feminism, gender, and sport, as well as the history of Canadian women in sport. Specific topics in history include the struggle for gender equity; the famous Canadian women's basketball team, the Edmonton Grads; and the professional nineteenth-century cyclist Louise Armaindo. Bruce Kidd contributed expertise as a policy analyst, policy adviser, and historian, and practical experience as the head of physical education for nineteen years at the University of Toronto. He also brings the comparative perspective of leadership on several international bodies, including the International Council of Sport Sciences and Physical Education and the Commonwealth Advisory Body on Sport. Patricia Vertinsky is a social and cultural historian at the University of British Columbia. She works across the fields of women's and gender history with a special interest in physical culture, physical education, and modern dance. She has played leadership roles on international learned societies that coordinate research into physical culture, including the International Society for the History of Physical Education and Sport, and the North American Society for Sport History.

While critical of its shortcomings and often advocates of reform, we have had mostly positive experiences in physical education, and admire the many brilliant innovators, practitioners, and colleagues who have devoted their lives to its provision. This book is neither a eulogy nor an obituary. We believe physical education needs to be strengthened, not abolished.

During the heyday of Canadian school- and university-based physical education in the 1960s and 1970s, there was an outpouring of books, articles, conference presentations, and theses on the history of physical education in Canada. The Canadian Association for Health, Physical Education and Recreation had an active history committee that held well-attended sessions at its annual conference. Maxwell Howell, in the Faculty of Physical Education and Recreation at the University of Alberta, was responsible for the creation of a doctoral program in sport history in the mid-1960s. He also encouraged students to write theses on various aspects of physical education and initiated a series of symposia on the history of sport and physical education to draw in scholars from other universities. Another important stimulus was the *Canadian Journal of History of Sport and Physical Education* created by Alan Metcalfe at the University of Windsor in 1970. However, "Physical Education" was dropped from the title in 1981 when the journal became the *Canadian Journal of the History of Sport/ Revue canadienne de l'histoire des sports*. According to Metcalfe, as faculties, schools, and departments changed their name to Human Kinetics, Human Movement, Kinesiology, and the like, keeping "physical education" in the title made it too restrictive.[14]

There have been several insightful theses in the intervening period, valuable reflections in published histories of childhood, higher education, and militarism, and useful case studies in specialist journals. Provincial governments, professional associations, non-governmental bodies, and United Nations agencies like UNESCO have published curricula, participation statistics, and important data for evaluation. The reader can see the array of sources we tapped in our extensive list of references. However, there has been no published, comprehensive history since Cosentino and Howell's slim *History of Physical Education in Canada* published in 1971.

One important source has been the personal records placed in archives by several leading innovators and commentators, including R. Tait McKenzie, a pioneer of compulsory physical education for university students, J. Howard Crocker, John Dewar, and Robert Osborne, leading figures at the universities of Western, Laurentian, and British Columbia respectively. Another invaluable source proved to be the interviews with fifty "pioneers" of physical education, sport, and recreation recorded in 1978–9 by Stewart Davidson of the University of Ottawa, and deposited in the Sound Archives of Library and Archives Canada in Ottawa.[15] Davidson's objective was to develop a history of sport and physical education in Canada through the memories and reminiscences of these pioneers. He sought to discover the "origins, growth and development of the field, the problems faced and solved, the cultural forces exerted, the movements that have waned and persisted, the changes in implements, facilities, and costumes, [and] the thoughts and deeds of the pioneer leaders who have shaped the profession over the years."[16] The interviews followed a similar format: schooling and education; early teaching/work experience; war service (in some cases); further education; volunteer experience and organizations with which they were involved; full exploration of their career; professional associates considered to have made significant contributions to physical education, sport, or recreation in Canada; opinions about significant accomplishments within the profession in Canada during the twentieth century; and thoughts regarding the direction the physical education profession should take in the future. Interviews usually lasted at least two hours and were most often conducted in the interviewee's home. Since all fifty interviewees have now passed away, it has been a fascinating experience to hear their voices again, appreciate their personal and professional lives, learn of their many accomplishments, and understand both their joys and their frustrations.[17] We have incorporated some of their stories and views into our text.

The chapters in *Educating the Body* follow a chronological, historical timeline beginning in the mid-nineteenth century to the present day. Chapter 1 describes Egerton Ryerson's vision for physical education within the free, non-sectarian, state-directed system of education he created in nineteenth-century Ontario, and what he was actually able to realize. We examine Ryerson's role in the creation of industrial schools, the beginning of the residential schooling system in Canada for Indigenous children and youth. He also advocated military drill, especially for boys, as a form of physical education. Other impassioned advocates, like Frederick S. Barnjum in Montreal and later E.B. Houghton in Ontario, were much more enthused about calisthenics and gymnastics for both boys and girls. Finally, we examine Indigenous schooling in late nineteenth-century Canada, especially the role of calisthenics, drill, and recreation in the residential schools.

Chapter 2 outlines the creation of a single, coordinated pan-Canadian curriculum for physical education in the early years of the twentieth century through the Strathcona Trust. We continue our discussion of Indigenous schooling and physical education, noting the appalling conditions in the residential schools, and the efforts by Indian Affairs to encourage calisthenics and games. The Strathcona Trust with its emphasis on military drill and Ling's Swedish gymnastics had its outspoken detractors, including Arthur S. Lamb, the influential director of Physical Education at McGill University and physical educator Ethel Mary Cartwright, also at McGill. We end this chapter with a discussion of the role of physical education in the early youth movements like the YMCA and YWCA.

Chapter 3 provides a case study of the Margaret Eaton School (1901–41) in Toronto, arguably the most important institution for women's physical education in Canada. We examine the history of the school through the philosophies and accomplishments of its three principals: Emma Scott Raff, Mary Hamilton, and Florence Somers. This chapter also provides an opportunity to discuss the new "kinesthetic of modernism" as represented by three movement theorists: François Delsarte, Émile Jaques-Dalcroze, and Rudolf Laban, whose theories and work challenged the more rigid system of gymnastics and calisthenics promoted in the public schools. Through its graduates, the Margaret Eaton School provided the YWCAs, private schools, settlement houses, summer camps, recreation centres, playgrounds, and other agencies across Canada with well-trained female staff.

In chapter 4, we analyse the fascinating efforts mounted during the Depression and wartime to move beyond the Strathcona Trust in the schools and to develop broadly based physical fitness programs for young adults outside the schools, and the creation of the national network for physical educators in schools and universities. We also continue our examination of physical education in the residential schools through a case study, namely, the Pelican Lake Indian Residential School, which opened in 1926 in northern Ontario.

In chapter 5, we examine the achievements and failings of school-based physical education during the 1950s and early 1960s, a time when the subject was compulsory from kindergarten to grade twelve, yet rapid postwar economic growth, growing suburbanization, and increasing leisure contributed to a perceived decline in physical fitness. Also discussed is the promotion of movement education, a more child-centred approach to physical education, especially in the elementary schools, brought to Canada by émigré physical educators from Britain after the war. Although it gradually gained popularity, it also provoked considerable controversy and debate. As for the Indigenous residential and day schools, we examine the efforts by Indian Affairs to include physical education as part of the curriculum and to provide equipment and facilities, although not always successfully.

The background to chapter 6 is the changing Canadian landscape from the 1970s through to the 1990s such as cutbacks to education, an ascendant nationalism in Quebec, the phasing out of Indigenous residential schools, a boisterous feminist movement, increasing immigration, and a renewed interest in physical fitness and sport. Following experiments in France, some schools and districts mandated the "1/3 system," where one-third of the weekly curriculum was devoted to physical education, leading eventually to quality daily physical education. University-based exercise physiology labs were established to study fitness, and ParticipACTION encouraged Canadians to adopt regular exercise. The growth of sports in schools, colleges, and universities also had implications for physical education, as did the continuing rise of kinesiology as research universities took more interest in this growing field than they did in preparing physical education teachers.

Chapter 7 analyses the energetic, sometimes contradictory developments of the early decades of the twenty-first century. First, we examine physical and health education curricula throughout the various provinces and territories noting the similarities and differences, but more importantly how political forces influence curriculum reform. Although the notion of "physical literacy" has a long history, it is now a powerful movement forcing changes, primarily at the secondary school level, in the activities taught in physical education programs, how they are delivered, and the type of pedagogy used. Of concern is the declining enrolment in physical education teacher education degree programs in universities, and the uneasy alignment with kinesiology. Of even more concern is the lack of equity, diversity, inclusion, and social justice within university-level physical education and kinesiology. We end the chapter with an examination of the reinvigoration of federal government funding targeted at promoting sport and physical activity well beyond the school. In the last chapter, an Afterword, we set out our vision for physical education in the future.

Finally, a word about the title, *Educating the Body*. The most frequently expressed epistemological perspective on physical education is that it is a regime for *schooling* the body. Educator and historian David Kirk argues that physical education is best understood as the social regulation and normalization of bodies. Schooling connotes the imposition of vested interests, ideology, and power, with control residing and exercised by the institution and the teacher, not the students. Writing about Australia, he suggests that even when the nineteenth- and early twentieth-century teacher-led mass exercises and drill were replaced in the latter twentieth century by sports and games, the result was "a form of corporeal regulation that may be looser than it once was, but that nevertheless enmeshes bodies in matrices of power."[18] While we accept that much of physical education has historically been mandated, delivered, and experienced as top-down "schooling," we believe that in schools, youth organizations, colleges, and universities physical education has been and can be imparted in ways that enable participants to define, pursue, and direct their own learning about their bodies, in ways that can be highly self-expressive and liberating, and also inculcate respect for other people.

CHAPTER ONE

Ryerson and His Vision

A system of instruction making no provision for those exercises which contribute to health and vigour of body, and to agreeableness of manners, must necessarily be imperfect.

Egerton Ryerson, 1847

Whenever there is a public meeting on sports, fitness, or recreation in Canada, someone will invariably call for strengthened, compulsory physical education in the public schools. One such occasion was the cross-country consultations on the *Canadian Sport Policy of 2012*, an agreement between the federal, provincial, and territorial governments. Even though the hearings were called to discuss a completely different subject – high performance and community sport – some participants insisted that the priority should be high-quality physical education in every school. They always received a round of applause. Those sentiments were subsequently captured in the final document as a call for "physical literacy ... as a precondition for the lifelong participation in, and enjoyment of, sport ... and a foundation for active living and health for everyone."[1]

The deep reservoir of support for universal physical education reflects the idea's long history in Canada, predating Confederation. While it has been fully and effectively realized at some times and marginalized during others, it has been a framing ambition for many ever since the first attempts to create an independent Canadian settler state in the mid-nineteenth century. It has always been closely associated with the ideals of accessible, high-quality education for all and the nation-building aspirations of Canada itself. It will be a continuous thread of this history to which we will return again and again.

The ambition for universal physical education was first popularized by Egerton Ryerson (1803–1882), the superintendent of education for that section of the Province of Canada known as Canada West (1844 to 1867) and then the new province of Ontario (1867 to 1876).[2] Ryerson was determined to create a universal, free, and public (i.e., state-administered) system of education as a strategy for developing a civic culture in the emerging settler society, and he advocated physical education as integral to that effort. That he did so meant that physical education eventually became universal, public, free, and associated with nation-building as well. Those familiar attributes raise the responsibility and the challenges of physical education to this day. This is why we begin our story with Ryerson.

While other contemporary states took different approaches, Ryerson proposed that physical education in Canada impart the knowledge and habits of health, discipline, and Christian values as well as physical strength and skills. He wanted it to be compulsory and taught in uniform, but gender-specific, ways through standard curricula and teacher training. Most other Canadian provinces subsequently embraced the structure he imposed.

Ryerson and His Times

It is important to understand Ryerson's character and the context in which he intervened, because those factors had a profound effect upon what became physical education in Canada. Ryerson was always physically active, and consciously understood the importance of physical activity for mental and physical health. As a boy and young man, he worked hard on the family farm near London, Ontario. At twenty-two, he became a "saddle-bag" Methodist preacher, riding on horseback through all sorts of weather to minister to families and communities in southern Ontario, including the Mississauga reserve along the Credit River. Subsequently he settled in Cobourg (to establish what became Victoria College), and then Toronto (to edit the Methodist newspaper, the *Christian Guardian*). Later, he became a civil servant and travelled to other parts of the Canadas, the United States, and Europe. Throughout his life, he walked, rode, and swam on a regular basis, and when ill, stepped up his exercise as a strategy of regaining health. In his late fifties, he took up rowing and sailing, often taking his skiff out solo on Toronto Bay. In 1863, he sailed it across Lake Ontario to Port Dalhousie, then had it shipped through the Welland Canal to Port Colborne on Lake Erie. From there he sailed (and when the wind died, rowed) to Port Dover, a distance of fifty-five miles, where he gave two lectures at an educational conference. He returned the same way, and later rhapsodized about "the wonderful sense of freedom and relief" the experience brought, and how it helped him "forget the sorrows, labours and burdens of more than two score years."[3] Ryerson had a lived appreciation for the joys and health benefits of physical activity.

As a minister of the Methodist church, Ryerson was an evangelical Christian. He vowed "never to rest contented until [Christ] becomes not only my wisdom, but my sanctification and my full redemption."[4] Ryerson's devotion gave his entire work a spiritual character. In the case of physical education, it was not just exercise he advocated, but activity with a moral purpose. He felt physical education should tame the unchecked appetites of the body, strengthen personal discipline and responsibility, and foster a love of country and its institutions. Methodism not only shaped his world view but propelled him into public life. It was a time when a small group of wealthy landowners, merchants, and Anglican clergy (known as the "Family Compact") dominated the colonial government, and powerful leaders like Bishop John Strachan sought to consolidate the Anglican monopoly on the most important positions in government and education. Ryerson's eloquent opposition to Strachan in speeches and newspaper articles made him a leading representative of Methodism and a prominent advocate of a more democratic approach.

Ryerson was also a loyalist, whose father and uncle had fought as British officers against the United States revolution and had received grants of land when they eventually settled in Upper Canada. During his childhood, his father and his three older brothers fought against the Americans in the War of 1812. Those family experiences gave him a deep attachment to the Canadian settler state, a strong commitment to the British connection, and an appreciation for the role of government in the affairs of the colony.

There was a broad consensus that education should be a priority for whatever faction controlled the government. Ryerson became a mediating figure in the swirling, bitter politics of Upper Canada in the decades prior to Confederation. While he was known as a reformer, he was out of the country, fundraising in England for what became Victoria College during the rebellions of 1837, when both Upper and Lower Canada erupted against the undemocratic character of the colonial government and the ruling elites. The government brutally suppressed the uprisings, executing and deporting the leading activists and forcing those it could not catch into exile. The British government then appointed the earl of Durham to find a solution to the expressed grievances. Durham in turn recommended the integration of Upper and Lower Canada into a single colony, and a gradual transition to responsible government. During the unstable governments that followed, Ryerson forged a middle position. He supported responsible government but opposed complete republicanism on the American model; he sought a measure of Canadian autonomy, but he also believed in an ongoing role for the British crown. It was in this context that in 1844

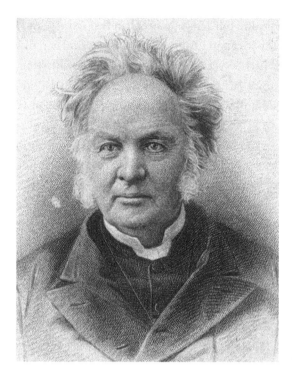

Figure 1.1. Rev. Egerton Ryerson, D.D., L.L.D., 1886 (Library and Archives Canada, acc. no. 3029964)

the British governor Charles Metcalfe offered him the position of superintendent of education, with a mandate to make schooling more relevant, accessible, and effective. It was not a political position: Ryerson would not be a member of the ministry. But his acceptance of the appointment signalled his support for the government. Ryerson quickly turned what seemingly began as an electoral expedient into the most stable position in colonial administration. With education a priority of all factions, Ryerson enjoyed almost complete authority and held the position through a long series of shifting ministries and the constitutional creation of Canada, until 1876. It gave him enormous scope to reshape public education.

It was not only a turbulent time politically. Social, legal, and economic changes were transforming everyday life and the way people thought. The liberal idea of the individual's right to property, popularized by writers like Adam Smith, advanced by the French and American revolutions, and pursued by a steady wave of European immigrants and speculators, accentuated the importance of land ownership and land for settlement. Despite the promises of the British Proclamation of 1763 to protect Indigenous title to land and the decisive military assistance that Tecumseh and the Indigenous nations provided the colony during the War of 1812, European and North American–born settlers put tremendous pressure on the colonial government to eliminate or remove the First Nations.[5] It was also a time of increasingly legal restriction upon women. As government expanded, the legislature codified masculine power over women in both the household and the public sphere. Racial distinctions between white and Indigenous women also hardened during this period.[6]

The Industrial Revolution in Canada was well under way, led by the extraction, production, and export of timber and agricultural surpluses, enabled by state-assisted investment in canals and railroads. A generation later, it was the possibilities for export-led growth, transcontinental trade and communication, immigration and western settlement, and the development of an internal market for manufactures stimulated by the railroad that fired the dreams of the Canadian nation.

The system of public education and physical education Ryerson created both responded and contributed to these broad social and economic changes.

Creating the Educational State

Ryerson did not begin from scratch – there were already about 2,000 common schools teaching literacy by the time he took over. Those schools operated under a wide variety of conditions, controlled by parents and local committees, financed by fees. They were not always available or accessible to every child, and school boards and parents struggled to keep them going. The same was true for the proprietary and religious voluntary schools to which middle- and upper-class parents sent their children and supported, in imitation of the private schools of Britain. These schools also struggled financially, and many failed in lean economic times.

Ryerson transformed the decentralized network of common and private schools into an integrated system, uniformly directed and administered, with the focus on a school for every child. He increased the number and quality of schools and made them free. As he wrote in his first set of proposals for public education, *Report on a System of Public Elementary Instruction for Upper Canada*, in 1847, "the first feature then of our Provincial system of Public Instruction, should be *universality*; and that in respect to the poorest classes of society … the rich can take care of themselves. The elementary education of the whole people must therefore be an essential element in the Legislative and Administrative policy of an enlightened and beneficent Government."[7] He brought in a uniform curriculum and ensured its consistent delivery through textbook publishing, teacher training, teams of inspectors to measure compliance and eventually compulsory attendance. He strengthened the grammar or secondary schools and made them more accessible.

Through these steps, Ryerson made the state schools attractive to the middle-class parents who had previously sent their sons and daughters to voluntary schools. They gradually realized that it was more financially feasible, sustainable, and educationally effective to send their children to a strengthened state system than continually struggle to maintain the fledgling private schools. While the colonial elite sought to emulate the system of private schools in Britain, it was too expensive to reproduce them on a widespread basis in Canada, and there was little support for the class hierarchy they encouraged. As Gidney and Millar argue, the financial and educational interests of middle-class parents played a significant role in legitimizing the system of state schools and the taxes they required from all classes for their support.[8]

Ryerson and a very small number of colleagues working in Toronto made most of the decisions themselves, communicating directly with supervisors, teachers, and parents in hand-written letters and published circulars. The archival record on his accomplishment and this period is rich and enormous. Under his leadership, the administration of schooling became one of the most important activities of the growing state. While critics complained about the top-down, highly centralized nature of the system, he succeeded in creating the universally available and accessible public school system we have known ever since.[9]

Ryerson's primary focus was strengthening moral character. At a time of rapid urbanization, fractious religious disputes, the emergence of an organized working class, and ongoing tensions with the United States, he set out to inculcate a new citizenry that would respect Canadian-British institutions and take pride in the new nation. He espoused the orderly development of society, a clear system of rules, respect for authority, and the preservation of loyalist traditions. He also sought to inculcate a new generation in the discipline and skills necessary for a flourishing economy. The "gospel of order" he advanced became a strong current of belief in the new nation. The British North America Act of 1867 (now the Constitution Act) entrusted the new Dominion government with preserving "peace, order and good government" – not the "life, liberty and the pursuit of happiness" of the American Declaration of Independence.

Developing Physical Education

Ryerson believed that public education "should develop all the *intellectual* and *physical* powers."[10] At the very beginning of his appointment, he travelled to England, Belgium, France, Austria, the German states, Switzerland, and the United States, at his own expense, to observe contemporary education first hand. He attended public and private schools, universities, and teacher training institutes, both Catholic and Protestant, and made detailed notes of beliefs, curricula, exercises, and apparatus. He interviewed educational, religious, and business leaders about their ideas, attended parliamentary debates and university lectures, and read everything he could on the subject. He concluded that a "system of instruction making no provision for those exercises which contribute to health and vigour of body, and to agreeableness of manners, must necessarily be imperfect ... To the culture and command of all the faculties of the mind, a corresponding exercise and controul [sic] of all the members of the body is next in importance."[11] He reinforced these ideas in his talks, correspondence, and newspaper articles over and over again.

Despite his British loyalties and his familiarity with the "games curriculum" of the all-male British elite schools and their Canadian counterparts such as Upper Canada College, Ryerson was most impressed with the nation-building benefits of free-standing and apparatus gymnastics as well as the military drill (i.e., marching in formation) advocated by Friedrich Ludwig Jahn in Prussia and Johann Heinrich Pestalozzi and Philipp Emanuel von Fellenberg in Switzerland. He extolled their ideas and recommended a composite of their systems, along with instruction in hygiene and military drill as the basis of the subject. In 1852, he published detailed instructions and illustrations of recommended exercises in seven consecutive issues of his *Journal of Education for Upper Canada*, 5,000 copies of which were distributed across the province. The modern reader will immediately recognize the principle of progression inherent in Ryerson's scheme. "Like the art of writing," he wrote, "they proceed from the simplest movement, to the most complex and difficult exercises, imparting a bodily activity and skill scarcely credible to those who have not witnessed them."[12] Historians debate how often they were actually read, but if any enterprising principal or teacher had kept and pasted them together, they would have had Canada's first effective manual of exercises.

Unlike field sports, which required large playing areas, the gymnastics Ryerson recommended had the advantage of being suitable for small spaces, even indoors and on rough grounds. The calisthenics and military drill could be taught and performed in a uniform formation, so they also became lessons in class discipline and coordination. In 1853, Ryerson hired Major H. Goodwin as "Master of Gymnastics" in the Toronto Normal and Model School to prepare teachers for delivering the subject. Goodwin thus became Ontario's first physical education instructor within the public education system.[13] Ryerson also encouraged the construction of playgrounds in every school. While it is difficult to determine the extent to which these ideas were taken up, several districts, notably Central Hamilton, began to teach the subject in earnest and constructed playgrounds for instruction and after-school activities.

Ryerson held to the "faculty psychology" of his day, which posited that the mind was composed of distinct faculties responsible for different mental tasks. The

PHYSICAL TRAINING IN SCHOOLS.
GYMNASTIC EXERCISES.
CONTINUED.
No. II.

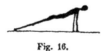

Fig. 16.

Action 25. The feet being placed close, the hands fixed on the hips, rise on the toes, then bend the knees, and lower the body gradually till the thighs touch the heels (see action 17): extend the arms in front, and fall forwards, so that the body forms a straight line from the head to the heels, and rests on the hands and the toes.

Fig. 17.

Action 26. The feet being placed close, the hands open, the arms straight upward, the palms in front, bend the body forward, and touch the ground with the points of the fingers. The knees are to be kept straight (fig. 17).

Action 27. This is the same as action 25, only springing up and clapping the hands.

Action 28. This action is performed by two, standing opposite to or facing each other. The left hand on hip, the right foot forward, the right arm in front; then grasp each other's hands, and try to bring the arm down to the right or left.

Fig. 18.

Action 29. The feet close, the hands on the hips: cross the legs, bend the knees gradually, sit down, and rise again (fig. 18).

Action 30. The reverse of action 28, viz., with the left arm, &c.

Fig. 19.

Action 31. The feet close, the arms extended in front, raise the left leg in front, bend the right knee gradually, and sit down on the ground, then get up again in the same position.

Fig. 20.

Action 32. This is performed by two persons facing each other. The left hand on the hip, the right foot in front, lock the middle finger on each other's right hand, and pull back (fig. 20).

Action 33. As action 31, performed with left leg.

Action 34. As action 32, with left hand.

Action 35. The feet close, the hands on the hips, jump up, at the same time spreading out the legs (fig. 21).

Figure 1.2. An example of Ryerson's gymnastic exercises (*Journal of Education of Upper Canada* 5, no. 6 [1852]: 83)

purpose of education, he believed, was not just to impart knowledge but strengthen the faculties. He believed that physical activity without self-discipline, including the abandoned love of sports and play, could dominate or distort the operation of the mental faculties. "A sensual man is a mere animal," he once wrote. "Sensuality is the greatest enemy to human progress."[14] He felt the same for entire societies: "In the arrangements of Providence, law, penalty meets us wherever we go. No wisdom or moral force in rulers or administrations was ever sufficient of itself to sustain an orderly government. Nations, States, armies, navies, need compulsion, as well as advice and persuasion ... If this is true of men, it is especially true of children, who are only men of smaller growth, and more uninformed and undisciplined."[15]

The risk for individuals, their families, and the entire society, was that playfulness and the unrestrained appetites of the body could lead to ignorance and illiteracy, which in turn led to idleness and delinquency, unemployment, poverty, and criminality. Such thinking reflected the fears of the rising urban middle class in a multitude of "others" – Indigenous peoples, non-British immigrants, and the growing working class – and the tumultuous changes of urbanization and industrialization. The solution was a rigorous system of exercises and performances that would tame the body and subordinate it to the discipline of the mind, thereby allowing for the full growth of the mental faculties. "To develop the mind of the pupil," the *Journal of Education for Upper Canada* quoted the superintendent of education in New Brunswick approvingly, "we must develop the power which the mind has govern, exercise his body, make him healthy and strong, that we may make him prudent and reasonable."[16]

Although Ryerson felt that girls' education should be conducted on a sex-segregated basis, focused on their future roles as housekeepers and mothers, and end after elementary school, here too he tempered these restrictive ideas with progressive proposals. He regularly called for girls' physical education in the form of ambitious calisthenics. The *Journal* favourably quoted the British feminist writer Harriet Martineau, who argued that girls and boys should learn and play together, and that girls especially needed vigorous exercise and games to enable them to strengthen their health and well-being, and resistance to disease.[17] Few schools could afford to teach girls and boys separately. Girls usually took the same gymnastics and calisthenics as the boys; they just did not participate in military drill.

Ryerson marshalled further support for physical education in the 1860s. In 1866, he published and distributed a consolidated manual of exercises, including formations and commands for military drill. It recommended that teachers devote three to four hours to the various exercises and drills. He enabled the Toronto Normal and Model School to add a well-equipped gymnasium and won approval for provincial grants to school boards for the construction of playgrounds and the purchase of equipment. In 1871, his ministry required all students in the province's teacher training institutes to take a course in physical exercise as it related to and facilitated the child's physical and moral development to prepare them for their responsibilities.[18]

A major stimulus for these investments was the changing political climate, as the Province of Canada and the Maritime colonies moved towards nationhood and had to think about their own defence. While once it could rely upon the British militia, Britain was in the process of withdrawing its regiments from Canada. At the same time, the United States was becoming more bellicose, with thousands of battle-hardened soldiers from the Civil War and eyes to the north. These worries intensified the importance of military drill. Previously marching in unison had been included in the curriculum as a means of inculcating the values and ambitions of the new nation. "Military drill is designed to foster in the youthful mind a love of country and its institutions," Ryerson wrote regularly.[19] Many normal and grammar schools formed their own voluntary associations. After 1866, military drill became a rudimentary form of national defence, and rose and fell in popularity and practice in the schools with the changing international context.

By the time Ryerson stepped down as superintendent of education in the new province of Ontario in 1876, the structures of physical education we recognize today were well established. While physical education would not become compulsory until 1887, and few school boards had the facilities and trained teachers to deliver it effectively to all students, it had become integral to the ideal of universal, free, and centrally administered public elementary and secondary education. The provincial ministry of education regularly endorsed it as necessary to effective learning, growth, and development, and a means of inculcating the values of the new nation. It also promoted a province-wide curriculum of gymnastics, calisthenics, and military drill through a common instructional manual, compulsory teacher training in the various normal schools, and capital grants for gymnasia and equipment. Physical education was not just exercise based, but incorporated instruction about health and hygiene, the values of respect and personal discipline, and loyalty to the settler state.

Ryerson, Industrial Schools, and Physical Education

As mentioned previously, the church appointed Ryerson as the first Methodist missionary to the Credit Mississauga in the fall of 1826. Assisted by Indigenous leader Peter Jones, a convert to Christianity, Ryerson set up a school in which children were taught in both Ojibwe and English. "I must now acquire a new language," he wrote in his diary, "to teach a new people."[20] He gained a basic knowledge of

Ojibwe and was given an Ojibwe name, *Cheehock*, meaning "bird on the wing" in reference to his going constantly among his flock. From his close contact with the Mississauga, Ryerson realized not only the complexity of their language, but also the strength of their culture.[21] Although his primary purpose was the conversion of as many as possible to Christianity, he earned the respect of the Mississauga through teaching their children and working beside them in the fields. The following year, the Methodist church appointed Ryerson to the Cobourg circuit as an itinerant preacher, where he travelled on horseback to various communities including the Indian missions at Rice Lake and Mud Lake. As he wrote in his diary on 3 January 1828: "I have this day visited the Indians of Rice Lake: all prosperity here. I have been much refreshed this evening in meeting my beloved brother and fellow-laborer in the Gospel, Peter Jones. These pleasing interviews bring to mind many refreshing seasons we have enjoyed together, when seeking the lost sheep of the house of Israel." Ryerson and Jones remained good friends until the latter's death in 1856, and as we have seen in the previous sections, although Ryerson's career was eventually in education, he never forgot his early days with the Indian missions.[22]

The origin of the Indian day school system was based on these early mission schools, which eventually led to the establishment of the residential school system. In 1828, for example, an Anglican missionary working for the New England Company (NEC) established a day school for Indigenous boys from the Six Nations Reserve at present-day Brantford, Ontario, called the Mohawk Institute. Chartered in England in 1649, for the purpose of propagating the gospel to the Indigenous peoples of New England, the NEC was also active mostly in Canada West. It held property and supported Indigenous students at various schools. The Mohawk Institute began taking boarders in 1831, and three years later started admitting girls, thus becoming the first residential school in Canada.

By this time, the overall purpose of the Department of Indian Affairs was directed at improving the prosperity of Indigenous communities, primarily in the southern part of the Upper Canadian colony "by encouraging in every possible manner the progress of religious knowledge and education generally amongst the Indian tribes." Supposedly this new "policy of civilization" called for Indigenous tribes to be located on "serviced settlement sites" on their reserves, complete with houses, barns, churches, and schools, and other amenities. Supposedly, they would also be provided with training in agriculture as well as the skills generally needed by settlers to achieve self-sufficiency.[23]

In October 1842, Sir Charles Bagot, the Governor General of British North America, appointed three commissioners to investigate the Department of Indian Affairs operations in Canada East (southern Quebec) and Canada West (Ontario).

Henceforth known as the Bagot Commission, its focus was to improve Indigenous living conditions and, at the same time, reduce operational expenditures within the department. Accordingly, the commissioners reviewed Indian Affairs' records, held public hearings, questioned the white officials responsible for overseeing the affairs of Indigenous people, and to a much lesser extent, sought the views of Indigenous leaders. Their final report in 1844 "painted a depressing picture of bungled departmental operations, deplorable Indian conditions, and unresolved policy questions." A new approach was needed that would "instill in Indian people the thirst for knowledge, and the qualities of industry and self-reliance."[24]

It was clear to the Bagot commissioners that Indian day schools were not satisfactory given the problems associated with parental influence, irregular attendance, and the few practical skills being taught. Instead, they recommended boarding schools with attached farms, referred to as manual labour schools, to teach Indigenous children about growing crops, animal husbandry, mechanical trades, domestic skills, and the like. They further recommended that religious groups should be encouraged by Indian Affairs to implement this new educational policy. Finally, the commissioners recommended separating Indigenous children from their parents and removing them from their homes as the best way to achieve assimilation, which they believed desirable. This led to the ongoing policy of assimilation through education.

Ryerson's 1847 report outlining a system of public education for Upper Canada, discussed previously, made no suggestions regarding the education of Indigenous children. While he commented favourably on practical or industrial education, he recommended it exclusively for Canadian children who were white. However, that same year he was asked by Indian Affairs to make recommendations "as to the best method of establishing and conducting Industrial Schools for the benefit of the aboriginal Indian Tribes."[25] In Ryerson's view, the purpose of these schools was to "give a plain English education adapted to the working farmer and mechanic." It is clear that he was referring only to boys here. He preferred the term "industrial" to what were normally called manual labour schools because their purpose was to make the pupils into industrious farmers. He admired the so-called industrial, trade, and agricultural schools he had observed in Europe, and especially Fellenberg's farm school at Hofwyl, his estate near Berne, Switzerland. For Fellenberg, "work on the land not only improved physique but also developed the mind."[26] These schools also exemplified Ryerson's strong belief that effective education should be practical. As he had argued in his *Report on a System of Public Elementary Instruction*, "the mere acquisition or even the general diffusion of knowledge, without the requisite qualities to apply that knowledge in the best manner, does not merit the name of education ... The very end of our being is practical, and every step, and every branch of our moral, intellectual, and physical culture should harmonize with the design of our existence. The age in which we live is likewise eminently practical ... Scarcely an individual among us is exempt from the necessity of living by 'the sweat of his face.' Every man should therefore be educated to practice."[27]

Ryerson insisted that students live together in order to provide for their "domestic education" and for the all-important Christian instruction provided by the denomination in charge of the school. It would also separate children from their parents and home reserves. During the summer, pupils would work eight to twelve hours a day, presumably outside in the fields or grounds, and study for two to four hours. During winter, time in the classroom would increase and their outside labour would decrease. His only reference to any form of physical training was to suggest that gymnastic exercises in the winter might replace the agricultural labour of summer, although circumstances would determine the time and kinds of recreation. He did not elaborate further.

The cooperation of the Indigenous bands was necessary for the success of these industrial schools, and especially to get them built. In Canada West, at regional meetings of Indian councils, virtually every tribe agreed to apply one-quarter of their annuities for a period of twenty-five years towards the construction and support of three new industrial schools. By 1851, two schools had been established with the cooperation of the Wesleyan Methodists, who were responsible for supplying books, supplies, and teachers' salaries, as well as the farm stock and equipment for the attached model farms. The Indian Department would maintain the school buildings and provide an annual per capita subsidy to defer food, clothing, and general education expenses. One school was located at Alderville on the Alnwick Reserve on the south side of Rice Lake, Ontario, approximately thirty kilometres north of Cobourg. The other was the Muncey Institute (later known as the Mount Elgin Industrial Institute), just southwest of London, Ontario, where boys were taught trades and farming, and the girls learned housewifery and tailoring.[28] Neither school followed Ryerson's suggestions to restrict training to farming, and to limit the school to boys (with girls remaining in day schools).[29]

By 1864, the Mohawk Institute could accommodate one hundred students of both sexes. In the annual report of that year submitted by Indian Affairs, it was observed that the "capacity of Indian children for learning is quite as good as that of whites."[30] At that time there were approximately thirty schools in Canada West reporting to Indian Affairs, but almost all were day schools either on a reserve or close to one, with the average number of pupils in each school ranging between twenty and fifty. There is no evidence of any form of physical training as part of the curricula of these schools. It would be some years before either the industrial or residential school system was well established within the Canadian provinces.

Physical Education after Ryerson

The creation of the new Canadian state gave further stimulus to Ryerson's vision of universal physical education. After decades of dreams and disappointments, the idea of a northern, transcontinental federation independent of Britain and distinct from the United States was realized in the mid-1860s. In September 1864, leaders of the British colonies of New Brunswick, Nova Scotia, and Prince Edward Island met in Charlottetown to discuss a Maritime union. When representatives of the uninvited Province of Canada showed up too, the discussion turned to the creation of a new state forged out of all the British colonies in North America. Subsequent meetings in Quebec and London produced a proposal to the British Parliament that addressed the delegates' major concerns, notably representation by population for the rapidly growing English-speaking population, protections for the largely Catholic *Canadien* minority, and a railway link with the Maritimes. The recommendations set out broad powers for both federal and provincial governments, enabling those who wanted a strong federal state and those who saw their interests best served by strong provinces, to say that they got what they wanted, thus setting the stage for a long history of federal–provincial disputes. With its passage as the British North America Act, the Dominion of Canada became a legal entity on 1 July 1867.[31] The British government then transferred the vast territory of Rupert's Land, over which it had given the Hudson's Bay Company a trading monopoly, to the new state, and Manitoba and British Columbia signed up. While Prince Edward Island did not sign the original agreement, it joined in 1873. Canada thus laid claims to territory covering the entire northern region of the continent, except for Newfoundland and Labrador, which did not join until 1949.

In none of these arrangements were the Indigenous peoples consulted. Despite the treaties they had negotiated with the British crown to share the lands and resources and learn from each other, the British government simply transferred the treaties to Canada. The new Canadian government ignored the intent of the original treaties, and in the years that followed used the form of the treaty process and the Indian Act to force most of the remaining Indigenous groups to relinquish their legal title and retreat to remote "reserves" in exchange for promises of protection and benefits that were rarely honoured.[32] Other groups were taken for granted in the creation of the new nation as well. For example, it would be decades before women won the vote and the rights to hold public office, control their own bodies and property, attend university, or practise one of the professions. In the rapid industrialization and urbanization that took place in the mid- to late nineteenth century, most workers toiled endlessly in difficult, often unsafe conditions, and lived day to day in crowded labour camps and urban slums with few rights. The history of Canada has always been a multiple narrative.

Among the white French- and English-speaking non-Indigenous populations, the prospects of expanded territory fired the ambitions and narratives of nation building in virtually every aspect of society. Civic leaders, entrepreneurs, and journalists promoted railways, new towns and cities, accelerated immigration and western settlement, while educators, churchmen, and artists formed distinctly pan-Canadian social organizations and new forms of cultural expression.

The hopes, responsibilities, and opportunities of the new nation inspired new interest in physical education. Three forms of instruction became prominent, namely, gymnastics, sports, and military drill.

Gymnastics

In Montreal, Canada's largest city – the crucible of industrialization and the jumping-off point for transcontinental migration, settlement, and trade – the English immigrant Frederick S. Barnjum single-handedly made gymnastic exercises and group routines a valued component of youth development and adult well-being among the urban middle classes. He promoted it for everyone. His journey followed an unusual trajectory. He arrived from England in 1859 with the intent to pursue landscape painting. His sketches and watercolours of rural landscapes are still collected today. Shortly after his arrival, he established the Montreal Gymnastic Club for young men, and from that base quickly became a persuasive voice for the importance of physical education. He also directed the construction of the first gymnasium at McGill, helped prepare thousands of teachers in physical education at the McGill Normal School, and persuaded McGill to include physical education in its curriculum, the first university in Canada to do so.

Barnjum added considerably to the exercises associated with gymnastics, designing new equipment and movements, including barbell drills that bore his name and a series of acrobatic routines he called "ladder pyramids." In these, gymnasts steadied a rank of ladders so they stood vertically on the ground or gym floor. Then other gymnasts would climb to the top, sometimes two or three on a single ladder, hanging on to the rungs and each other to realize handstands, pyramids, and other elaborate poses. In performances before spectators, they would hold poses for several seconds, then shift to other positions and then still others, creating a continually

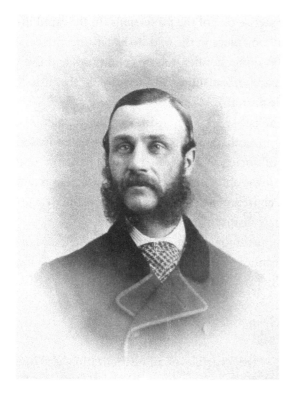

Figure 1.3. Frederick S. Barnjum, 1863 (McCord Museum, I-9604.1)

moving choreographed kaleidoscope of strength, agility, and beauty. Barnjum designed some 250 such poses. They must have been spectacular to watch.[33]

Barnjum was an impassioned advocate of physical education. In public meetings and articles in the press, he decried the indifference to the physical development of students in many schools. "The mind and body are so intimately connected that the health and well-being of the one must re-act upon the other," he wrote. "But for some reason or other, people appear willing to trust to *chance* in the vital manner of health and strength of body, whilst at the same time they spare no means to cultivate and develop the mental powers. The why and wherefore of this state of affairs it is hard to understand … physical education ought to be no longer relegated to a back seat, but is entitled to an equally honourable place with mental education, and until it is so, the number of properly qualified and educated teachers will be few."[34]

Barnjum also railed against the "conventional rules of society" that denied girls and young women the "same opportunity for romping as boys" and forced them into "one of those instruments of death called corsets, binding up the naughty muscles that are begging and praying to be let loose and have an opportunity of strengthening themselves … I do not hesitate to say that any young lady placed under the care of an intelligent, well-educated teacher cannot fail to attain a degree of health which otherwise she would have only dreamed of."[35] He recommended that young women exercise with light wooden dumb-bells, wands, and rings, and march to music. Barnjum was assisted in the classes he conducted for girls and young women by his sister Helen. She continued his work after his death, at the age of fifty-nine, in 1887.

Barnjum's disciples carried his ideas across North America. Two of them became famous physical educators in their own right. R. Tait McKenzie shaped university physical education and athletics at both McGill and the University of Pennsylvania, and he set the groundwork for what became the field of exercise rehabilitation. James Naismith, who took over Barnjum's classes at McGill before teaching at the YMCA college in Springfield, Massachusetts, invented and promoted the game of basketball. McKenzie compared Barnjum favourably to Frederick Ludwig Jahn and Per Henrik Ling, the fathers of German and Swedish physical education respectively, and others called him the Canadian Dio Lewis (after the well-known American physical educator.)

Other progressive educators began to incorporate physical education into their own fledging institutions. At the Collège Joliette, which was affiliated with the Université Laval, principal and Catholic priest Cyrille Beaudry included courses in hygiene and physical education in the curriculum, and in 1899 built a swimming pool for the students.[36] At Acadia College in Wolfville, Nova Scotia, president Artemas Sawyer opened a gymnasium in 1890 and required every male student to take exercise. A female seminary at Acadia was headed by principal Mary Elizabeth Graves, who also introduced physical education to her students and made certain they had their own gymnasium.[37] Thomas Burgess and John Mackieson insisted upon physical activity for the psychiatric patients in the institutions they supervised in Ontario and Prince Edward Island, while Alfred Dymond encouraged physical education in the Ontario Institute for the Blind.[38]

Sports

Another charismatic Montreal innovator was George Beers. A dentist by profession, Beers appropriated the Mohawk game of *tewaarathon*, which he learned as a young man in games with and against men from Kahnawake, and turned it into the sport of lacrosse with a different set of rules and equipment. He stamped it with the identity of the new nation, calling it "Canada's national game." Just as the new government claimed the entire northern region as their territory, so did Beers claim all of Canada for lacrosse, even though it would be years before first transcontinental

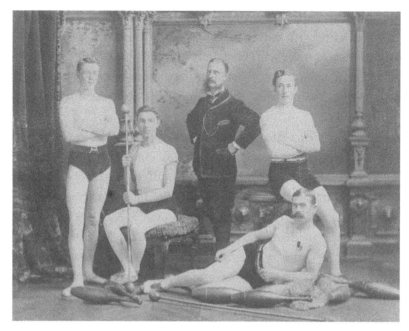

Figure 1.4. Competition for the Wickstead Medals, McGill University, 1886–7. L-R: R. Tait McKenzie, G.A. Brown, Fred Barnjum, and W.A. Cameron. Reclining is James Naismith. (University Archives and Records Center, University of Pennsylvania)

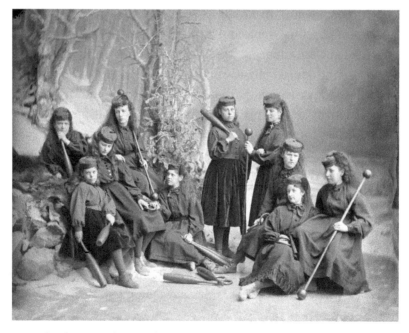

Figure 1.5. Frederick Barnjum's women's gymnastic group, Montreal, Quebec, 1870 (McCord Museum, I-45615)

railway was completed and players and officials were able to travel across the country. Beers promoted the new game whenever and wherever he could. In 1883, he staged exhibition matches between Canadian and Indigenous teams across the British Isles. The outcomes were predetermined to show off the superiority of the new Canadian society to that of the original inhabitants. To encourage immigration, he distributed 150,000 pieces of promotional literature along the way.[39]

Beers and middle-class men in other cities and towns sought to marshal the emerging practice of sport as a training ground for youth, and to impart Canadian nationalism and muscular Christianity, the belief popularized by the British Christian socialist Thomas Hughes that health and manliness strengthened secular Christianity.[40] These men created the clubs and associations that became the basis of amateur and professional sport in Canada, including the umbrella Amateur Athletic Association of Canada. Those first sporting organizations were based entirely in the anglophone middle class, and they excluded women, Indigenous peoples, francophones, and the working classes, who had to create competitive opportunities and form organizations on their own.[41] Upper-class girls and women gradually began to play sports like tennis in private clubs and church organizations during the 1880s, but it would take another generation before they were able to create a structure that could include other girls and women.[42] It was only in the 1890s that French Canadian middle-class men began to form their own clubs and competitions, notably the Association Athlétique d'Amateurs Nationale, and gradually, unions and immigrant associations began to organize their own clubs.[43]

From their early inception in the 1840s, sports were an integral component of the curriculum in the colleges, universities, and elite private schools for boys, such as Upper Canada College in Toronto. They were subsequently introduced to the state schools as an after-school activity by the students themselves. By the 1880s and 1890s, teachers and principals began to recognize their educational benefit, and gradually assumed control, organized competitions, and assigned teachers to provide leadership. What began as a trickle quickly became a flood. By the end of the nineteenth century, after-school sports flourished in most schools and communities. Girls as well as boys were involved, even playing games against boys' or representative teams from other cities. In 1904, for example, the Vancouver College girls' basketball team won the North Pacific Coast championship by defeating girls' teams from Seattle High School and the University of Washington.[44]

The Young Men's Christian Association (YMCA) in Canada has a long history going back to the middle of the nineteenth century when the first associations began to appear. Some made provision for interested members to make use of an "exercise room," although fully equipped gymnasiums rarely existed until the mid-1880s. In Montreal in 1883, for example, arrangements were made for members to enter classes in physical culture in Frederick Barnjum's private gymnasium. Opened in Toronto in 1888, a new YMCA building provided the first extensive facilities for physical education in Canada. It was highly successful in attracting new members, thus establishing physical "work" as a permanent feature of other evolving Canadian YMCAs. By 1890, H.C. Thompson, the gymnasium director at the Toronto Y claimed that the physical department attracted more young men than any other in the association. He also laid down a series of principles – how to make the most of their physical work, while at the same time making the most of their moral and spiritual influence – which other YMCAs soon followed. "Christian manhood" meant the equal development of the mental, social, spiritual, and physical attributes, the basis of the now-familiar four-fold YMCA philosophy.

The activities of young boys were not an important aspect of YMCA work in this period since their primary focus was on young men. However, as child labour, vagrancy, and crime became increasingly challenging in a growing industrial society, boys' departments were organized, and those YMCAs with gymnasiums often allowed some time each week for boys' activities. In Truro, Nova Scotia, one physical director took a group of boys on a five-day camping trip in 1890, and the following year he organized the "Annual Boys Summer Encampment," probably the first of its kind in Canada.[45]

Military Drill

The challenges faced by the new state gave renewed emphasis to military drill as a component of physical education. Both circumstances and prominent advocates encouraged it. Within the far-flung British Empire, with colonies in every corner of the globe, many of which had been militarily imposed on people of very different cultures, the need for troops and the martial spirit was never far from the public agenda. Many English-speaking Canadians identified with the empire and encouraged their sons to enlist in the imperial armies. In the early 1860s, as frictions arose with the United States during that country's bloody Civil War, fears rose that whichever army won might turn next to Canada. With Confederation, the British government announced that it would withdraw all garrisons by 1871. Moreover, the Fenian raids, a series of cross-border armed attacks between 1866 and 1871 by Irish Patriots intent upon capturing Canada and trading it for Irish independence, had exposed the inadequacies of the Canadian militia. Clearly, Canadians had to do a much better job of fending for themselves.

The most popular idea was a citizen army, inspired by the mistily remembered courage of volunteer forces during the War of 1812. To train that volunteer army, advocates felt that the rudiments of military formation and discipline should be taught to every male student in both state and private schools. It should be practised in "drill associations," after-school clubs where boys could march in unison, practise rifle shooting, and otherwise hone their military skills.[46] As Egerton Ryerson wrote in his *Journal of Education for Upper Canada* in 1866: "At the end of ten or twelve years from the first inauguration of such a system in Canada we should have, probably, half a million youths who had undergone a regular course of drill; a very large proportion of whom would be capable of bearing arms, and, should the emergency arise, could be readily converted into good and serviceable soldiers. Our common schools would thus be made the nurseries of our militia."[47]

An added concern was the "boy problem," the fear that the transformation of traditional masculine roles by urbanization and industrialization had left many boys and young men purposeless and psychologically adrift. Parents and churchmen worried that compulsory schooling and the rapid growth in the number of female teachers – in Ontario, they outnumbered male teachers by 1871 – had robbed young men of their physical toughness and inner strength.[48] Military drill offered a remedy. A succession of governors general, members of the House of Commons, newspaper editorialists, and other influencers proclaimed the advantages of drill to education, personal responsibility, and strengthened manliness. "If boys were to be put through a short military drill at school – lasting three hours a week – many benefits would accrue," the (London, Ontario) *Daily Free Press* argued in 1874. "The boys would not only become more tractable as scholars, but they would acquire a manly bearing, a brave and soldier-like disposition, which would prove of excellent value in national affairs. Education in Canada … leans too much to book learning."[49]

There were also practical advantages to military drill. It could be taught in the absence of equipment and facilities, and teachers were available from local regiments, certainly a consideration in impoverished communities or where the local school board was reluctant to pay teachers properly or invest in physical education. It was no coincidence that the very first "master of gymnastics" at the Toronto Normal School, Henry Godwin, was a retired soldier, a veteran of the Battle of Waterloo. Drill was also easier to organize for large numbers of students of different abilities, and for harassed teachers, it offered the promise of obedience. Egerton Ryerson would likely have preferred the ambitious gymnastics he witnessed in France, Germany, and Switzerland, or even a curriculum of sports and games along the lines of the English elite and Canadian private schools. But he reluctantly concluded that they were unrealizable in the conditions experienced by most Ontario schools, so he needed to promote military drill in their place.[50] Ryerson also had another motive for his support of military drill – it reinforced the sex segregation of pupils – although that turned out to be a losing battle.[51]

Military drill thus became a central component of physical education for boys and young men in the schools of Canada until the 1960s, waxing and waning with political and social conditions. While the British North America Act of 1867 declared education a provincial responsibility, given the implications of military drill for national defence, the federal government took an active interest. In 1868, for example, in response to the Fenian raids, the federal government passed a Militia Bill with the intention of creating a 40,000-volunteer army, members of which would be available to train students in the schools. But the legislation required would-be soldiers to buy their own uniforms and contribute to their other expenses, so it had a completely opposite effect. It discouraged the formation of cadet corps while taking the provincial government off the hook, so the net effect was the rapid evaporation of enthusiasm and the disappearance of cadet corps. The lesson was that both levels of government needed to act in a coordinated fashion for full effectiveness. This would not occur until the next century. When the Treaty of Washington of 1871 established peaceful relations between Canada, Britain, and the United States, it put an end to the concern for military preparations. While leading educators and influencers continued to call for military drill in the schools, and it continued to be taught in the normal schools, private institutions, and a few grammar schools, overall instruction fell dramatically.

Expanding Physical Education in the Schools

In 1871, the Ministry of Education reported that only 10,198 students in the publicly funded schools in Ontario received physical education at a time when 290,175 were taught writing. Morrow observed that "The dearth of equipment and the lack of readiness of a taxpaying public to support such a system combined with the paucity of trained teachers who could advocate such a physical training system prevented Ryerson's ideas from being crystallized."[52] The difficulties were understandable. As table 1.1 illustrates, between 1847 and 1876, the province's school-age population more than doubled through natural increase and immigration. Even though the provincial government doubled the number of schools and teachers between those years, it could not keep up, and the teacher–pupil ratio fell from 41.2 to 75.2, a challenge for any school and teacher. Most teachers were female and generalists, with little training and actual experience in the stipulated gymnastics and marching drill. In the Ministry of Education's annual report for 1876, 335,265 students were reported to have been taught writing, but only 14,835 drill and gymnastics. That is less than 5 per cent of the students reported to have been taught one of the three "Rs."

Table 1.1. Growth of the Ontario school system, 1847–76

	1847	1876
School-age children (5–16)	203,975	502,250
Public school attendance	124,829	465,243
Public schools	2,727	4,875
Number of teachers	3,028	6,185
Male teachers	2,365	2,780
Female teachers	663	3,405
Length of school year	8½ months	10¾ months

Source: *Annual Report of the Normal, Model, High and Public Schools of Ontario 1876.* Toronto: Minister of Education, 1876.

But slowly, the province moved to make physical education universal. The most effective innovation proved to be the introduction and widespread distribution in 1886 of E.B. Houghton's *Physical Culture: First Book of Exercises in Drill, Calisthenics, and Gymnastics*. It provides the best early example of what has become a tried-and-true strategy for Canadian schools, an easy-to-use, hands-on guide for teachers, with daily lesson plans and easy-to-assess assignments. Houghton was a retired physical educator from the Chatham area, who well understood the challenges, including the rudimentary facilities and days of wet and cold weather. "In the fall and spring," he wrote, "the drill should take up most of the time; in the winter, calisthenics and gymnastics."[53] The book was divided into different sections for drill, calisthenics, and gymnastics. Drill closely followed the regulations of the Queen's Own Rifles of Canada. Calisthenics constituted free-standing exercises beginning with easy stretching and flexibility positions, and then moving to handstands, stork stands, pushups, running, and rope jumping. Gymnastics involved primarily light dumb-bell exercises and rope climbing. The instructions followed the principle of progression from easy, elementary movements and exercises to the more complex. There were detailed illustrations, and Houghton offered a model lesson plan for each grade and season. The book concluded with an entire section, "For Girls," the largest in the book. After opening paragraphs arguing for the necessity of physical education for girls, Houghton prescribed modified drill, calisthenics (a series of stationary dance positions for flexibility and balance), and gymnastics (light dumb-bell and Indian club exercises).

Houghton was the first physical educator in Ontario to provide guidance for girls. It was a complicated, contested terrain. His encouragement of female-specific physical education reinforced the legitimacy of girls and young women in public schools. On the other hand, many of the exercises stipulated for girls were different and generally less demanding or strenuous than those for boys. The differences

Table 1.2. Growth of physical education in Ontario, 1871–1901

Years	Reported enrolment in writing*	Reported enrolment in drill and calisthenics	Percentage (%)
1871	290,175	10,198	3.5
1876	335,265	14,835	4.4
1881	355,627	65,422	18
1886	381,869	117,841	31
1891	379,405	184,717	49
1896	369,767	193,643	52
1901	407,080	245,094	60

Source: Ontario, *Annual Reports of the Minister of Education, Province of Ontario*.
* Along with reading and arithmetic, writing was one of the most widely taught subjects.

in prescribed exercises and the exclusion of girls and young women from marching and after-school sports perpetuated the myths of "female frailty" and a sexual division of labour that disadvantaged women at every turn. Yet it could have been worse. Some physicians and moralists sought to keep girls and women out of education altogether so that they could conserve all their energy for reproduction. To send them to school, such alarmists argued, would be to risk "race suicide."[54] Universal, free public education enriched the lives of girls and young women in many ways. Houghton's text was favourably reviewed in many newspapers and adopted for use in the normal schools. It enabled the Ministry of Education to make physical training compulsory in 1887. Each student in the early grades was to receive ninety minutes of drill, calisthenics, and gymnastics every week, and each student in the upper grades sixty minutes. While making any subject mandatory does not automatically lead to its instruction, Houghton's textbook helped many schools and teachers realize the requirement. As table 1.2 illustrates, the five years immediately following its introduction stimulated the largest single jump towards mainstreaming the subject in the nineteenth century. By 1891, 184,717 students were reported to be receiving drill and gymnastics, almost half the number of students taught writing.

Indigenous Schooling in the Late Nineteenth Century

The British North America Act gave the federal government the responsibility of legislating for Indians, and the lands reserved for Indians, which meant that Indigenous children were expected to attend schools established under the auspices of the federal Department of Indian Affairs, which in turn relied on the cooperation of the major Christian churches to maintain these schools. In post-Confederation

Canada, there were three categories of Indigenous schools: day, boarding, and industrial. Usually located on reserves, day schools enrolled most children, but they struggled with finding and keeping competent teachers, which no doubt contributed to student reluctance to attend. Boarding or live-in schools were also located on or near reserves and isolated children from parental and cultural influences. These schools were the property of the missionary organizations that built them, and operating costs were subsidized by an annual per capita grant from Indian Affairs.[55]

By the late 1870s, there were no fewer than a dozen boarding schools for Indigenous students sprinkled throughout Ontario, Manitoba, British Columbia, and the Northwest Territories.[56] In 1879, Prime Minister Sir John A. Macdonald asked Tory backbencher Nicholas Flood Davin of Regina to investigate similar residential institutions, specifically industrial schools, in the United States and to make recommendations for the Canadian situation. Davin's report made it clear that the day school did not work because "the influence of the wigwam was stronger than the influence of the school."[57] After consultations in Washington, Davin laid out the costs and benefits of a typical industrial boarding school managed by the government through an agency, and he recommended that at least four schools be established, all in western Canada. Parliament voted to establish three new industrial schools – only for boys – at Battleford, Qu'Appelle, and St. Albert in the Northwest Territories.

Over the next twenty years, educational institutions for Indigenous children expanded dramatically. By 1896, just under 10,000 students were enrolled in a day, boarding, or industrial school throughout the country, although this was probably little more than half of all Indigenous children of school age in the country. Still, the majority (238) of these institutions were day schools with obviously the most students (7,112), followed by thirty-four boarding schools (1,322), and fifteen industrial schools with 1,280 students. Almost all schools were run by a Christian order – Roman Catholic, Church of England, Methodist, Presbyterian, or some other denomination. As expected, the enrolment versus attendance ratio was higher for the industrial and boarding schools (87 and 85 per cent respectively), but still lower for the day schools (44 per cent).[58]

The students' daily existence at these schools, especially the boarding and industrial institutions, was severely regimented. For example, at the Shingwauk Home, an industrial school located in Sault Ste. Marie, Ontario, which at that time housed some sixty-five boys, their routine began early in the morning and ended twelve to fourteen hours later (see box 1.1).[59] Wednesday afternoons were reserved for the inspection of everyday clothing, mending worn clothes, and dispensing new clothes as needed. The student dormitories were also inspected. On Saturdays, mornings

BOX 1.1. DAILY SCHEDULE AT SHINGWAUK HOME FOR BOYS, 1886

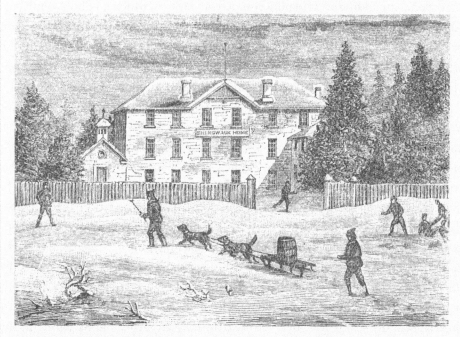

Figure 1.6. Shingwauk Home for Boys, Sault Ste. Marie, Ontario, 1886 (The General Synod Archives, Anglican Church of Canada, P2010-07-03)

6:00	Rise, wash, dress, and make bed
6:45	Roll call and prayers in school room
7:00	Assemble (where appointed)
7:05	Breakfast, march in order, stand for grace
7:30	Rise, grace, workers to work, others to preparatory class
8:30	Morning pupils assemble in school room
8:35	Roll call by classes, morning school
10:30	Fifteen-minute recess
12:00	Close school, workers quit work, wash, assemble
12:05	Dinner, march in order, stand for grace
12:30	Rise, grace, dish washers remain, others to play
1:00	Afternoon workers to work.
1:30	Afternoon pupils to preparatory class, workers to work.
1:35	Roll call by classes, afternoon school
3:00	Fifteen-minute recess
5:00	School closes
6:00	Assemble (where appointed)
6:05	Supper, march in order, stand for grace

6:30	Rise, grace, march in order, dish washers remain, others to play
7:00	Assemble all
7:05	"English" roll call, prayers in school room
7:15	Pupils who have to report go to superintendent's office, junior pupils to bed (preceded by monitor), evening preparatory class (under monitor)
8:00	Medium sized pupils to bed
9:30	Senior pupils to bed, dormitory gates locked

were reserved for cleaning and chores, afternoons were free, and evenings reserved for baths. Sundays were taken up with church, Sunday school, and bible study.

Shingwauk was typical of industrial schools of this era in that the half-day system was used to maintain the school by having students work in the gardens and fields, in the barns with the animals, or in the carpentry, blacksmith, or shoe shops. If girls were attending the school, they worked in the kitchen, sewing room, or laundry. Regardless, they all laboured for half the day and went to school for the other half. This left little time for play or recreation. Nothing like this occurred in the state schools for white children.

Calisthenics, Drill, and Recreation in Indigenous Schools

In the standard course of study for Indigenous schools outlined in the year 1889 by the Department of Indian Affairs, ten subjects were listed. They covered English and its various aspects (reading, spelling, grammar, writing, dictation, and conversation), as well as arithmetic, geography, music, and religious instruction.[60] The program of studies for 1894 included four significant additions: courses in history and general knowledge, as well as ethics, which at the first level included the practice of cleanliness, obedience, respect, order, and neatness. At the sixth and final level, ethics was concerned with "Indian and white life" and the "evils of Indian isolation." Most importantly for our purposes, calisthenics was defined as "exercises, frequently accompanied by singing, to afford variation during work and to improve physique."[61]

A few years later the schools for Indigenous children were presumably catching up to the public schools regarding the inclusion of calisthenics in the curriculum. But were they? A medical officer based in Manitoba was concerned about the lack of calisthenics in the Indigenous schools within his jurisdiction: "The teaching of calisthenics so beneficial in developing the chest and guarding against consumption and other diseases, should form part of the duties of all the teachers, as I have found it carried out only by two or three."[62] More positively, other schools reported that dumb-bells and what were called "Indian clubs," implements that originated on the Indian subcontinent in Asia, were used with calisthenics, which were thoroughly enjoyed especially when accompanied by music of the school's brass band.

Calisthenics and drill seemed to go hand in hand, especially if there was a brass band at the school. The principal of St. Boniface Industrial School in Manitoba, for example, reported that "lessons in calisthenics, gymnastics, drill, dumb-bell exercises and singing, are given to the children. In music the pupils take a very active interest, the band progresses rapidly under its skillful instructor. Many invitations have been received to play in public."[63] However, no sort of drill or military structure was mandated by Indian Affairs at this time, and if it existed at all in the Indigenous schools, it was at the initiative of individual school administrators. For instance, Robert Ashton, a schoolmaster from an industrial school in England, was hired in 1872 as the first full-time superintendent of the Mohawk Institute near Brantford, Ontario. Shocked by the lack of discipline at the school, he proceeded to set up a strict, military-style system. Over time, he devised a comprehensive set of rules, organized the boys into squads with corporals and sergeants who acted as monitors, established good-conduct badges, and constructed cells for the solitary confinement of offenders. There was also a modified, but less strict, system for girls. As time went on, regular instruction in drill became mandatory for the boys, a brass band was added, and the school often put on military displays for visiting officials and the Brantford public.[64] However, the Mohawk Institute was an exception, and although it provided a model for similar institutions, there is little evidence of military drill in Indigenous schools prior to 1900.

The Battleford Industrial School was located in the capital of the Northwest Territories in what is now Saskatchewan. After a visit to the school in the spring of 1888, an inspector commented on the role of games at the school. "They are rapidly acquiring an interest in the ways of white people in their mode of dress and thought … A noticeable feature of this school is its games. They are all thoroughly and distinctly 'white.'" He also noted that the "boys use the boxing gloves with no little science, and excellent temper, and play good games of cricket and football with great interest and truly Anglo-Saxon vigour. The girls dress dolls, make fancy articles of dress, and play such games as white children do. From all their recreation Indianism is excluded."[65] Next year, yet another inspector praised the Battleford principal and governess for their efforts in engaging the students during their hours of recreation in sports and pastimes such as cricket, baseball, boxing, swings, lawn

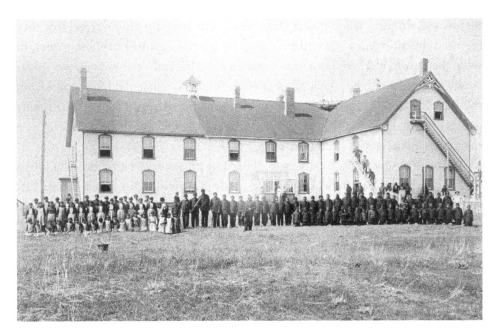

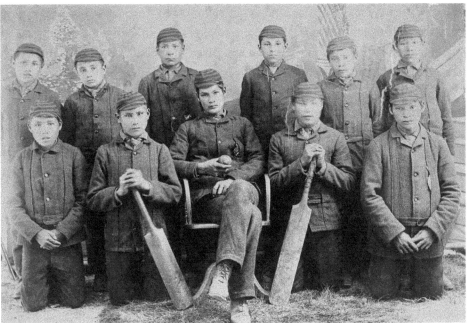

Figure 1.7. Annual sports day at the Battleford Indian Industrial School, Saskatchewan, 1895 (Library and Archives Canada, acc. nos. PA182265 and PA182266)

tennis, and croquet. "Their object," he wrote, "is to make the children feel that they are no different from white children; and, by interesting them in these games, to wean them from their wild habits and traditions."[66] Indianism, therefore, was undesirable and needed to be ameliorated or eliminated altogether. An 1895 report from the Rupert's Land Industrial School in Manitoba noted approvingly: "The manly games of cricket and football, introduced and practised by the principal, have done much to take the 'sneak' out of the boys."[67]

Although students, especially in the boarding and industrial schools, had little time for active recreation, when they did, it too was rigidly controlled and far different from the traditional games and contests they would have experienced in their home reserves. By far the most popular sport for boys was football (soccer), which could easily be played on a rough field with makeshift goal posts. Ice hockey, likely played on a frozen lake and rarely in a proper rink, was the most popular sport in winter, along with skating. Cricket and baseball were also common in the summer months. Girls simply did not play rough-and-tumble sports, but in some cases, they were allowed to row in summer and skate or toboggan in winter. Swings and croquet were also popular among girls along with summer walks and picnics. Little or no instruction or coaching was provided in these sports and activities, and students were left mostly on their own except for the occasional boys' team, which became skilled enough to compete with local line-ups.

By the turn of the century, physical education was well established as a subject in the state and private schools and less so in the Indigenous schools of Canada. Military drill, calisthenics, gymnastics, and some sports were the major activities, although the actual instruction varied widely among provinces and institutions, and girls' instruction differed significantly from that given to boys.

CHAPTER TWO

Towards a Pan-Canadian Curriculum

While physical training and elementary drill should be encouraged for all children of both sexes attending public schools, especial importance is to be attached to the teaching of military drill generally to all boys, including rifle shooting for boys capable of using rifles.
Constitution of the Strathcona Trust, 1909

By the beginning of the twentieth century, despite significant economic, cultural, and political differences between provinces and regions, as well as provincial autonomy in education, free publicly funded primary and secondary schools had been established for the settler population across Canada in much the same way. The overwhelming majority of non-Indigenous, school-age children attended state-funded elementary schools for at least some portion of the year, compelled by law and the wishes of their parents. While secondary education was still inaccessible for most children, some high school attendance would soon become an expected part of every child's development.[1] At every level of schooling, the participation rates of girls and boys were roughly the same. Where there were differences, they were more likely to be between urban and rural systems rather than provinces.[2] To be sure, there was an ongoing push and pull between the directives of the provincial departments of education and the local school boards that built the schools, hired the teachers, and implemented the curricula. Some schools in Quebec, Ontario, and New Brunswick were operated by religious organizations. But most schools across Canada were funded, regulated, and supervised by the state.

In part, such convergence was imposed from the top, the result of personal links between senior officials in different provinces. The first superintendent of education in British Columbia, John Jessop, explicitly sought to emulate the work of Egerton Ryerson, and educational leaders in other provinces often took inspiration from Ontario.[3] But the most powerful motivation came from middle-class parents who realized that it was more financially feasible, sustainable, and educationally effective to support the idea of an ongoing state system paid for by all taxpayers than continually struggle to maintain the fledgling voluntary schools of the colonial period. While some scoffed that state-subsidized schools constituted "a monster system of education for the middle and upper classes," they provided the basis for the idea of public services for all.[4]

By contrast, it was clear that separate Indigenous schooling throughout Canada was in serious difficulty. Irregular attendance, especially at day schools, was a persistent problem, along with considerably reduced government funding. Another issue was the inability to find and retain competent teachers. Abominable health conditions and escalating death rates especially in the industrial schools troubled students, parents, and school officials alike. In order to keep up student numbers, unhealthy children, often suffering from tuberculosis, were enrolled in these schools, thus infecting others. Too many children were crammed into unheated and poorly ventilated dormitories and were never fed enough to maintain their growing bodies. A 1902 survey of industrial schools across the country confirmed the devastating results: "there had been 2752 pupils admitted and of these 1700 had been discharged. Of the latter number 506 are known to be dead; 249 lost sight of; 139 in bad health; 86 transferred to other schools; 121 turned out badly and 599 said to be doing well."[5] The mistreatment of children, and high rate of disease and death, especially in the industrial schools, intensified Indigenous hostility. Most parents refused to send their children away, preferring instead the day and boarding schools closer to their reserves.

By 1900, physical education had become an accepted subject in the settler school systems, at least in expectation if not in practice. Every province had its well-known advocates, schools, and facilities, an instructor devoted to it in the normal schools, and a widely distributed manual to assist classroom teachers. In most provinces, the curriculum centred around calisthenics and marching drill, with after-school sports increasingly popular. Despite the fears whipped up by "moral physiologists" against female physical activity, most girls fully participated in calisthenics and after-school sports. But actual implementation varied widely, complicated by poor or non-existent facilities, inadequate instructors, and the feeling among school boards that physical education, like music and drawing, was a "frill" or "outer" subject.[6] In Ontario, despite its compulsory status, it was taught only 60 per cent as often as writing. In Nova Scotia, the weekly provincial average was only twenty minutes a week.[7] In Manitoba, public school inspector Charles K. Newcombe complained that the education system paid "scant attention ... to the needs of the physical organism."[8] It was, as one educational historian concluded, "generally conducted in a perfunctory way and occupied minimal space in the academic curriculum."[9] That would all change in 1911 with the Strathcona Trust.

Canadian Imperialism and Lord Strathcona

While Confederation brought Canada considerable political autonomy, it did not sever ties with the mother country entirely. In fact, Britain controlled Canadian foreign policy, citizenship, and final legal appeals to the Judicial Committee of the British Privy Council for many subsequent decades. It was not until 1931 that the British Parliament finally relinquished the right to make laws for Canada, 1949 that the Supreme Court of Canada became the final legal authority, and 1982 that Canada fully repatriated the power of constitutional amendment. The ties of empire were maintained by immigration and sentiment. In the late nineteenth and early twentieth century, as Britain and the other European powers vied with each other for colonies and trade by arming themselves heavily, Canadians hotly debated their place in the British Empire. English-speaking conservatives were prepared to support Britain carte blanche, while Quebec nationalists, pacifists, and non-British immigrant groups argued for neutrality. Prime Minister Wilfrid Laurier sought a middle way, specifically a commitment to Canadian support of the British Empire but the right to determine the nature and extent of Canadian contributions. In 1899, he sent a small Canadian contingent in support of British troops to the South African Boer War.

A well-connected group in these debates was composed of Canadian "imperialists." The term has other, more familiar, uses. For some, it connotes a political system in which one powerful state controls one or more colonies by military and political means, for example, the British Empire in the nineteenth century. For others, it means an economic system in which the capitalist interests from one country or region control the economies of other countries to ensure access to raw materials at low prices and to enjoy markets for finished goods, such as American imperialism in Central and South America. The Canadian "imperialists" had still a different idea: Canadian independence within a federation of all British countries and colonies. They believed in the worth of British (as opposed to American) political institutions, respect for the social hierarchy, and Christian social Darwinism.[10] Strategically placed in senior positions in schools and universities, the imperialists sought to impart those ideas and values in

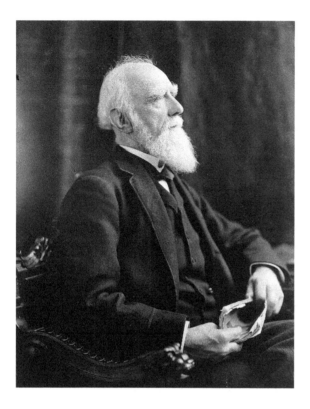

Figure 2.1. Sir Donald Smith, Lord Strathcona, 1895 (McCord Museum, II-110266)

the young through a system of military drill and cadets. One of the most influential was James L. Hughes, chief inspector of Toronto public schools between 1874 and 1913, and a prominent sports leader. In 1879, he wrote the first Canadian textbook on physical education, *Manual of Drill and Calisthenics*, to make it easier for teachers to conduct classes. Hughes's overarching goal was to strengthen obedience, discipline, and loyalty to British values. "Where we have so many foreign lads," he declared, "I am sure the quickest and best way we can make them respect the British flag is to march them through the streets in uniform behind that flag."[11] Another well-known imperialist was Maurice Hutton, principal of University College at the University of Toronto, who wrote that military training is "in itself a safeguard against physical degeneracy and that physical decadence which industrialism continually brings in its train."[12]

Another prominent supporter of Canadian imperialism was Sir Donald A. Smith, Lord Strathcona, a successful fur trader, railroad magnate, and philanthropist with financial interests around the world.[13] He served as Canada's High Commissioner to the United Kingdom from 1896 to 1914. As chancellor of McGill University, he created scholarships for women and established Royal Victoria College, a residential school for women where the students were known as the "Donaldas." In 1907, at the request of Laurier's minister of militia, Frederick Borden, Strathcona donated £500,000 to create a trust fund to finance improvements in physical education, military training (including the creation of high school cadet corps), and patriotism in Canadian schools. The annual interest from the Trust would provide each province an allotment proportional to its school enrolment. The Trust established local committees in every province (and one Catholic and one Protestant in Quebec) to oversee the program and administer the funds. While it gave each provincial committee latitude in how it spent the money, it also stipulated that physical training form an integral part of the curriculum in every school; a certificate of ability to instruct in physical training be part of every teacher's certificate; and that the Education Department encourage the formation of cadet corps. Furthermore, it suggested that the system of physical training adopted be the same as the elementary public schools of Great Britain, "with such modifications therein as the local conditions of any Province may show to be necessary."[14]

At first, not every province embraced the plan. Some were concerned about their autonomy. Others faced protests from teachers as well as labour, church, and peace groups who feared that the military and paramilitary training included in the plan would contribute to the worldwide preparations for war.[15] However, there was precedent for federal–provincial cooperation in cadet training through an 1896 agreement the federal Department of Militia had forged with the Ontario Department of Education. Physical education was also promoted through a 1907 pilot program Borden undertook with his home province of Nova Scotia. By 1911, every province had signed on. The Trust published and distributed across the country a teacher's manual, the *Syllabus of Physical Exercises for Schools*, for use in elementary schools. As noted in a prefatory memorandum, the *Syllabus* was, in the main, a reprint of the "latest official Syllabus authorized for use in the Public Elementary Schools of England which is based on the Swedish system of educational gymnastics, already adopted by several European countries." It also noted that "freedom of movement and a certain degree of exhilaration being essentials of all true physical education, games and dancing steps have been introduced into many of the lessons."[16] With no requirements for specialized equipment, the curriculum could be delivered virtually anywhere there was open space – aisles, corridors, and schoolyards as well as gymnasia – no small consideration given the wide variety of facilities and conditions that existed in Canadian schools at the time. The *Syllabus* carefully spelled out every step of the lesson, with illustrations and photographs, from the arrangement of the class and the best manner of command to the warm-up, progression of developmentally appropriate exercises, and "suitable dress for girls" (tunic, jersey, or blouse and knickers). It gave the generalist a comprehensive framework for planning and conducting a year's sequence of lessons and exercises of increasing difficulty and fitness. Copies found in second-hand bookstores are full of underlining and hand-written marginal notes that indicate the *Syllabus* was well used.

In 1920, the Trust authorized a new version of the *Syllabus* for elementary schools, one that had been revised by the British government in 1919. The circumstances reflected the times. The previous year, a conference of ministers of education and normal schoolteachers from the four western provinces had been highly critical of the original *Syllabus* and proposed major changes. Before their recommendations could be considered, let alone implemented in a made-in-Canada manual, a visiting physical educator from England, "a certain Miss Brackett," was "discovered" to be teaching in a Montreal school using a much-improved 1919 version of the *Syllabus*.[17] Although there was neither a Canadian preface nor a French translation, Ethel Mary Cartwright at Royal Victoria College in Montreal, and others, persuaded the Trust to authorize its use. There was limited free distribution, but copies quickly became available in stores and most teachers bought their own. Among the improvements, commands were significantly rewritten to enable teachers to instruct students in movements rather than static positions. The revised *Syllabus* recommended that not less than half the lesson be devoted to active free movement, including games and dancing; and that the classroom teacher be allowed more scope for personal initiative, freedom, and enterprise.[18] The Trust also lengthened the course of physical training for teachers in normal schools to forty-five hours (from the previous thirty) to strengthen the training in hygiene, anatomy, and physiology.

The Strathcona Trust was remarkable in the history of non-Indigenous Canadian education. A small amount of money – the cost of publishing and distributing the first edition of the *Syllabus*, and annual grants to the provincial committees – gave the federal government a determining voice in the elementary physical education curriculum in every province, therefore overcoming provincial jealousy over their constitutional autonomy in education. Full credit should be given to Frederick Borden because, according to historians, "there can be no doubt that he was the prime mover" behind the plan.[19]

The pan-Canadian mobilization necessitated by the First World War, the accessibility and convenience of the *Syllabus*, the requirements for teacher training, and the financial incentives for teachers and students all gave physical education a significant boost. In Ontario, for example, it was at a low ebb before the *Syllabus* was introduced, yet within a decade, it was the most widely taught subject in the province, with the number of students enrolled surpassing those taking composition, which was often used as a measure of the total student population (see table 2.1). In 1914, the first year of full reporting, 5,757 teachers-in-training across Canada received the basic training. In Ontario, virtually the entire normal school enrolment

40

(iii) *Arm Stretching Upward.* (*Upward Stretch Position.*)

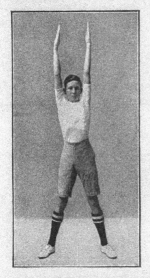

FIG. 39.

The arms are bent and then stretched upward to their fullest extent, the hands being the width of the shoulders apart, the fingers and thumbs straight and close together, and the palms turned in. The hands should be in line with the arms. (*See* Figs. 39 and 40.)

COMMANDS:
  ARMS UPWARD—*stretch.*
  ARMS DOWNWARD—*stretch.*

[*Common faults*:
  Hands not in line with the arms.
  Hands and arms brought too far forward.
  Head carried forward.]

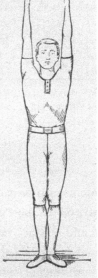

FIG 40.

(iv) *Arm Stretching Forward.* (*Forward Stretch Position.*)

The arms are bent and then stretched forward at the shoulder level, keeping the body erect. The fingers and thumbs must be straight, the palms turned in, and the hands and arms should be at least the width of the shoulders apart. (*See* Fig. 41.)

COMMANDS:
  ARMS FORWARD—*stretch.*
  ARMS DOWNWARD—*stretch.*

[*Common faults*:
  Bringing the shoulders forward.
  Bringing the hands too close to one another.
  Rounding the back.]

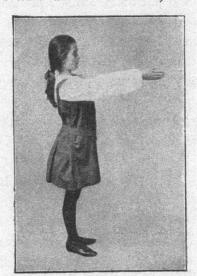

FIG. 41.

Figure 2.2. *Syllabus of Physical Exercises for Schools*, 1911 (published by the Executive Council, Strathcona Trust, 1911, 40)

Table 2.1. Influence of the Strathcona Trust in Ontario, 1911–31

Years	Reported enrolment in composition*	Reported enrolment in physical culture	Percentage (%)
1906	320,806	225,434	70
1911	339,577	327,491	96
1915	391,967	403,752	103
1921	438,849	476,449	109
1926	479,627	504,166	105
1931	462,686	527,652	114

Source: *Annual Reports of the Ministry of Education, Province of Ontario.*
* The Trust was introduced in 1909.

received the training. The grants for prize money for outstanding teachers and students also provided stimulus. The first competition invited teachers to submit essays on "the best method of introducing and developing a general system of physical and military training in the public schools throughout the Dominion on the principle set forth in the rules of the Strathcona Trust."[20] Later, prizes were awarded to both teachers and pupils for the performance of designated exercises from the *Syllabus*, presented after well-attended public competitions in arenas and stadia like Arena Gardens in Toronto and Lansdowne Park in Ottawa. The net effect was to make physical education a prominent subject in elementary schools. As George Tomkins, an educational historian at the University of British Columbia, once observed: "I am convinced that for all our bewailing the lack of a national curriculum in Canada (a dubious ambition), we effectively had one by the 1920s. Physical education was the most successful example – if success is defined as every Grade 6 kid from Victoria to Halifax doing the same number of push-ups on the same day. The 'school promoters' would have had them doing them at the same hour, but for time differences, I am sure."[21]

Indigenous Schooling and Physical Education

Dr. Peter Bryce, the Chief Medical Officer for the Department of Indian Affairs, inspected thirty-five industrial and boarding schools in Manitoba and the Northwest Territories (Alberta and Saskatchewan) during 1905–6. He was particularly interested in the condition of the schools and the health of the pupils, which of course were related. He obtained statistical data from fifteen industrial and boarding schools regarding the history and present health of the children who had been pupils at these institutions. The results were shocking. Of 1,527 pupils in these schools, all of which had been in operation for an average of fourteen years, 7 per cent were sick or in poor health, and nearly one-quarter were reported dead.[22] In one school, 69 per cent of ex-pupils had died, and in all schools, the most common cause of death was tuberculosis. Literally, these schools were killing the young Indigenous population.

In his report, Bryce blamed the lack of ventilation in schoolrooms and dormitories, especially through the long winter months, as the main cause for the high tubercular infection rate. Interestingly, he also commented on the "almost complete absence of any drill or manual exercises amongst the boys or calisthenics or breathing exercises amongst the girls." He went on to say: "One would suppose that in boarding schools the need for such exercises would be looked upon as an elementary necessity; but it was found that it was only in some isolated cases that it had ever been heard of or put into practice. And yet the disciplinary value of such exercises, apart wholly from their health value, is so obvious ... it may be expecting too much to suppose that so elementary a necessity of school hygiene as physical exercise should have been a part of the course in these schools."[23] Dr. Bryce was probably the first public health official to recommend the need for regular physical exercise among Indigenous students in the industrial and boarding schools. His report was leaked to journalists, and the resulting publicity prompted more intense criticism of these schools as well as support for his recommendations. Bryce's colleagues in government and in the field were also initially supportive, but church leaders whose denominations ran the schools, were critical, pointing to the lack of federal funds.

Duncan Campbell Scott had been with Indian Affairs since its establishment as a separate department in 1880. Starting as a junior copy clerk, he had progressively climbed the bureaucratic ladder, and in 1909 was appointed Superintendent of Education. As one biographer has noted, his "avoidance of conflict in the workplace, and his embracement of the status quo, aided greatly his steady career advancement."[24] He too claimed a lack of federal monies, which masked his strong personal and political preference for the aggressive assimilation of the Indigenous population as quickly as possible. Scott's solution was to phase out the large industrial schools and replace them with cheaper and smaller boarding schools located mostly on reserves. The "industrial" component of the industrial schools had never been very successful since farming and carpentry for boys and housewifery for girls were usually the only skills taught. The curricular differences between the industrial and boarding schools were also insignificant so that these terms were phased out, and by 1923 had been replaced by the all-encompassing "residential" term. Scott also wanted new, improved day schools with qualified teachers that would supply footwear and clothing to deserving students, and a warm meal in the middle of the day. He also mandated "to vary the school exercises by games and simple calisthenics; these are the best means to banish the idle teacher and the empty schoolroom, and they are being gradually introduced whenever they are needed."[25] By 1930, there were 78 residential schools and 272 day schools in operation across the country, with a total enrolment of just over 15,000 Indigenous students and a 74 per cent attendance record – the largest ever in terms of both enrolment and attendance.[26]

In 1910, Indian Affairs distributed a small booklet to encourage calisthenics and games, suitable for children between six and sixteen, in schools under its jurisdiction. "As Indian children show a tendency towards pulmonary disease," wrote the author in an introductory note, "special attention to the several deep breathing movements should be given."[27] The exercises were to be taught daily, in the open air in spring, summer, and fall, and usually in a large and well-ventilated room in winter. Students should be arranged in columns with adequate space to allow the free movement of arms and legs, and then "command the squad to take the correct standing position." Whoever wrote this probably had a military background because the fundamental standing position should correspond to the position of a soldier when at "attention," followed by marching on the spot, to assist in "obtaining the attention and prompt discipline so necessary before real work can be commenced."[28] There were exercises to be used appropriately especially after prolonged sitting or if there was any tendency towards chest contraction and deficiency in breathing. Also included were jumping movements to increase circulation and quicken respiration. The final section of the booklet contained suggestions for indoor and outdoor games and sports suitable for both boys and girls: "Running, jumping, ball games and similar sports are vitally important as a means of moulding the child's character and for general exercise."[29]

The following year, Indian Affairs sent a directive to all teachers in its schools stating that the "department desires to give special prominence on the curriculum of studies for Indian schools to the subject of hygiene and, with this object in view, it has been decided to adopt for use the textbook recently authorized by the Department of Education for Ontario."[30] A copy of the textbook was sent to all schools, and teachers could order enough copies required for their students. Not less than twenty minutes each day was to be devoted to the subject, and no portion of the textbook should be neglected, with special prominence given to chapters dealing with sanitation, food, the use of alcohol, and tuberculosis. "One of the problems that confront all workers in their efforts to ameliorate the home conditions of the Indian," stated the memorandum, "is his indifference to the matter of sanitation and to a wholesome diet."[31] Tuberculosis, assured the memorandum, is curable in its early stages, and its spread preventable through fresh air, nourishing food, sanitary homes, and exercise to improve the physical condition of the students.

Within the schools, there was an almost immediate increase in reports of calisthenics but less so in military drill. Most principals indicated that they had received the booklet outlining calisthenics and games, and were implementing some sort of exercise program in their schools. In 1911 there were twenty-eight references to calisthenics and thirty-nine in 1912, the majority of schools, in the annual reports from Indian Affairs. For example, a report from the Kenora Boarding School, situated on Lake of the Woods in Ontario with nearly forty students, and run by the Sisters of the Roman Catholic Church, was typical:

> The class rooms are under the charge of Sisters Audette and McAvoy, who are qualified teachers, earnest and devoted to their work. The progress made during the year was excellent, in all branches of the studies, as prescribed by the department, including calisthenics and games. Good practical instruction is given the boys in farming and care of stock, and the girls in domestic housework. They have a fine hockey team and skating rink where the pupils enjoy themselves during recess and evenings, which is of much benefit to their health. All rooms and premises are kept scrupulously clean and well ventilated. The management of this institution is first class in every respect.[32]

The first reference to "physical education" in the Department of Indian Affairs annual reports appears in 1924: "A special effort has been made in the matter of physical education and in the correlation of classroom exercises with vocational training and home interests."[33] In 1925, there was a similar comment that again a "special effort" was being made with regard to physical education, which seemed to mean a comprehensive medical inspection and more attention to physical education within the school curriculum. However, the Department no longer provided individual reports from the many day and residential schools so that it is almost impossible to know what this special effort entailed or how it was being accomplished. We can only assume that as physical education was becoming more organized and recognized within the regular school curricula, the same might be occurring in the Indigenous schools.

Cadet Movement and Militarism

The Strathcona Trust injected new energy and resources into the flagging cadet movement as well. In addition to the stimulus Borden sought to provide to physical education in the elementary schools, he and Strathcona wanted to place military training (marching and rifle shooting) in the secondary schools "as a potential benefit to the Militia Department."[34] This was ensured by loaning military officers to the schools and appointing military men to the leadership of the national and provincial committees, where they could award grants for cadet corps. The Trust stimulated competitions and parades in many cities and towns, especially during the First World War. A smartly uniformed, well-disciplined student corps could excite great acclaim and patriotism among schools, parents, and communities. In Quebec, Henri-Thomas Scott taught physical education in the French Catholic schools of Montreal, and organized boys in both cadets and gymnastics, taking teams to competitions across the province and to Europe. He became the chief recruiting officer of the 57th Infantry Battalion during the First World War.[35] The Ontario champion of the cadet movement was James L. Hughes, still the chief inspector of Toronto schools after thirty-four years. In 1911, Hughes's younger brother Sam became the Minister of Militia in the Conservative government of Robert Borden. From the creation of the Trust, Hughes was secretary of the committee responsible for administering the grants in Ontario. He served in that role for fourteen years and stayed on the committee for another ten. Critics suggest that he used his influence to ensure that the cadet programs had more in common with militarism than with the educational objectives of the school.[36]

At the beginning of the war, several Canadian universities instituted military training for male students, often accompanied by a medical examination that determined their fitness for military drill, and relegated the unfit for compulsory physical training.[37] Some universities, like Queen's for example, had initiated compulsory physical education and medical examinations for all first-year students prior to the war. In 1914, the University of Alberta introduced compulsory "physical drill" (two periods a week) for all first- and second-year students, although in the case of male students, military drill could be substituted.[38] At McGill University, although a required program of physical education for women (at Royal Victoria College) had begun in 1907, it wasn't until 1916, following an intervention by the Graduates' Society, that male students were required to attend two hours of physical education classes per week during their first three years.[39]

Although the Department of Indian Affairs supported cadet programs in general, it refused to finance them. By 1914, the Canadian government had sanctioned only three school cadet corps in Indigenous schools. They were at the Mohawk Institute, near Brantford, Ontario, which was the original (1828) residential school in Canada; the Elkhorn Indian Residential School (1888) in Manitoba; and St. Paul's Indian Residential School (1889) on the Blood Reserve in Alberta.[40] However, as discussed earlier in this chapter, the addition of drill and military structure to a particular school came from individual school administrators. A good example was Rupert's Land Industrial School on the banks of the Red River near Winnipeg, Manitoba. Opened in 1889, it almost immediately established a drill team for boys, and entered local school drill competitions. A few years later, the principal called upon a drill sergeant from the Boys' Brigade to provide instruction in military drill, but the expense was too great, and it had to be discontinued.[41] By 1901, the school, now called St. Paul's Industrial School, had a fully functioning cadet corps and brass band for the boys, in addition to a calisthenics club for the girls. Also available, especially in winter, was a "commodious drill hall" for practice. The military aspect of the school was discontinued in 1904 because there was no leader for the band and few instruments; nor was there an available drill instructor. "We think the time given to both," explained the principal, "can be devoted to those things which will be more beneficial to those having to make their way in the world when they leave the institution."[42] However, the following year, the cadet company was reorganized with an ex-sergeant drill instructor training it two nights a week. Unfortunately, a serious fire erupted sometime in 1906 and much of the school burned down. It was never rebuilt.

The Mohawk Institute near Brantford, Ontario always had a military-style system for disciplinary purposes (see chapter 1), and the boys especially received regular instruction in drill with wooden muskets. In 1909, they were organized into a proper cadet corps (No. 161) and supplied with new Ross rifles by the Militia Regiment.[43] The Mohawk Institute Honor Roll lists eighty-three former students who enlisted in the First World War, with six staff and students making the supreme sacrifice. After the war, many residential schools discontinued their participation in government-sponsored cadet corps due to the anti-war sentiment and growing peace movement. The Mohawk Institute's cadet corps was officially disbanded in 1925, although the militaristic organization of the school continued.

While both contemporary and recent observers have judged the cadet corps and the military spirit they exemplified harshly, they also had strong supporters. A survey of British Columbia education in the 1920s found that school principals held widely different views on their value. About half approved and the other half were either opposed or lukewarm. Some objected on the grounds that the training was too militaristic, but others defended military drill because it instilled "good carriage and valuable discipline" in the boys.[44] More recently, the eminent American historian William McNeill, who participated in cadet marching as a young man, challenged us to rethink the educational power of "muscular bonding," in other words, the essential activity of military drill: "Words are inadequate to describe the

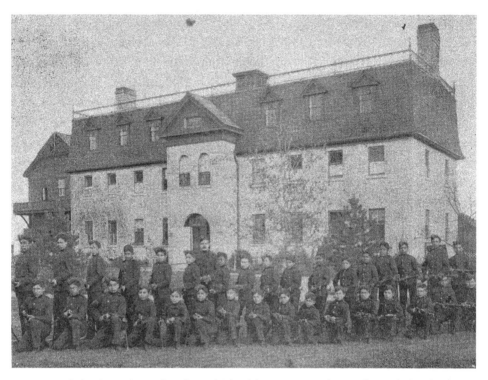

Figure 2.3. Cadet Corps, St. Paul's Industrial School (near Winnipeg), 1900 (United Church of Canada Archives, 1993.049P/2022)

emotion aroused by the prolonged movement in unison that drilling involved. A sense of pervasive well-being is what I recall; more specifically, a strange sense of personal enlargement; a sort of swelling out, becoming bigger than life, thanks to participation in collective ritual."[45] He concluded that "large and complex human societies, in all probability, cannot long maintain themselves without such kinesthetic undergirding. Ideas and ideals are not enough. Feelings matter too, and feelings are inseparable from their gestural and muscular expression."[46]

Challenging the Military Drill Approach

The Strathcona Trust was not without its detractors, both within and outside the school system. After the war, some returning soldiers became teachers. Teaching what they knew best, they placed a heavy emphasis upon marching and cadet training to the neglect of the *Syllabus of Physical Training for Schools 1919*. In the survey of British Columbia education mentioned earlier, Drs. J.H. Putnam (senior inspector

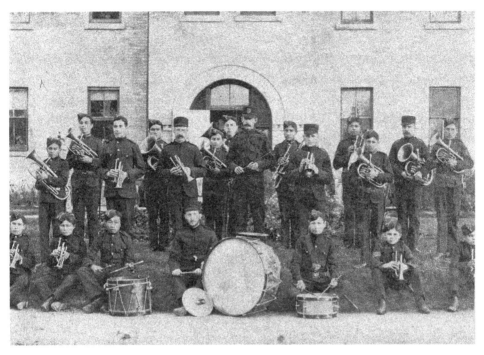

Figure 2.4. Band of St. Paul's Industrial School, 1900 (United Church of Canada Archives 1993.049P/2023)

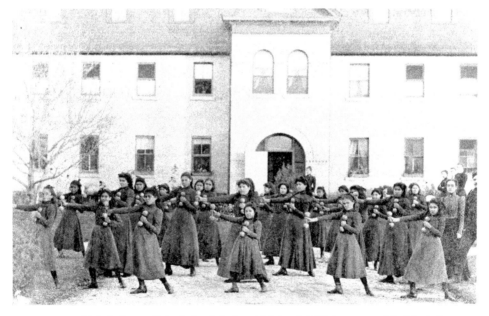

Figure 2.5. Girls' Calisthenic Club, St. Paul's Industrial School, 1900 (courtesy of the Manitoba Museum, Winnipeg, MB, EP 3189)

of schools in Ottawa) and G.M. Weir (a professor of education at the University of British Columbia, who later became the provincial education minister) noted complaints that "too much emphasis is placed upon cadet training and that boys are sometimes coerced into taking military drill." They concluded that "the schools would suffer no real loss if every vestige of military training was eliminated from the school programme."[47] They also attacked the method of instruction at the normal schools: "The smack and atmosphere of the drill sergeant and military camp are too prominent, where the initiative, spontaneity, and joy of the recreational side of life should be in more evidence."[48] These methods, they argued, were better suited to the parade ground than to teacher training institutions. Instead, they recommended that the physical education course at normal schools be "humanized" through the introduction of more group games and organized activities, and as well through the hiring of female physical education instructors to teach women students. They also recommended that the qualifications for school physical education instructors be equivalent to the academic and professional training of regular teachers. Putnam and Weir were not opposed to physical education. On the contrary, they condemned the futility of "attempting to erect a vigorous intellectual structure on a weak physical foundation."[49] They just wanted it more educationally focused. They called for daily exercise and a new emphasis upon student-directed organized games.

These critiques, which grew in number and intensity during the 1920s, contributed to a much more child-centred, educationally focused approach to physical education, especially in the emerging university-based schools of physical education and in private institutions like the Margaret Eaton School in Toronto (see chapter 3). One of the strongest and most persistent critics was Arthur S. Lamb, who had studied physical education at the YMCA Training School in Springfield, Massachusetts, and in 1912 arrived at McGill University to study medicine. He was also appointed Physical Director, and after graduation, followed by a stint in the military during the war, he returned to McGill in 1919 as Director of the Department of Physical Education. Lamb became a commanding presence in Canadian physical education and athletics, known far and wide as "Dad" Lamb. According to biographer John Douglas Eaton, he acquired the nickname when he became a father while attending medical school.[50]

In a speech to the 1923 annual convention of the Ontario Educational Association, Lamb laid out his philosophy of physical education: "Education differs from training in that education has a much broader ideal than training which, in my opinion, may only mean training for some definite, particular objective. And so to-day we speak of physical education rather than physical training or physical culture,

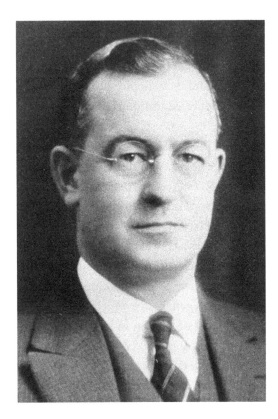

Figure 2.6. Arthur S. Lamb, 1926 (*Old McGill*, 1926, p. 218; courtesy of McGill University Archives)

and ... the application of that meaning is one that physical educators must strive to uphold, and they must strive to relate their activities towards general education."[51] Physical education, he lamented, is looked upon as merely formal drill and gymnastics, when it is so much more – including medical examinations, instruction in health education, and participation in physical activity for its physiological, social, and moral benefits. Therefore, in Lamb's opinion, the aims of physical education were corrective, educational, hygienic, and recreative. He saw no educational value whatsoever in the "arms raising sideways" type of physical exercise, represented by the content in the *Syllabus of Physical Training for Schools 1919* and distributed through the Strathcona Trust. "I fail to see very much value, except an ability on the part of the child to jump at the word of command when given," he reasoned.[52] Basically, there were few educational advantages to formal gymnastics, and these could only be obtained through activities like games, natural gymnastics, and dancing. For Lamb, the present-day systems of physical exercise and training were entirely inadequate because they were not designed for the growing, living child. Rather, he argued, they were devised with a military end in view. He was also highly critical of the short, forty-five-hour, summer training course in physical education, as laid down by the Strathcona Trust, and designed for elementary school teachers. Rather, prospective teachers should receive instruction in anatomy, physiology, hygiene, public health, and preventative medicine, and they should study psychology, sociology, and biology, which would require higher education studies in physical education.

Ethel Mary Cartwright, the British-educated physical director of Royal Victoria College at McGill, took another tack. In 1907, she had established a compulsory physical education program for all first-year McGill women students and soon expanded that to 140 hours of physical education as a requirement for graduation. In 1912, she helped start the McGill School of Physical Education (MSPE) to train women as teachers and leaders. What began as a short summer course had by 1919 expanded to a full, two-year program recognized by the university. By 1921, MSPE had graduated eighty students, many of whom were working far afield.[53] She was not prepared to criticize Lord Strathcona's generosity, which had financed the creation of her college. She valued his support of women in higher education and probably sought his additional contributions. Instead of criticizing it, she positioned the Trust as an opportunity to advance both the subject and the profession of physical education as a body of knowledge and practice dedicated to the healthy physical growth and development of all children and youth. As she told a colleague: "If you can't beat them, join them and work to improve them from within."[54]

In a series of speeches and articles presented between 1913 and the end of the war, Cartwright commended Lord Strathcona on his foresight and generosity, thanked the military for their leadership and financial support, and then turned the topic towards what should be done to enable physical education to fully realize its promise.[55] First, it was necessary to recognize that considering the demands made by those who have to teach physical education, their "training has been limited and not sufficiently in touch with educational procedure." Then she stated: "emphatically and unreservedly ... the military teacher, be he ever so good, is not the right person to teach physical exercises to women. Nor is his training the best preparation for one who is to instruct men teachers ... for it is inevitable that his experience should have been with men, whereas the fundamental problem of the school is the adaptation of physical exercises to the varying needs of boys and girls in the successive stages of their growth."[56] From that starting point, Cartwright declared that the "expert" physical educator "is not one who can perform and teach a few exercises, but one with an intimate knowledge of applied anatomy, physiology, school and public hygiene, physiology of exercise, physical diagnosis, medical gymnastics, psychology, folk dances, games and athletics for all ages, and the recognized

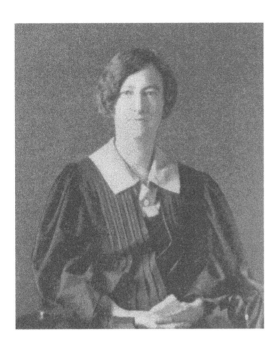

Figure 2.7. Ethel Mary Cartwright, 1927 (*The McGill News* 8, no. 3 [1927]: 5; courtesy of McGill University Archives)

systems of physical education."[57] This knowledge, she argued, cannot be obtained at a six-week or two-month course. She then proposed a national, university-based college of physical education where women and men could receive thorough training for other than military purposes. She also persuaded the Militia Department to provide grants to McGill University to train physical education teachers to replace military instructors in the schools, and to appoint her an instructor and examiner.[58]

It would have been fascinating to see where Cartwright could have taken her diplomatic, constructive approach to the ambitions of physical education in the immediate aftermath of the war. Unfortunately, she never had the chance. In 1919, Lamb was given sole authority over an integrated School of Physical Education at McGill, and despite appeals from Cartwright and her supporters, he denied her (and other women) any recognition or position of influence in the academic program. Lamb seemed to regard Cartwright, an experienced teacher, organizer, and eloquent advocate of women-led education and sport, as a threat to his early leadership.[59] While he always supported women's participation in sport and physical activity, he did so in the protective, paternalistic way associated with distinctive, restrictive rules for girls and women.[60] In 1929, Cartwright was appointed to the University of Saskatchewan with the mandate to establish a School of Physical Education, where she was finally able to resume her visionary leadership and contribute once again to the development of physical education in Canada.

Another strong and reasonable voice was that of Ruth Clark, who like Cartwright had been trained at the Chelsea College of Physical Education in London, England. She first came to Canada in 1913, when she was invited by Cartwright to teach at the McGill Summer School in Physical Education. She returned in 1919 to organize physical education for women students at Queen's University in Kingston but stayed only a year before returning to her teaching position at Chelsea College.[61] Aside from her important work at McGill and Queen's, she also left a written record of her views about school physical education. Like Lamb and Cartwright, she maintained that a short, six-week summer course was far too limited to train a physical education teacher properly, and what was badly needed was a three-year university-level program. It was also absurd, she argued, "to expect every teacher to be sufficiently interested or temperamentally suited to teach physical work successfully."[62] Not only must teachers be more fully trained, but better facilities and equipment should also be provided in schools. At the very least, there must be a gymnasium fitted with Swedish gymnastic apparatus, and complete with a dressing room and showers, as well as an outdoor playground for games. All students (especially girls) should wear special uniforms for both games and gymnastics; and in all cases, girls should be taught by women.

In the 1920s, more universities began to institute compulsory physical training programs although they tended to mirror those established prior to the war, which mainly included gymnastics, folk dancing, and remedial posture exercises. Although more women were entering university, they still only constituted less than 20 per cent of the undergraduate population. Universities were also more likely to initiate a physical training program for women before they did so for men because of the general view that women were less able to tolerate the strains and stresses of full-time study (and the endless socializing), and therefore needed the strengthening more. The course for students at Mount St. Bernard College for women at St. Francis Xavier University, for example, consisted of "March Tactics, Setting Up Exercises, Folk Dancing, and Formal Gymnastics."[63]

In 1926, at the Third Congress of the Universities of the British Empire, held in London, England, R. Tait McKenzie (now a professor at the University of Pennsylvania) opened a session about "The desirability of making Provision for the Physical Welfare and Training of Students and the Organization of Athletics with a view to securing more general participation."[64] Although he was speaking only about male students, he argued for a progressive and systematic course of physical education for which they should be given credit. Also attending the congress were two Canadian representatives, one from McGill University and the other from the University of Toronto, who provided detailed reports about physical training/

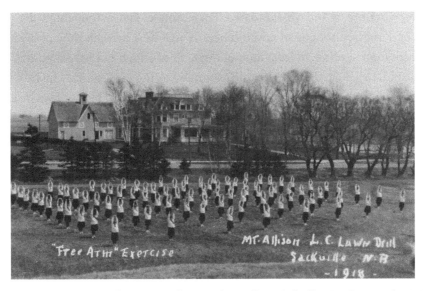

Figure 2.8. Exercise lawn drill at Mount Allison Ladies College, Sackville, New Brunswick, 1918 (Mount Allison University Archives, 2010.29/3)

education and athletics at their respective universities. At McGill, all students entering the university for the first time were medically examined and placed in one of the following categories: fit for all exercise, fit for limited exercise, fit for gymnasium work only, required to do "remedial gymnasium," or unfit for any form of exercise.[65] In 1925–6, 1,134 men and 316 women were examined with 80 per cent of males found to be fit for all forms of exercise (no information was given about the females). At the University of Toronto, physical training was compulsory for the first- and second-year students, all of whom were medically examined to decide the form and amount of exercise best suited to their needs. All students were taught to swim. Only 2 per cent of students were found to be unfit and were exempt from any form of physical training.

Early Youth Movements and Physical Education

The modern concept of "adolescence" was relatively unknown until American psychologist G. Stanley Hall popularized the term and gave it scientific authority through his two-volume opus, *Adolescence: Its Psychology and Its Relations to Physiology, Anthropology, Sociology, Sex, Crime, Religion, and Education* published in 1904. In many ways, Hall's views of adolescence were enlightened and progressive, especially for the early twentieth century, yet others were repressive, even bizarre, certainly by today's standards. For example, Hall wrote about the prevalence of depressed moods in adolescence, as well as it being a time of crime and high sensation seeking, at least among boys, all of which hold true today. On the other hand, he equated adolescent development to the evolutionary history of humanity; he had puritanical views of adolescent sexuality; and he was convinced that religious conversion in adolescence was normative and universal.[66] Nonetheless, his work about the importance of physical exercise in character formation provided a new and theoretical framework that some founders of early youth movements used to justify their programs, especially those for boys and young men.[67]

At the beginning of the twentieth century, there was growing concern in Canada, and many countries in the Western world, that young people – men and boys in particular – were becoming less manly or virile, more prone to indolence or even hooliganism, and consequently more in need of new experiences. One cure for their moral and physical deterioration was to remove them from the unhealthy, stifling city and entice them to explore nature through camping and woodcraft. Another was to bring them into a Christian religious environment through new youth clubs. The main purpose of these early movements was to save a generation of *boys* (girls would come later) from godlessness and degeneracy. Overall, and to varying degrees, the youth movements of the nineteenth and early twentieth centuries preached virility, discipline, love of nature, Christianity, patriotism, and imperialism.[68] Certainly, physical training and, more accurately for some, physical education played a major role in the philosophies, programs, and activities of these movements. It should be noted that the membership of the movements discussed here consisted almost entirely of non-Indigenous youth except where occasionally the Boy Scouts or Girl Guides were organized at a residential school.

Between the last decade of the nineteenth century and the first two decades of the next, the most rapid growth within YMCA programming was in physical education and sport. By 1914, a YMCA was considered incomplete if its building lacked a gymnasium and swimming pool. Rough statistics suggest that participants in physical activities numbered just under 4,000 in 1900 and by 1920 had jumped to nearly 23,000.[69] The indoor gymnasium classes of exercises and games were the most popular. Other physical activities included wrestling, fencing, track and field, swimming and lifesaving, and gymnastics as well as leagues in basketball and other sports. YMCAs without indoor facilities promoted outdoor activities with organized leagues in lacrosse, baseball, football, and track and field. Men with training, often graduates of the YMCA Training College in Springfield, Massachusetts, were employed to head these physical departments and to ensure that their purpose was to develop Christians, not pugilists. The necessity of training leaders was

BOX 2.1. J. HOWARD CROCKER (1870–1959)

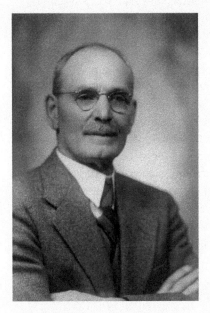

Figure 2.9. John Howard Crocker, L.L.D., University of Western Ontario, 1950 (R.K. Barney Image Collection, International Centre for Olympic Studies, Western University)

As the firstborn of an old United Empire Loyalist family, John Howard Crocker was born in St. Stephen, New Brunswick, on 19 April 1870. At sixteen, he was employed in a lumber camp to earn money to help support his mother and four younger siblings. This adventure into manhood was cut short by a bout of rheumatic fever that left him partially crippled. He was learning to be a machinist when the YMCA was organized in Amherst, Nova Scotia, where he lived, and he began a program of physical training to rebuild his body. In a few years, he had won the all-round athletic championship of the Maritimes.

Determined to become a YMCA secretary, Crocker attended Dalhousie University in Halifax as an undergraduate, earning a Bachelor of Arts degree in 1897. He began medical studies but discontinued them in 1899 in order to become the Physical Director of the Toronto YMCA. At some point he earned a master's degree at the YMCA Physical Education Training College in Springfield, Massachusetts. After gaining experience at several Canadian YMCA branches, and holding positions of ever-increasing responsibility, including a stint in Shanghai, China, Crocker was appointed the YMCA National Physical Education Director in 1921, a position he held until 1930.

During his career with the YMCA, Crocker was selected to manage Canada's first official Olympic team (all male) in London, England, in 1908. He was also affiliated with the Amateur Athletic Union of Canada from 1896 until his death in 1959. He was secretary of the Canadian Olympic Committee from 1922 until 1947 and named honorary manager of Canada's Olympic teams from 1912 to 1956.

In 1930, at age sixty, Crocker took on the position of Director of Physical Education at the University of Western Ontario (UWO) in London, seeing the university through two periods of financial crisis – the Depression and the Second World War. He worked hard to develop a fieldhouse on campus to house intercollegiate, intramural, and recreational athletics (Thames Hall officially opened

> in 1949, after his retirement). Crocker's idea of a degree course in physical education was the second phase of his developmental plans for UWO, envisioning a course in physical education and another in recreation. At age seventy-six, he realized the necessity of choosing an associate as a possible successor following his retirement from UWO. Together with W. Alex Dewar, he outlined a course of study advanced for its time – a four-year honours degree program, which began in the fall of 1947, following Crocker's retirement from UWO on 30 June 1947.
>
> In 1948, Crocker received one of the first R. Tait McKenzie Honour Awards from the Canadian Physical Education Association. In recognition of his years of service to UWO and his promotion of athletic excellence, the university awarded him an Honorary Doctorate of Laws in 1950. At age eighty-nine, Crocker died on 27 November 1959 in Victoria, British Columbia. Since 1991, the International Centre for Olympic Studies at Western University has dedicated an annual lecture in his name.
>
> For more information, see Mary E. Keyes, "John Howard Crocker, LL. D, 1870–1959," MA thesis, University of Western Ontario, 1964. Also published as *Western Ontario History Nuggets*, no. 32, March 1966.

also recognized. Howard Crocker, who in 1901 was appointed physical director at the Toronto YMCA, organized a volunteer leaders' corps, many of whose members went on to become physical directors themselves. Crocker also ran a summer school in Toronto especially for physical directors.

The early Young Women's Christian Associations (YWCAs) benefited greatly from the example and assistance of the YMCAs, whose arrival in Canadian cities invariably preceded that of the women's organizations.[70] The first Canadian YWCAs appeared in major cities such as Toronto, Montreal, Quebec City, and Halifax as early as the 1870s. Middle-class religious and social reformers, concerned about the increasing numbers of young, single women seeking out employment and educational opportunities in the city, saw this as a "girl problem" and campaigned to do something about it. Their primary objective was to provide wholesome and affordable recreational opportunities as an alternative to the commercialized saloons, dance halls, and movie theatres. Usually beginning with a leased house on a residential street, most YWCAs originated as boarding homes for these women. New programs and services, such as educational classes, physical culture, and religious instruction, were often made possible through the rental of additional rooms in the downtown business district. Clearly, the YWCAs required their own buildings, and in this regard the YMCAs offered advice and assistance with fund-raising and the

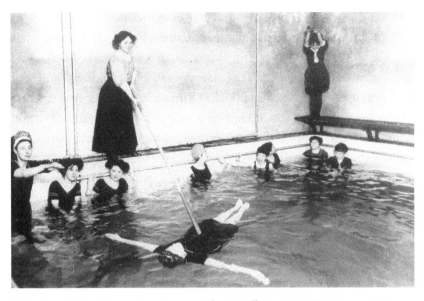

Figure 2.10. Mary Beaton instructs swimmers at the McGill Street YWCA, Toronto, 1910 (City of Toronto Archives, Fonds 1244, Item 2558)

purchase of property. By the end of the century, Canadian YWCAs, beginning with Toronto in 1894, were financing the construction of buildings especially designed to meet their needs.

As was the case with the YMCAs, the lack of a gymnasium was often the principal reason for undertaking the construction of a new YWCA building, followed where possible by a swimming pool. By 1900, with fourteen branches established across the country, many in their own buildings with a cafeteria, gymnasium, and sometimes a swimming pool, the YWCA effectively became a women-centred athletic club. Attendance statistics consistently demonstrated the preference for gymnasium and swimming classes over Bible study. Since the Physical Department was attracting more women than any other program, it was also the most profitable. Between 1907 and 1916, for example, the number of YWCA registrants for "physical culture" saw more than an eight-fold increase in part because of new swimming pools or the possibility of using one in the nearby YMCA.[71] These numbers continued to increase into the 1920s to such an extent that the YWCAs began seeking full-time women physical education directors. Many of these early specialists were trained at the Margaret Eaton School, a private women's physical education college in Toronto, whose origins and influence we discuss in the next chapter.

In 1902, a seven-part series on "American Woodcraft" written by Ernest Thompson Seton appeared in the *Ladies' Home Journal*, a leading women's magazine. The articles were clearly aimed at boys and taught them how to track animals, use a bow and arrow, build a teepee, make a council fire, and what to do if lost in the wilderness.[72] The same magazine also serialized Seton's novel, *Two Little Savages*, about the adventures of boys who lived as "Indians" and what they learned. Seton used his articles and books to promote his boys' movement, namely, the Woodcraft Indians, which enjoyed a relatively brief period of nation-wide popularity, but more importantly, set a precedent for other youth movements that followed, especially in Canada.

Who was Ernest Thompson Seton? Born in England, he was six years old in 1866 when his family immigrated to Canada, settling on a homestead near Lindsay, Ontario. A few years later they moved to Toronto, where they remained. Seton spent hours exploring and sketching the wild areas of the Don Valley within reach of the city. His artistic talent led him to study at the Royal Academy in London, but ill health and impoverishment forced his return to Canada. By the 1880s, he was in Manitoba studying prairie wildlife, and from there he travelled, lectured, and wrote about what he learned. It was also on the Canadian prairies that he first came to appreciate the pre-colonial Indigenous way of life, by then under serious threat, and especially their "arts and tricks of tracking, stalking and survival" in the wild.[73]

Seton's growing reputation as a naturalist and wildlife artist led him to pursue his career in the United States. As he studied Indigenous culture and history more intensely, his ideas for a youth movement took shape. Taking his lead from progressive educational theories of the day, including those of psychologist G. Stanley Hall, Seton argued that the essential activity during childhood was "not learning to work, not learning to be a scholar, not learning to be a citizen, not learning to be a soldier, – but play."[74] He also realized the importance of channelling the play instinct into guided peer group activities, given boys' natural inclination towards gang loyalty. He opposed the new emphasis on team sports arguing that eventually they would divide the nation into mostly spectators and a small group of paid gladiators. However, he encouraged physical activities like canoeing, swimming, and running. Finally, he wanted to inspire city boys to explore the outdoors, and to learn how to survive in that environment, by teaching them simple woodcraft and camping skills, and most importantly, how to "think Indian." Seton's movement was built on two cornerstones, namely, the celebration of outdoor life and the appropriation of Indigenous culture.

By 1910, about 200,000 boys in the United States had joined the Woodcraft Indians. Within inner cities, they were renamed "Indian Scouts," and tribes sprang up among playground and church groups, YMCAs, and independent private academies. The movement also spread to Canada, but it has been difficult to locate any specific evidence except to note that Seton was an occasional visitor to Ahmek, one of Canada's oldest (1921) boys' private summer camps, where he showed campers how to make sweat lodges, perform Indian dances, and conduct a Council Ring.[75]

Sir Robert Baden-Powell, military hero of the Boer War (1899–1902), first heard of the Woodcraft Indians in 1904, when Seton visited England to promote his movement. Baden-Powell was immediately interested, and in the summer of 1905, he attended one of Seton's camps at Seton's estate in Connecticut. Back in England, Baden-Powell began working on his own scheme and in 1908, he published *Scouting for Boys: A Handbook for Instruction in Good Citizenship*. It has been described as "gunny-sack of a book" that "spoke compellingly to boys cooped up in the suburbs of the mushrooming new twentieth century town and city (not only in Britain) inviting them to get on with things, find a 'backwoods' for themselves, and go adventuring," by which Powell meant they should help expand the colonies. "Wishy-washy slackers without any 'go,' patriotism, or manliness," he predicted, "will lose the Empire for Britain."[76] There was also an emphasis on woodcraft and the outdoors, although he anglicized many of Seton's woodcraft principles to fit his own movement's patriotic emphasis, and he allowed for more adult supervision.[77]

Scout troops began to spring up in Canada well in advance of Baden-Powell's cross-country tour in August and September of 1910. Ties to England, certainly among recent immigrants, were central to the rapid spread of Scouting across the country. During his tour, Baden-Powell made clear that Scout training was designed to turn all of Canada's boys – French Canadians, those of British descent, and the sons of "foreigners" – into useful citizens of the great empire in which the Dominion of Canada was "a rising nation."[78] In Ontario, for example, the movement mushroomed in 1911 with more than a hundred troops founded in small villages and major urban centres. However, the rapid growth of Scouting across the country revealed serious organizational weaknesses, which were somewhat ameliorated by an appeal for funds from prominent Canadian businessmen (including a $15,000 gift from Lord Strathcona) and the federal incorporation of the Boy Scout movement in 1914.

Although church and YMCA leaders had been initially enthusiastic about the Boy Scouts, they soon parted ways because early Scout leaders, many of whom came from the military, were not primarily oriented towards religion. Also, with Scouting's primary focus on younger boys, they failed to recruit older boys in whom the churches and YMCAs were most interested. In 1912, the YMCA established the Canadian Advisory Committee on Cooperation for Boys' Work to promote a new plan for boys. Awkwardly named the Canadian Standard Efficiency Training (CSET), it was designed by Taylor Statten, the YMCA's National Boys'

Work Secretary.[79] CSET bundled a series of tests and awards under the YMCA's original four-fold formula – spiritual, mental, social, and physical. Separate programs were also developed for the two age groups: Trail Rangers (ages 12–14) and the Tuxis Boys (ages 15–17). The physical tests, for example, pushed boys to learn a variety of athletic skills in the gym, swimming pool, and out of doors. Ideally, a boy would grow in "efficiency" by working to raise his scores as he passed from one stage to the next.[80] By 1919, almost 13,500 boys were registered in the CSET program, but within a few years it proved too costly and time-consuming for most YMCAs, and the program was turned over to the churches. By 1926, there were 28,152 CSET enrolments, whereas the Boy Scouts were at 28,817, but by the end of the 1920s, it was clear that the churches preferred Scouts to the Trail Rangers.

Following their sisters in Great Britain, English Canadian women and girls first started forming Guide companies in 1910. Baden-Powell and his sister Agnes jointly wrote *The Handbook for Girl Guides or How Girls Can Help Build the Empire*, which was published in 1912. That same year, Baden-Powell, now in his mid-fifties, married twenty-three-year-old Olave St. Clair Soames, who as Lady Baden-Powell gradually took over responsibility for the Guides. In 1923, at the annual convention of the Ontario Educational Association held in Toronto, Lady Baden-Powell, Chief of the Girl Guides, explained how the movement develops character in girls and how they learn to be leaders. Wearing a uniform and earning badges are important, she pointed out, but so is training in health: "We take them into the open, take them out to camp, give them healthy, wholesome jolly games, and point out to them that it is their business to be healthy."[81]

The original handbook was replaced with *Girl Guiding: A Handbook for Brownies, Guides, Rangers, and Guiders* reflecting the different age groupings in the Guide movement: eight to ten for Brownies, eleven to sixteen for Guides, and over sixteen for Rangers. The movement was designed to provide training in character and intelligence, skill and handicraft, service for others and fellowship, and, most relevant to our discussion, physical health and hygiene. Clear and simple instructions with many examples were provided in the three age groupings on how to keep oneself healthy and fit. Badges were also designed to test knowledge and skill in this area. Even Arthur Lamb praised the Boy Scout and the Girl Guide movements for their educational values and advantages: "we get them through games, through natural gymnastics, folk and characteristic dancing, club and camp crafts."[82]

When Guiding was first introduced into Canada, the YWCA had found its program and international character sufficiently attractive to sponsor several Guide companies. However, among YWCA leaders there were growing concerns that Guiding's badge system was too competitive; the leadership too authoritarian with little opportunity for girls to participate in decision-making; and, most importantly, Guiding was not devoted to Christian education.[83] The YWCA established the Canadian National Advisory Committee for Cooperation in Girls' Work, and out of this developed the Canadian Girls in Training (CGIT) program utilizing the now familiar four-fold standards – physical, intellectual, religious, and service. The physical standard was clearly defined: "As health is the first essential in a girl's normal development, and as present-day business conditions make it necessary for many girls to spend much of their time in-doors, thus depriving them of regular exercise, the importance of emphasizing the 'Physical Standard' is self-evident."[84] They had also rejected the competitive nature of the comparable CSET program for boys, arguing that girls were in many respects different from boys. Adult CGIT leaders were to adapt the four-fold program in consultation with girls in small, church-controlled groups, which were encouraged to alternate sessions among the four standards. Therefore, a physical session would stress health standards and good sportsmanship, and possibly might include a hike or group sports. It is difficult to assess the role of physical culture within the CGIT except at its summer camps, which were by far the most successful of CGIT activities. By 1925, nearly 3,000 girls (9.8 per cent of the membership) had attended a CGIT camp with the usual outdoor activities such as swimming, boating, and hiking.[85] It was also estimated that by 1927, more than 75,000 girls, aged twelve to seventeen, had participated in CGIT in its first decade.[86]

In the YMCA and YWCA, physical training/education was vital to their programming and membership, and indeed was often the primary reason that kept boys and girls, young men and women returning to these institutions. Within most other youth movements there was a focus on active games and sports for boys, but not for girls. Where girls gained the most physical activity was likely at summer camps often sponsored by these same organizations.

At the outbreak of the Second World War, a common curriculum for physical education was taught in the state schools of every province in Canada, while calisthenics, sport, and military drill were offered sporadically to the Indigenous children in residential schools. Despite the complaints of educators like Lamb, and Putnam and Weir about military drill, the Strathcona Trust legitimized drill as an integral component of physical education for most of the interwar period. Through its executive council that oversaw the plan, the Trust created links among the provincial departments of education. During the 1920s, physical education grew in importance, as school boards constructed new facilities with elaborate gymnasia, swimming pools, and playing fields, extended opportunities for after-school sports, and hired teachers with specialist certificates. Several universities, including Toronto, McGill, and Saskatchewan offered diploma programs in physical education, as did the YMCA and private institutions like the Margaret Eaton School. The rapid growth of youth organizations, women's and men's amateur sports, public and private investment in parks, playgrounds, and sports facilities, as well as media concern about the state of children's health all contributed to the legitimacy of school-based physical education.

Those dedicated to the development of physical education as a profession took advantage of these circumstances to strengthen their links with each other, share research and ideas, and affirm acceptable and ideal practice. In 1921, those teaching the subject in Ontario formed their own organization, the Ontario Physical and Health Education Association (OPHEA). A few years later in Montreal, Arthur Lamb initiated the Quebec Physical Education Association (QPEA) with an even wider (but almost entirely anglophone) membership – McGill; the YWCA and YMCA; the Protestant Board of School Commissioners; Montreal Parks and Playgrounds; Montreal Amateur Athletic Association; MacDonald College; the schools of Westmount, Montreal West, St. Lambert, and Outremont; and several physical education students from McGill.[87] QPEA soon affiliated with the American Physical Education Association. In 1933, during the harsh conditions of the Depression, Lamb would team up with Ethel Cartwright in Saskatchewan and other leaders to form the Canadian Physical Education Association (see chapter 4). Stressing their professionalism as educators, they gradually wrested control of the subject away from the retired soldiers whom the Strathcona Trust advanced after the war.[88] A pan-Canadian movement was well under way.

CHAPTER THREE

The Margaret Eaton School: Forty Years of Women's Physical Education

It is this unique emphasis upon a body-centred education – an education which included the uneven and at times contradictory experiences of both elegance and expression, sweat and strength – which offers a distinctive point of entry into the analysis of the socialization and embodied experience of "the Margaret Eaton girl."

Anna Lathrop

In this chapter we return to the early twentieth century to explore the history and influence of arguably one of the most important Canadian institutions for women's physical education. Founded in Toronto in 1901, the Margaret Eaton School, as it was eventually called, was a remarkable innovation, providing a new kind of training in physical culture for young women from well-off families. The activities of the school over its forty-year history are especially interesting for the light they shine upon institutional, artistic, and professional developments in Canadian physical education during the first half of the twentieth century. They illustrate what was perceived to be an appropriate education at this time for affluent women during their years between school and the responsibilities of marriage. They also highlight the ways in which physical education came to be viewed (at least by some) as a worthy career for women in a rapidly modernizing and industrializing society.

The school's notable teachers, and many of its students, had a far-reaching impact upon the structure and gender dynamics of Canadian physical education, sport, and recreation, although the struggle for gender equality was hard fought and the results uneven. The school was also Canada's first truly national institution to prepare teachers of physical education. As one historian observed: "one cannot emphasize too strongly the tremendous influence that the Margaret Eaton School and its staff had on the development of professional education in health and physical education in Canada."[1] During its existence, the school provided a comprehensive program in physical education training to over 250 women, and upon graduation many were employed in YWCAs, private schools, settlement houses, summer camps, recreation centres, playgrounds, and other agencies across the country.[2]

Over four decades, the Margaret Eaton School was directed by only three principals, each of whom brought her own unique vision to the primary purpose and curriculum of the school. For founder and longest-serving principal, Emma Scott Raff Nasmith (1901–25), the emphasis was on expression, elegance, and appropriate feminine deportment. Influenced by the new European systems of body culture, she sought out individuals for her staff to bring these innovative ideas to the curriculum. She was followed by Mary Hamilton (1925–34), whose pragmatic belief that the school must prepare graduates for the developing field of physical education saw a shift away from the dramatic arts and dance to an exclusive emphasis on physical education. Hamilton firmly believed in the benefits of outdoor summer camping, and as the founder of Camp Tanamakoon for girls, she incorporated this aspect into the school's curriculum. Finally, American-educated Florence Somers (1934–41) brought the "play for play's sake" philosophy of women's athletics to the school – the enjoyment of sport and the development of good sportsmanship and character, rather than the breaking of records and the winning of championships. She also adhered to the doctrine of innate biological and physiological differences between the sexes and its implication for women's sport. Somers was instrumental in seeing the Margaret Eaton School amalgamate with the University of Toronto, thereby bringing the school's history to a close. During these years, the image of the "Margaret Eaton girl" changed considerably. The initial training in elegance and expression, primarily for the theatre and the drawing room, shifted to training in athletic skill and pedagogic knowledge in the growing field of physical education.[3]

The women who attended the Margaret Eaton School were the very essence of what historians call Modern Girls, the metaphorical daughters of the earlier New Women, and by the 1920s this included most young women. Generally speaking, they endeavoured to make themselves modern through popular culture and consumerism. They were likely reasonably well employed, making a living for themselves between school and marriage, after which they were expected to leave employment to look after husband, house, and children. Modern girls helped define and shape the modern, female, sexed body, and, as one historian has argued, they often bore the brunt of developing standards for a woman's body.[4] Just as the modern girl was predominately white, so too were the Margaret Eaton girls. As we have seen in the previous two chapters regarding Indigenous peoples in Canada, increasing government control, the reserve system (which severely restricted movement), residential schools, disease, poverty, and cultural dislocation meant that an Indigenous modern girl would have a very tough time indeed. It was far more prevalent to see and depict Indigenous girls and women as antimodern relics or not represent them at all. "Indigenous modernities," as one historian noted, "were discounted by the very absence of their presence."[5] Certainly Indigenous modern girls existed but they were not fairly represented in the popular media, advertising, or nation-building projects. In other words, whiteness was firmly associated with modernity. They never were, nor could they become, Margaret Eaton girls.

The Female Tradition in Physical Education

Although the Margaret Eaton School was by no means the only female-organized enterprise established to provide training for well-placed women in the broadening range of physical cultures at this time, it was unique in Canada. In England, for example, Madame Bergman-Österberg, a Swedish woman trained in Ling's gymnastic system, founded a small empire of female physical education training schools, which had an enormous influence upon girls' education and physical culture for well over half a century. So well received was her system that by 1914 six female institutions in England and Scotland had organized around her movement philosophies – namely, Dartford, Anstey, and Bedford, followed by Chelsea, Liverpool, and Dunfermline. It was a model, based mainly on Ling's gymnastics, that would reach Canada from England, as well as from Europe and the United States, through teacher-training approaches to girls' physical education. Ling's achievement had been to ground gymnastics in anatomy and physiology, thereby opening the remedial and educational possibilities of exercise. Madame Österberg also added games to her training methods in Swedish gymnastics and developed a female physical education tradition that went unchallenged by men until after the Second World War.[6]

In the United States, Ling's system was brought initially from Sweden by Hartwig Nissen and Baron Nils Posse.[7] Posse's Normal School of Gymnastics in Boston, for example, was one of several that trained female physical educators such as Vendla M. Holmstrom. A native of Sweden, she graduated from Posse's school in 1891, and immediately moved to Halifax, Nova Scotia, setting up a private gymnasium and physical education school. She also gave lectures to public school teachers on the scientific and medical aspects of gymnastics, especially for girls, and introduced them to fencing and basketball.[8] In 1899, she moved to Montreal to become the physical director at Royal Victoria College (see chapter 1), a women's school with some 150 students and affiliated with McGill University. At their disposal was a large gymnasium, fitted with the apparatus required for the Swedish system, and since Holmstrom had been a "student under the best masters" she was welcomed enthusiastically. She also introduced the women students to basketball, which the student paper predicted "bids fair to occupy as high a place in their conversation and affections as football does in those of their brothers."[9] Before entering the gymnastic course, all women students underwent a physical examination under the supervision of R. Tait McKenzie, who at the time was a lecturer in anatomy at McGill.

Holmstrom left Royal Victoria College at the beginning of the 1904–5 session, although she continued to teach at the High School for Girls in Montreal with glowing reviews: "she has gained for herself the reputation of being in the very front rank of specialists in knowledge of her subject, and those of us who have seen the work of her girls in the regular classes, in entertainments, and 'Parents' Afternoons' are thoroughly convinced of the effectiveness of her training."[10] Holmstrom also instituted a medical examination for senior girls at the school to determine who could undertake the physical work with safety, and to prescribe corrective exercises for those requiring special treatment. A special costume – sailor blouse, bloomers, stockings, and running shoes – was adopted for all gym classes. She taught at the school until 1912, and after this seems to have returned to Boston. She became an expert in the art of physiological breathing and provided instruction for health and physical development, speech defects, and preparation for artistic singing and dancing.[11]

The New Kinesthetic of Modernism

Although Ling's Swedish system held the promise of a more liberated, active notion of femininity, with its attention to functional health and therapeutic movement, it was challenged by a series of new approaches to movement and by the realization that gymnastics could be expressive as well as functional and corrective. The early decades of the twentieth century saw a nudging aside of Ling's remedial gymnastics in a multi-pronged search for real expression in movement. It was generally described as the new kinesthetic of modernism, and one that "demanded sincerity, the loving accommodation of the force of gravity, fluid movement flowing out of the body centre, freedom of invention and natural transitions through many fully expressive positions."[12] As such, it influenced the fields of dance, art, and drama, as well as methods of physical training. It also found expression in modernist artistic and theatrical movements in English Canada, becoming an important aspect of body training for dancers, actors, and public speakers.[13]

At the heart of this new enthusiasm for expression through gesture, modern dance, and rhythmical movement were the ideas, practices, and schools of three important movement theorists: François Delsarte (1811–1871), Émile Jaques-Dalcroze (1865–1950), and Rudolf Laban (1879–1958). Their common philosophy was that human movement was a critical component of artistic expression. In many respects their ideas were a reaction against the perceived negative regimentation of industrialization and mechanization upon the body in work and play in the late nineteenth century. There was a general sense of having lost touch with the natural rhythms of daily life as industrial work began to dictate workers' movements.[14] In response to these anxieties, innovators developed a series of physical culture innovations, each attempting to liberate the body by defining appropriate and meaningful exercise and movement patterns that could be taught in different national arenas and a variety of institutions.

The movement principles of François Delsarte formed an important core of this transatlantic traffic, and helped revolutionize approaches to gymnastics.[15] In France, Delsarte had originally studied as a singer, but soon became more interested in drama and elocution. His major contribution was to create a system of body training designed to integrate speech and gesture, and to counter the stilted, artificial, and stylized body actions used by actors in early nineteenth-century dramatic performance. It was a field of study known as "expression" and it included physical culture, pantomime, and dramatics as well as training in public speaking.[16]

Delsartism was transplanted to the United States by his only known American student, Steele McKaye (1842–1894), an actor, director, and playwright. He promoted Delsarte's theory in addition to practical training procedures, known as harmonic, or sometimes aesthetic, gymnastics. Primarily intended for actors and public speakers, these gymnastics were designed "to give symmetrical physical development, and to take out the angles and discords, to reduce the body to a natural, passive state, and from that point to train it to move in harmony with nature's laws."[17]

American Delsartism was also promoted by a variety of teachers and performers, primarily women, such as Genevieve Stebbins (1857–1934). Originally an actor, she studied with McKaye and others, became a noted lecturer and teacher, and in 1893 established the School of Expression in New York. Through her leadership, Delsarte movement or harmonic gymnastics became popular among women of the upper and middle classes, essentially as a form of training in posture and gracefulness. It also helped to combat the stiffness imposed by women's clothing (such as corsets) and limiting codes of behaviour. Stebbins had many students and imitators across North America and Europe who spread her influence and choreographed movement sequences widely. She publicized her system in numerous books, including *The Genevieve Stebbins System of Physical Training* (1913), which was a manual of exercise and drills geared mainly for teachers of physical education. They often added a musical accompaniment integrating folk dance steps, rhythmic marching, and traditional dances. Stebbins also organized statue posing compositions where her pupils, each draped in a loose flowing gown, were instructed to stand in front of a mirror and move through a series of poses in harmony with the gestures of classical Greek statues. Group tableaux were another popular innovation, as were yoga breathing exercises. Her aim was "to teach and preach physical culture and aesthetics to middle- and upper-class women, educating them to appreciate bodily motion as a healthy and pleasurable part of life."[18] Delsartism, concluded Stebbins, brought together all the elements essential to evolve beauty in form, graceful motion, and artistic presentation.

By the turn of the century, Delsartism had branched into two directions – modern dance and physical culture. In the United States, modern dance pioneers such as Isadora Duncan (1877–1927), Ruth St Denis (1879–1968), and especially Ted Shawn (1891–1972), studied and drew upon Delsartean theory and practice in their performances, and thus significantly influenced their students and followers. However, the impact of Delsartism on physical culture/education was more controversial, and Stebbins herself was well aware of the debate between what she called "the defenders of artistic grace" versus "the advocates of muscle."[19] For instance, when Delsarte teachers Emily M. Bishop and Franklin H. Sargent presented their papers before the American Association for the Advancement of Physical Education in 1892, they were met with vociferous criticism, especially from influential physical educator Dudley A. Sargent: "The exception which we take to the Delsarte system as a system of physical training is that it is simply an anomaly. It is not a system of physical training and you cannot make it so in any way. Our friends the Swedes are either fundamentally wrong or our friends the Delsartians are. They are diametrically opposed. If the Swedish system is a system of physical training designed to bring out bodily vigor, then the system of Delsarte exercises is designed ... to do the opposite."[20] On the other hand, the highly respected Canadian physical educator R. Tait McKenzie observed: "Delsarte may be said to have been the greatest influence in directing attention to economy of muscular action in expressing thought, and his principles continually crop out in such schemes of gymnastics."[21] By this point, the Delsarte culture in North America was almost totally a women's movement that provided them with a rationale to engage in physical activity and

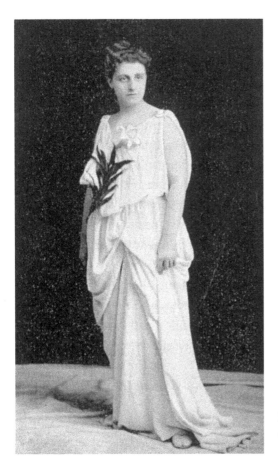

Figure 3.1. Genevieve Stebbins, principal of the New York School of Expression, 1892 (Library of Congress)

expression as well as a relatively easy form of physical training. Teachers like Emily Bishop, who taught at the Chautauqua School of Expression in western New York, offered summer courses easily available to interested Canadians. It was the Delsarte system of expression, filtered through one of its American teachers, that would strongly influence Emma Scott Raff's early studies of drama and elocution as well as her approach to teaching physical culture as the first principal of the Margaret Eaton School.

As for the systems developed by Émile Jaques-Dalcroze and Rudolf Laban, they had far less impact on the curricula of the Margaret Eaton School, but we discuss them briefly here because they were very much a part of the new kinesthetic. Swiss composer, musician, and music educator Dalcroze developed eurythmics, which was an approach to learning and experiencing music through movement.[22] By introducing the importance of music and rhythm to expressive movement forms,

Dalcroze's system became especially useful for physical education, expressive dance, and gymnastics practices. At the 1913 International Congress of Physical Education in Paris, for example, Dalcroze and his students gave a performance of rhythmic gymnastics at the amphitheatre of the Sorbonne. With Dalcroze at the piano providing the music, his students (all girls), wearing short purple tunics, performed their rhythmic gymnastic interpretations in groups or solo.[23] Although Dalcroze did not lecture at the conference itself, several presenters discussed the educative importance of his system of eurythmics, especially for girls and women, as a form of rhythmic gymnastics.[24] Rudolf Laban, an Austro-Hungarian dancer, held similar views to Dalcroze, although his influence was mostly through modern dance. After the Second World War, Laban and his students were central to the development and spread of children's dance and movement education, discussed in chapter 5.

As we have seen, these European systems – represented in the work of Delsarte, Dalcroze, and Laban – advocated natural, spontaneous, and rhythmic movement through the promotion of modern dance, eurhythmics, and expressive gymnastics. They were considerably different from the more rigid system of Ling's Swedish gymnastics promoted in the public schools across Canada through the Strathcona Trust and various versions of the *Syllabus of Physical Exercise for Schools* discussed in the previous chapter.

Emma Scott Raff: Elegance and Expression

In 1900, Emma Scott Raff opened the School of Expression in a small studio over a bank at the corner of Toronto's Bloor and Yonge Street, to offer classes in literary interpretation, voice culture, and the art of expressive movement. Born in 1869 in Watertown, Ontario, Emma Scott was the daughter of a Methodist minister.[25] After finishing school, she studied art and then went off to Colorado to paint and teach, where she met her husband, William Raff. Sadly, by 1897 she was a widow with a one-year-old daughter.[26] Returning to Toronto, she pursued a variety of eclectic and artistic studies before being appointed in 1902 as Director of Physical Culture at the new Annesley Hall women's residence of Victoria College, affiliated with the University of Toronto. Annesley Hall was designed to provide a separate and protected space where the women students' health was safeguarded through appropriate regimens of exercise and rest. Scott Raff's task was to offer them brief, twice-daily physical culture classes in Delsartean aesthetics and Swedish gymnastics. She also gave classes in voice culture, which in the end were her undoing because of concerns among female students that Victoria College might narrow its academic offerings and be reduced to a school of elocution, rather than an academic institution.[27]

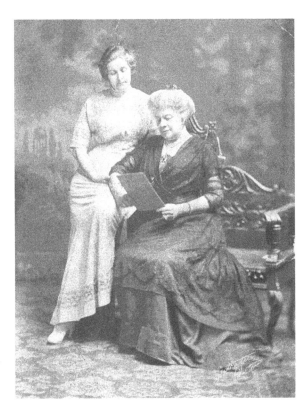

Figure 3.2. Emma Scott Raff (left) and Margaret Wilson Beattie Eaton (image used by permission of the Margaret Eaton School Digital Collection, Redeemer University, Ancaster, Ontario)

To train her own students in the School of Expression, Scott Raff drew especially upon Delsarte's system by emphasizing aesthetic movements and deep breathing exercises. The focus, she said, was on the freedom of body movement rather than the development of muscle. As she put it: "Where the voice is trained to express what the soul feels; while the body, by reverential, assiduous care, is made obedient to the mind; where self-reverence, self-knowledge, and self control are essentials; where gentleness and grace of thought, bearing, and action are imparted."[28] It was a system Scott Raff had learned when training with Samuel Silas Curry (1847–1921), professor of elocution and vocal expression, at his School of Expression in Boston. Her challenge was to bring modern methods of dramatic training into a form considered suitable for a female education, and at the same time add to this remedial work in the gymnasium in order to foster poise and grace. In this sense, she could bring literature and voice culture together in the curriculum with physical culture and household science to educate her students in developing the body *and* keeping the home. The school, therefore, was especially attractive to the young daughters of Toronto's elite during their years between adolescence and marriage.

Scott Raff was fortunate to find a wealthy sponsor in the wife of Timothy Eaton, founder of Eaton's department store, namely Margaret Beattie Eaton, who began studying at the school in 1903. Although the school's purpose was not intended to train students for the platform or stage, Margaret Eaton had long cherished an interest in theatrical activity. Scott Raff's school offered her a space to enjoy otherwise frowned-upon activities due to her strict Methodist background and follow her passion to study literature and the theatre. She persuaded her husband to donate a larger building for the school and she remained deeply involved in the school's management and activities. Indeed, she personally underwrote all the expenses of the school as well as paying off its accumulating debt.[29]

In 1907, the school moved to a new location and was renamed the Margaret Eaton School of Literature and Expression. "Looking like a relic from another land," observed one historian, "with its Greek temple design, genie motif and cryptic motto [it] never seemed quite at home sandwiched between two anonymous homes on North Street, just south of Bloor."[30] Inscribed on the architrave was the Greek phrase meaning: "We strive for the good and the beautiful." The building was equipped with a large theatre auditorium, studio, classrooms, and appropriate antique fittings. Scott Raff enhanced the environment with her flowing velvet gowns, exotic jewellery, and suede sandals.

The curricular emphasis of the school was still voice culture, literature, and physical culture. Slowly, the literature and dramatic study streams merged and became entirely distinct from the physical culture stream with the students referring to themselves as either "the physicals" or "the expressions." Helen Ward Armington, a graduate of the Sargent School for Physical Education in Boston, and Constance Wreyford, an early Canadian graduate of Sargent's Harvard Summer School of Physical Education, were the first two instructors to teach physical culture at the school between 1907 and 1910. Dudley A. Sargent's influence on American physical education during these years was immense through his training schools and comprehensive system of individualized exercise programs, which numerous Canadian teachers experienced. In his training regimes, Sargent claimed to incorporate a variety of systems: "the strength-giving qualities of the German gymnasium, the active and energetic properties of the English sports, the grace and suppleness acquired from the French calisthenics, and the beautiful poise and mechanical precision of the Swedish free movements, all regulated, systematized, and adapted to our peculiar needs and institutions."[31] While he included aesthetic dance in his female training systems, as well as various sports, he saw dance primarily as a form of exercise to attain suppleness and good posture, not as an art form. His theory courses were almost all centred on the natural and health sciences, and *Gray's Anatomy* was

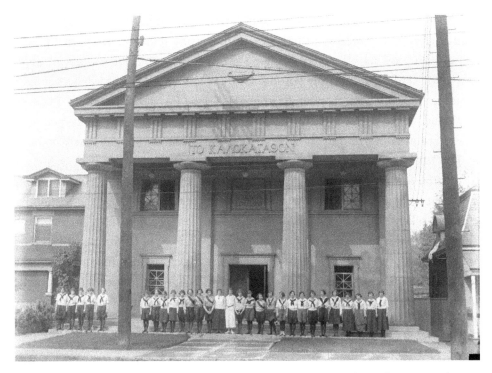

Figure 3.3. Margaret Eaton School of Literature and Expression, c. 1908 (City of Toronto Archives, Fonds 1244, Item 2405)

often used as a textbook with a focus on preventive medicine through exercise and good health habits. The curriculum in its detail and scope was not very different from other similar normal schools of its time, but what differentiated the Sargent School was its large student body and extensive influence upon the direction of physical education in North America.

Although Scott Raff's interests were clearly in literature and drama for self improvement, students became more interested in obtaining employment before they married. Her own views were changing on the subject when in 1916, Scott Raff was remarried to George G. Nasmith, deputy health officer with the City of Toronto. Despite popular sanctions against marriage and work for women, she continued as principal of the school.[32] Her earlier view of exercise for personal improvement also changed to a more vocational emphasis with courses offered in anatomy, physiology, hygiene, anthropometry, and remedial gymnastics, as well as practical instruction in Indian clubs, dumb-bells, wands, elementary fencing, aesthetic gymnastics, and games. As she put it, "the teacher of to-day wants not so much the student who can stand on her head and perform with her feet, but the student who can stand on her feet and perform with her head."[33] For students studying physical education, there was an increasing focus on vocational preparation with growing placements in the YWCAs, settlement houses, playgrounds, recreation centres, and private schools. By 1923, students were awarded a teacher's diploma in either Literature and Dramatic Art or Physical Education. Between 1908 and 1925, the school averaged twenty-eight full-time students per year, reaching a peak of over fifty in 1920. Also, part-time study was extremely popular, and by 1924–5 involved over one thousand students.[34]

In 1924, the city of Toronto widened Bay Street, where the school's Greek temple stood, necessitating the removal of the front of the building and the distinctive entrance pillars. This set off a series of events that led to diminishing financial and administrative support from the Eaton company, the need to shift locations, and Scott Raff Nasmith's angry resignation over these issues. In the summer of 1925, the Margaret Eaton School of Literature and Expression closed, but reopened a couple of months later in a building at the corner of Yonge and McGill Streets, which since 1918 had been used by the school's Physical Education Department. Formerly an old YMCA, it had been purchased by Eaton's to house the Eaton's Girls Club – a recreation centre for their women employees – and included a gymnasium, swimming tank, library, cafeteria, and sitting rooms. Margaret Eaton students used it during the daytime, and the Eaton workers in the evenings. The facilities were renovated to include an enlarged swimming pool and new theatre. Although Margaret Eaton wanted nothing more to do with a school devoted more to physical education than to theatre arts, the school's name was changed to the Margaret Eaton School (MES), which Mrs. Eaton allowed on a temporary basis. It was also apparent that the school needed to become more self-financed and less dependent on the largesse of the Eaton family. For the latter, the question was how to rid themselves of the school and yet still preserve a positive name for their company.[35]

Mary Hamilton: Beauty and Fitness

Born in Fergus, Ontario, in 1883, and raised as a staunch Presbyterian, Mary Hamilton enjoyed an athletic childhood in the outdoors before attending the Sargent School for Physical Education for two years as a diploma student. Following her training in Boston, Hamilton moved back to Ontario to work at the Kingston YWCA, and then to teach physical education at Bishop Strachan and Branksome Hall, private girls' schools in Toronto, before joining Scott Raff at the Margaret Eaton School of Literature and Expression in 1910 as director of physical education. She was a quiet woman of practical vision who opted for a professional life

BOX 3.1. MARY ROSS BARKER (1905–2004)

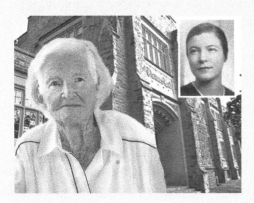

Figure 3.4. Mary Ross Barker (John P. Metras Sports Museum, Western University)

Born in Toronto in 1905, Mary was the only child of Wesley E. Barker of Springfield, Massachusetts, and Christine Ross of Little Bras d'Or, Cape Breton. She attended Branksome Hall, a private school in Toronto, where gym mistress Mary Hamilton convinced her to study at the MES from 1923 to 1925. Mary returned to Branksome as the junior school's gym mistress until 1929 when she moved to another girls' school, namely Loretta Abbey in the Catholic system. In 1935, the University of Western Ontario was looking for someone to replace Joyce Plumptre, head of women's physical education, who was getting married. Florence Somers suggested Mary to director Howard Crocker, who hired her immediately. She was responsible for the required physical education courses taken by all women students at Western, which included an extensive array of physical activities: archery, golf, tennis, soccer, swimming, hiking done outside, while badminton, gymnastics, folk and square dancing took place indoors.

The Second World War interrupted Mary's physical education career when she was asked to join the newly established Canadian Women's Army Corps (CWAC) as a staff officer with the rank of Major. Her job was to establish CWAC centres across Canada to enable recruiting and training, and she also served overseas. Returning to Western after the war, she stayed for a couple of years but became disillusioned when the university decided to eliminate the required physical education course for all students. Never at a loss for what to do next, she joined the staff of the national YWCA in 1949 as National Secretary of Physical Education. Again, her job required a great deal of travelling throughout the country assisting and consulting with local branches from Newfoundland to British Columbia.

She remained with the YWCA until 1957, when in her early fifties she decided to retire to Ingonish on Cape Breton Island, Nova Scotia. She did so with her lifelong companion Irene Gettas, whom she had known since her days at Western. Mary was remarkably active in community affairs, sports promotion, and youth activities, while Irene tended to their home and garden.

In recognition of her life's work, Mary became a Member of the Order of Canada in 1999 and was posthumously inducted as a builder into the John P. Metras Sports Museum at Western University in 2012. She died in 2004 at age

> ninety-nine leaving her estate to Irene. When Irene passed away in 2016, she left both estates to the community of Ingonish, therefore providing a lasting legacy to assist community recreation groups.
>
> For more information, see a taped interview with Mary Barker conducted by Stuart Davidson in 1978 (Stewart Davidson fonds, Library and Archives Canada, Item number 435197).

of education and service, wanting her students to be competent in organizing and taking charge of all forms of physical training for girls.[36] Her desire was to bring the MES to the leading edge of professional preparation for women so its graduates would be competent to organize and take charge of every branch of physical activity for girls. It was not surprising, therefore, that when Hamilton succeeded Scott Raff Nasmith as the principal early in 1926, she changed the school's motto from "striving for the good and the beautiful" to a more functional focus on "beauty and fitness." By then, Hamilton had accumulated a wealth of experience, spending her vacations each year at various summer schools in order to study the latest trends in physical education. "If it was not Harvard," she said, "it was Chautauqua or New York, or perhaps England at Stratford or Cheltenham where I found Cecil Sharp and his work on the English Folk Dance particularly fascinating."[37]

The two-year Normal Course in Physical Education led to a teaching diploma adequate to teach in private schools, settlement houses, and the YWCA, although it was still not sufficient to enable students to teach in the public school system. In 1901, the University of Toronto had initiated a women's diploma course in physical training, taken in conjunction with a Bachelor of Arts degree, but it attracted few students. In 1912, Miss Ivy Coventry, a graduate of the Sargent School, was appointed Director of Athletics for Women at the University of Toronto, and one of her responsibilities was to revitalize the diploma program. It was discontinued during the First World War but reinstated in 1924. Graduates of the program could then attend the Ontario College of Education, qualify for a Specialist Certificate, and subsequently teach in a public high school. Similarly, in chapter 2 we discussed the all-women McGill School of Physical Education, headed by Ethel Cartwright, and the first Canadian school of physical education affiliated with a university. Many of its graduates found teaching jobs as physical education specialists in the Protestant schools of Montreal. MES graduates could not do this, unless they took the time to obtain a degree; nonetheless, the MES consistently attracted more students.

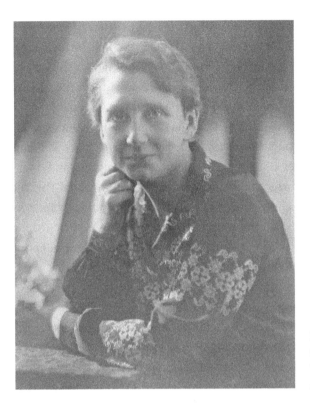

Figure 3.5. Mary Hamilton, c. 1925 (Violet Keene photographer, Camp Tanamakoon fonds, Trent University Archives)

In addition to their physical training classes, physical education students at the MES were required to take classes in voice training, rhythm, and expression offered by the Department of Literature and Dramatic Art, while dramatic arts students studied classic and aesthetic dancing, folk dancing, and physical training with instructors in the Department of Physical Education. Included as part of their intensive training, all students were expected to attend cultural events such as local performances of the Russian ballet and the Isadora Duncan dancers. However, by 1925–6 there were thirty-nine first-year students in the Department of Physical Education, but only nine in the Department of Literature and Dramatic Art. This did not bode well for the latter, and that department was soon closed with the MES now completely focused on training students in physical education.

Hamilton brought in the best qualified instructors with speciality training, many from afar. The gymnastics and games instructors generally came from Britain by way of the physical education training colleges (see earlier discussion about the female tradition), and the dance and educational theory teachers were drawn primarily from the United States. She also hired faculty who specialized in either new or internationally renowned areas of study, usually on shorter-term appointments.

Madeleine Boss Lasserre, for example, a eurythmics specialist from the Dalcroze School in Geneva, offered classes between 1924 and 1926, the first of their kind in Canada. Leon Leonidoff from the Imperial Russian Ballet taught at the school at the same time. Hamilton also continued some of the courses from the former Literature and Dramatic Art department such as public speaking and voice.

Hamilton's leadership brought the introduction of a camp training course for all students enrolled in the normal course in physical education. It took place at Camp Tanamakoon, the private summer camp for girls she founded, owned, and operated some two hundred miles north of Toronto in Algonquin Provincial Park. It was during a visit to the Sargent School summer camp near Boston when Hamilton recognized that camping could be a rich and effective socializing experience for young girls, and indeed for herself. "It … was becoming increasingly evident at the Physical Education Conferences in the United States," she wrote, "that summer camps had come to stay and that schools of physical education would have their part to play in the training of counsellors."[38] Beginning in 1925, her camp training course continued annually every September until 1948, including a mandatory three- or four-day overnight canoe trip as part of the curriculum. Young women, Hamilton insisted, needed to learn to be "staunch and rugged, unwilling to acknowledge defeat by weather or circumstances." In a program she described as "Spartan regimentation," each day would begin at seven in the morning with exercise and a swim, and continue with students "learning to wield an axe and handle hammer and saw" to help in the camp's building projects.[39] The students worked and suffered together, but they also had fun and emerged triumphant as counsellors.[40] She also believed that Septembers spent at the camp produced a lasting loyalty to the school. Such was Hamilton's dedication to Tanamakoon that when she retired from the MES she devoted herself entirely to the affairs of the camp and became involved in the formation of the Ontario Camping Association in 1933, which held its first conference at the MES in 1939.

One unfortunate aspect of Camp Tanamakoon was the appropriation of Indigenous customs and culture, which was a common practice at this time (see also the discussion in chapter 2 about the origins of the youth camping movement).[41] In *The Call of Algonquin*, Hamilton wrote: "The love of Indian adventure led us to adopt some Indian customs as well as names in those early days, customs such as pinning on a blanket and going to council fire, stalking home from council fire in silence, and using the Indian expression of applause, 'How! How!'"[42] The camp itself was divided into "tribes" – Chickasaw (juniors), Ojibway (intermediates), and Cree (seniors) – and each tribe elected a "little chief" by secret ballot. Also, each cabin chose an "Indian" name such as *Ehawee* (laughing maid) or *Okokoho* (owl), which

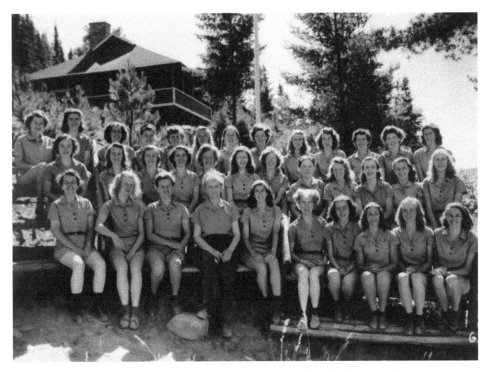

Figure 3.6. Counsellors at Camp Tanamakoon with Mary Hamilton (in long pants), 1946 (Algonquin Provincial Park Archives and Collections, 6464)

were more representative of Native American culture than of Canadian Indigenous peoples. Since Tanamakoon was exclusively a girls' camp, they were encouraged to emulate a different sort of "Indian," one appropriately feminine, through the development of artistic abilities such as weaving and painting Indigenous themes, rather than through more masculine, primitive activities as might be found in boys' camps. In Hamilton's view, acting "like Indians" subtly encouraged a more active and assertive womanhood.

Most summer camps of this era, and certainly those like Tanamakoon located in Algonquin Park, employed Indigenous people as indispensable canoeing and woodcraft instructors, trip guides, maintenance workers, and kitchen staff, thus providing jobs and income. Idealistically, Hamilton defended her use of Indigenous themes as functional and inspiring, but also something belonging to the past. "The North American Indians' way of life," she wrote, "has offered much of the inspiration for the organization of today's camps, living as they did in tribal communities, dwelling in huts or teepees, travelling on foot or by canoe, settling their affairs at the council ring."[43] When describing "Indian Day" at the camp, she also wrote: "The

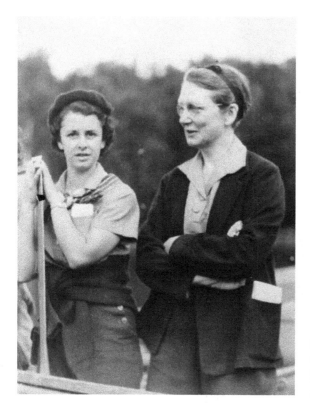

Figure 3.7. Mary Hamilton and a counsellor at Camp Tanamakoon (Algonquin Provincial Park Archives and Collections, 3152)

day, with its campfires, dances and songs, in no way caricatured the Indian, but rather proved quite educational in showing the greatness of these early inhabitants of our country."[44] Here, as elsewhere, there was absolutely no recognition (or perhaps even knowledge) of Canadian government policies of the day to aggressively assimilate Indigenous peoples, nor of the thousands of Indigenous children and youth suffering in residential and day schools across the country.

Another aspect of Hamilton's training for camp counsellors was her focus on interpersonal relationships, and more specifically emotional "crushes," which was an oblique code for lesbianism. In her book, *The Call of Algonquin*, she warned of these sorts of attachments especially among campers by commenting: "above all, do not allow it to develop into an exclusive friendship."[45] Hamilton and her staff used both formal and informal means to instil a white, middle-class, heterosexual model of gender in their students, campers, and counsellors. Improper friendships, whether casual or intimate, could ruin a young teacher's career and stain the profession, and teachers/camp directors worried even more about lesbianism.[46] Hamilton remained single all her life, which was unusual, certainly among MES students and graduates, where the general expectation was that after working for a short period, they would marry and raise a family. Indeed, according to a 1992 study of all living MES graduates, approximately 15 per cent remained single. On average, students graduated at twenty-one years of age, worked for about five years, and then were married.[47]

Hamilton's practical and vocational vision strongly influenced her leadership as did her deeply held religious beliefs, which together created an atmosphere of moral integrity and careful student guidance. She was not someone who expressed her thoughts in words, and she spoke in public only when absolutely necessary. Nevertheless, dedicated to her work, she demanded perfection from her students, excusing no one from the attempt to achieve it, while also inspiring a fierce loyalty from those who came to call her "Ham" or "Mary G." She would also play a role in helping develop the Canadian Physical Education Association in 1933 (see chapter 4), serving for two years as its vice-president. When Hamilton left the school, Florence Somers said about her: "Generous, unselfish, just, open-minded, progressive, you and I are the richer for having known her. She has made the Margaret Eaton School known throughout the length and breadth of Canada for its high standards."[48]

Despite the MES's ambitious and well-designed program, the one continuing major drawback to the school's success (and eventual survival) was that it lacked provincial authority to award a teaching degree to its students. Even the transition of leadership in 1935 from Mary Hamilton to Florence Somers, former Associate Director of the Sargent School and eminent American educator, was unable to effect this, leaving the YWCA as the most important, indeed critical, hiring destination for most MES graduates. At the same time, Hamilton had begun talks with the University of Toronto to share faculty resources and courses with the MES, and to exchange students for particular courses. The development helped increase the school's legitimacy within the broader academic community, which would be further enhanced with Hamilton's successor.

When Hamilton took over the principalship in 1926, it was understood that the MES needed to become completely self-financed, or receive only minimal assistance from the Eaton Company. By and large throughout Hamilton's tenure this was the actual situation. The student residences, for example, became a money-maker for the school, although as the Depression dragged on, some students could not pay their tuition fees. Robert Y. Eaton, a nephew of Timothy Eaton and now the representative on the MES board, was responsive to periodic requests for money, such as furnishings and the like. Nevertheless, from the perspective of the Eaton Company, there was increasing talk of closing the school or finding a suitable solution so that it could get rid of the financial burden and at the same time preserve its positive name.

Florence Somers: Femininity and Charm

Florence Somers came to the MES with an impressive academic and administrative history, including a BA from Boston University, an MA from New York University, and a diploma from the Sargent School. She also had a depth of experience working as both Assistant Director of the Department of Education in Massachusetts and Associate Director of the Sargent School. Canada increasingly looked south for its educational experts in addition to its reliance on teachers from the United Kingdom and Europe. Canadian education was becoming increasingly professionalized in the 1920s, a trend marked by the growing tendency to commission experts from the United States for advice, to draw on their pedagogical research, and to utilize opportunities for graduate study south of the border.

When Somers arrived at the MES, she brought with her a rather different philosophy from the previous two principals, one laid out in her influential book *Principles of Women's Athletics*. Her attitude regarding women's participation in sport and athletics was conservative and essentially maternal; femininity and charm with a zest for action was the stated goal for her students. She wanted them to enjoy "appropriate" female fitness development and the joys of sport's participation, but they were also expected to be ladies first. She did not want them to develop muscles, have their sexuality exploited, or their personal health damaged in competitive athletic arenas. Therefore, she endorsed the idea that the pursuit of strenuous competition and vigorous sport was a masculine quality, and one inappropriate for "proper" females.

The best athletic program for girls, according to Somers, was educational rather than competitive; activities should involve skill and neuromuscular control rather than strength, speed, or endurance; after puberty, girls should play only with girls, especially in the more vigorous, competitive games, and all aspects of competition should be carefully controlled and monitored. "Standards measure success in athletics," she wrote in an article published in a Canadian journal, "not in terms of scores, not in terms of pleased audience, not by winning teams or broken athletic records or championship victories, but in terms of the *welfare of the girl* who is taking part in them."[49]

Much has been written about this era when female physical educators, especially in the Toronto region of Ontario, readily adopted the biologically deterministic platform of the Women's Division of National Amateur Athletic Federation in the United States.[50] As mentioned previously, their "play for play's sake" philosophy stressed the enjoyment of sport, the development of character and sportsmanship, rather than the seeking of records or championships. Their creed – "a team for

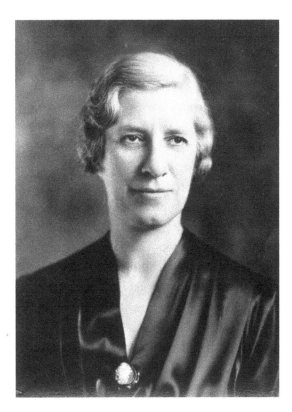

Figure 3.8. Florence A. Somers (University of Toronto Archives, 2008-26-2MS)

every girl and every girl on a team" – was best accomplished through broadly based intramural programs and "play days" where everyone, no matter how skilled or unskilled, could compete and have fun. In their drive for professional authority in this era, female physical educators were increasingly pressed to articulate exactly how their programs might best meet the unique physical and personal needs of girls and young women. To authenticate their claims, they worked to develop the "premise of sex differences into a coherent philosophy of active womanhood connecting female bodies, character, and exercise."[51] The twin beliefs about "women's unique anatomy" and their "special moral obligations" disqualified girls from the same treatment that boys received and instead prescribed for them a different physical education.[52] Interscholastic competition for girls was discouraged in schools; all teaching, coaching, and officiating were placed in the hands of competent women teachers.

Someone who agreed with Somers and her approach to girls' physical education and sport was Helen Bryans, who from 1929 until the mid-1960s taught at the Ontario College of Education (OCE) in Toronto. After completing a university degree, all would-be teachers spent either a winter or summer session at OCE to become qualified to teach in an Ontario high school. Bryans was an undeniably powerful and influential physical educator who for many years virtually dictated the hiring of female physical educators, certainly in Ontario, although her influence was wider.[53] Born just at the end of the nineteenth century, she attended Jarvis Collegiate Institute in Toronto, followed by the University of Toronto in the early 1920s, where she was a noted swimmer. She returned to Jarvis Collegiate as a teacher in 1921, and used her summers to attain further qualifications, including a master's degree, at several universities in the United States, where she came to understand and firmly believe in the American philosophy towards sports competition for girls. In her view, the purpose of a secondary school physical education curriculum for girls was to ensure that "every girl should carry herself erect and with body pride, moving with grace and poise; she should know how to play two or three team games and two or three individual games with skill and enjoyment, be able to participate in a folk-dance group with confidence, swim with safety and be prepared to assist others when necessary."[54]

Although Somers was the director of the MES for only a few years, her considerable impact affected students, staff, curriculum, and in the end, the institution itself. The social life and values presented at the school clearly mandated heterosexual attractiveness, marriage, and motherhood as the only acceptable life choices possible for its graduates. As an example, the school began to publicize marriage rates alongside employment statistics. Not only were MES students expected to graduate with marketable skills, but they were also anticipated to be traditionally suitable for marriage. By 1941, the statistics showed that since 1926, the MES had graduated 236 young women with the relevant percentages: 42.7 teaching, 41.1 married, 8.4 in other occupations, and 5.5 unemployed.[55] Despite this pressure, a remarkable 20 to 25 per cent of graduates during the last fifteen years of the school remained unmarried.

Somers also made an effort to strengthen the academic legitimacy of the school through changes to the courses offered, and by formalizing facility and personnel links with the University of Toronto. Specifically, more "scientific" theory courses, such as sociology, kinesiology, and physiology of exercise were added to the curriculum. Gymnastics courses were considerably reduced and replaced with more forms of dance including children's, tap, and certainly modern. Marion Hobday, a graduate of the Sargent School in Boston, who had also trained at some of the best schools of modern dance, was hired to teach the subject, which students found highly enjoyable yet challenging. They were required to wear a costume of red silk jersey with long sleeves and a mid-calf length flowing skirt, just like the famous dancer Mary Wigman, which made them feel especially empowered. Increasingly, there was greater reliance on instructional personnel from the University of Toronto such that by 1940–1, the MES calendar listed more staff affiliated with the university than with the school.

One of the first changes made by Somers was to extend the camping experience beyond Tanamakoon. Students alternated between attending the Ontario Athletic Commission camp at Lake Couchiching (see more about this camp in chapter 4) in 1936, 1938, and 1940, and Tanamakoon in 1935, 1937, and 1939. Those who attended the camp at Couchiching had a different experience because the setting was more open and designed for sports, especially track and field, than the wilderness of Tanamakoon. Somers believed that students should understand the basics of most games and sports so that they could teach and referee them in various community settings. In keeping with Somers's philosophy of women's sport, it is not surprising that the MES encouraged intramural games and play days with other schools, rather than regularly scheduled competitions.

As early as 1927, Robert Eaton was approached by the University of Toronto with a proposal to affiliate the MES with the university so that it could establish a "school for physical training." Obviously, such a school would require a new building, and along with the proposal came a request for $400,000. The Eaton Company refused because Margaret Eaton, devoted as she was to literature and the dramatic arts, wanted nothing to do with a university department focused entirely on physical education.[56] Another request for affiliation was made in 1931, but again rebuffed by the Eaton Company for much the same reason. When Margaret Eaton died in 1933, the Eatons were still adamant that a school for physical education would not be a fitting memorial to her memory. In 1934, when Mary Hamilton had announced her pending retirement, Robert Eaton wondered "if we should not just let it close up and be through with it when Miss Hamilton quits."[57] The Board of Directors of the Eaton Company did in fact decide to close the MES, but Florence Somers convinced them to allow the school to continue for another two years while she worked to make it more financially secure. By the end of the 1936–7 school term, she had accumulated a small surplus primarily by increasing the school enrolment.

Somers held out for several more years while negotiating with the University of Toronto, and at the same time allowed some of the MES courses to be taken at the university. Finally, on 1 September 1941, the MES became part of the new School of Physical and Health Education at the University of Toronto, which offered the first undergraduate degree program (Bachelor of Physical and Health Education) of its kind in Canada. It was headed by Dr. E. Stanley Ryerson, an assistant dean of medicine and grandson of Egerton Ryerson. The school had nine male faculty, who were joined by three women: Somers, former MES staff member Dorothy Jackson, and Jean Forster, the last remaining faculty member from the University of Toronto women's diploma program.

Once the merger was complete, the curriculum for the new university school of physical and health education needed to be restructured, which from Director Ryerson's perspective was to "give a sound knowledge of health from a scientific point of view."[58] It soon became clear that Ryerson knew nothing about the pedagogical and practical orientation of the former MES curriculum, nor was he interested. From his standpoint, the purpose of the new degree program was primarily to focus on health education, with some arts and sciences courses for general education, and all physical activity courses (one-third of the degree experience) came under "physical education." Gone were courses in how to teach dance, gymnastics, and sport activities, as well as the practice teaching experience. By the third year, students were taking courses in functional anatomy, applied physiology, health assessment and promotion, and hygiene and preventative medicine.

Fearing the loss of the camp experience, Mary Hamilton donated $2,000 to the university requesting that the money be used to launch the camp counsellor course for women students in the new School of Physical and Health Education. In 1942, Dorothy Jackson proposed that such a course be held during the first three weeks of September at Camp Tanamakoon in Algonquin Park. The purpose was to prepare students wishing to qualify for positions as camp counsellors, and it would be open to any female university students. There would be no cost to the students, except for the railway fare to the camp and living expenses of twelve dollars per week. Despite the efforts by Hamilton and Jackson to keep the camp course a compulsory part of the physical education curriculum, by 1948 their efforts had failed and it slowly disappeared.

As for Florence Somers, she continued to seek ways to develop physical education: for example, she was the first female president of the Canadian Physical Education Association in 1939. She continued to teach at the University of Toronto, where students remembered her as kind yet firm, understanding but distant, and always demanding a proper attitude. She retired in 1948 and returned to the Boston area, where she died in 1977.

The Margaret Eaton School in Retrospect

The MES played an important and effective role in a rapidly modernizing society to create and enable female demands for more freedom of movement and greater leisure opportunities. It stimulated a growing appetite among girls and young women for sport and physical activity of all kinds, and at the same time provided a growing number of opportunities for leadership and training activities. In this sense the MES directly stimulated the professionalization of the discipline of female physical education, shaping its content and purpose, and opened the curriculum to a transnational swirl of creative ideas around body culture.

It was a story of neither success nor failure, but rather one of agency and compliance, and of autonomy and co-optation. It was an example of a narrowly restricted, woman-centred educational space that opened emancipatory possibilities and yet reinforced hegemonic notions of class, race, gender, and sexuality.[59] It was also an example of a transitional phase in the history of women in higher education at a time when women were introduced to the broader and more expressive forms of body culture. At the same time, what the history of the MES illustrates over four decades of leadership in female physical education was the extraordinary number of ways in which individual women enhanced female health, mobility, and creative expression in the face of economic hardship, tepid institutional support, and restrictive gender ideologies in society at large. Between 1901 and 1942, the MES graduated over 250 students with an average of eighteen graduates per year (although between 1939 and 1942, that number rose to twenty-eight graduates per annum).[60] Although most graduates were from Ontario, they also represented almost every province. By today's standards this is a small number, yet the MES chartered a unique terrain for Canadian physical education and contributed in important and useful ways to female professional advancement.

Vestiges of the MES still remain today primarily in the Faculty of Kinesiology and Physical Education at the University of Toronto. For several years, the Margaret Eaton Library, endowed by the Eaton family, existed in the Athletics Centre, although by the early 1990s many of the books were donated to other libraries and the space turned into a faculty lounge. Margaret Eaton's portrait still hangs in this room. Also, the Margaret Eaton School Digital Collection, housed at Redeemer University College in Hamilton, Ontario, consists of 17,500 archival materials collected from alumnae. Many of these items are available through the Internet Archive.[61]

CHAPTER FOUR

Fit for Living

I believe that it is much wiser to develop a race of people who will be *fit for living*, than wait until we are required to make them fit for national defense.

Arthur S. Lamb, 1933

In October 1929, the Wall Street stock market crashed, ushering in the Great Depression of the thirties. A widespread drop in world commodity prices, along with a sudden decline in economic demand and credit, led to a rapid deterioration in global trade coupled with rising unemployment. Like many countries Canada was severely affected by these events but more so because of our dependence on primary industries like farming, fishing, mining, and logging. Across the country, farmers, young people, small businessmen, and the unemployed bore the brunt of economic hardship, and there was a widespread loss of jobs and savings. By 1933, some 30 per cent of the labour force was out of work – one in five Canadians became dependent upon government relief for survival. Along with crippling drought and the fall of wheat prices, the Prairie provinces faced the worst economic conditions especially in rural areas, where two-thirds of the residents went on relief. Immigration to Canada was curtailed, while deportations increased, and birthrates plummeted as children were postponed until families could afford to support them. Women who worked were encouraged to leave the labour force especially when they married.

The Depression also triggered the birth of social welfare, which proved woefully inadequate, as well as the rise of populist political movements. The federal government, for example, set up unemployment relief camps, run by the Department of

National Defence, primarily for single, homeless men who worked on construction projects. The rise of working-class militancy, organized primarily by the Communist Party, led to numerous strikes and protests, and often violent clashes with police. Canadian unions became more forceful and powerful.

Within the educational sector, school budgets diminished although enrolments increased because dropouts could not find employment. To save money, school districts consolidated schools, postponed new construction, and increased class size. Married women teachers were let go and not replaced by new teachers, so that teachers' average age and experience increased, but salaries decreased. Since less than 3 per cent of the twenty- to twenty-four-year-old age group attended college in 1930, universities served a comparatively small portion of the population, most of whom were from middle-class backgrounds. Although university budgets were drastically cut, they survived the Depression and no institutions were closed.

The Depression era was particularly difficult for students in Indian residential schools, where hunger and malnutrition were even more severe due to less funding and support from Indian Affairs. This department also cut back on its provisions for unemployment relief, which meant that throughout the Depression, per capita expenditures on relief were consistently between two and three times higher for non-Indigenous Canadians than they were for Indigenous peoples.[1]

By 1937, the worst of the Depression had passed, although it had left its mark on all sectors of the Canadian economy. Recovery proceeded slowly while employment increased but productivity remained sluggish. All this changed with massive state expenditures necessitated by the onset of another world war, which by 1942 had reduced unemployment to minimal levels. The war, of course, brought heartache and misery to many, especially those who lost loved ones on the battlefields of Europe and elsewhere.

In this chapter we examine the growth of physical education in Canada through the formation of regional and national associations; school physical education across the provinces; Dominion–Provincial physical training programs; the wartime National Physical Fitness Act; physical education in the various youth movements during the Depression and war; and Indigenous schooling through a residential school case study. The historical period discussed begins in the early 1930s and continues to the end of the Second World War in 1945.

Creating a National Association for Physical Education

In 1931, at the annual meeting of the Quebec Physical Education Association, Arthur Lamb invited members to undertake the formation of a similar Canadian association (CPEA for short). If they agreed, the McGill University School of Physical Education would underwrite the costs of compiling a list of physical education leaders in other provinces and sending out notices. Some 196 replies were received from 464 letters sent out across the country with more than 80 per cent from Ontario and Quebec.[2] Toronto was chosen as the site of the first national conference because the city had an active physical education association that would perhaps guarantee a more positive response from potential members. Mary Hamilton of the Margaret Eaton School, along with Fred Bartlett, Supervisor of Physical Education for the Toronto Board of Education, and Mary Barker of the Toronto Physical Education Association were enlisted to do the convention organizing. Lamb's joint initiative in promoting a national association with the Toronto and Quebec Physical Education Associations was based on his belief that there were enough educators devoted to physical education across the country to come together and share common concerns. "Its platform must be basically sound," he declared, "its vision broad, its ideals high, its enthusiasm boundless, and its courage great."[3]

What is interesting is that the highly organized and active School Health and Physical Education Section of the Ontario Education Association was not included in these early plans for a national association. Indeed, in 1933 it had over 400 members, but the association accepted only teachers. Lamb had encouraged the formation of an Ontario Physical Education Association to attract not just teachers, but also physical educators working in youth movements, especially the Y's, and also in Parks and Recreation and other related organizations (see chapter 2). During the Depression years, teachers took on heavy teaching loads for little money, and most considered the Ontario Educational Association more helpful and useful for their needs. In later years, the timing of the national convention, usually in June, prevented schoolteachers from attending. This division between school physical education teachers and other professionals in related fields as well as university-based physical educators would become a larger problem, especially in Ontario, as the CPEA tried to grow across the country.[4]

At the CPEA's first annual conference in April 1933, 168 people met at the Margaret Eaton School in Toronto to approve a constitution and elect executive officers and a legislative council. The purpose of the new organization was to stimulate universal, intelligent, and active interest in health and physical education; to acquire and disseminate knowledge concerning it; to promote interest and strive for the establishment of educative programs under the direction of adequately trained teachers; to set the standards of the profession; and to cooperate with kindred interests and organizations in the furtherance of these aims.[5] Newly elected president Arthur Lamb lambasted the current view of physical education within the country's school systems: "It is often looked upon as an addendum, a frill, an extra, and all that is necessary is to have some ignoramus snap out a few commands, strut about like a pouter pigeon, and treat children like so many automatic tin soldiers." He placed considerable blame on the Department of Militia and Defense, and especially the Strathcona Trust, for promulgating "false and imbecilic notions" regarding the role that physical education should play in education. It was vitally important, he argued, to stress the noun "education" and not the adjective "physical." Moreover, the negative attitude, the parrot-like repetition of established tradition, and the meaningless prescription of "tables of drill" must give way to a program adapted to the needs of the individual and society, based upon sound principles that enrich living, stabilize character, and improve citizenship. "We must demonstrate," he urged his listeners, "how a modern programme in health and physical education can transform a community." To his audience, the founding members of the CPEA, he implored them to aspire towards thorough professional training, wider scholarship, richer experience, and higher standards to inspire the children and youth whom they teach.[6]

Despite the initial interest, the CPEA had a slow start, especially in becoming established across the country. A year after its founding, there were eighty-six paid-up members, with only fifteen of these outside Ontario and Quebec. The association had little to offer its members but a "vision of hope" and a mimeographed *Bulletin* published three to four times a year. By the time of the second convention in Montreal in 1935, the CPEA was in serious difficulty. Lamb's address to the gathering was as bleak as the membership statistics: "Little if any progress has been made in Canada in the last 25 years towards a broad national programme for improving the physique of our people. Our Provincial and Federal Governments are apathetic and indifferent – content to allow people to wallow along in physical illiteracy. Some Departments of Education have been content to continue subscribing to a twenty-five-year-old moss-covered agreement whereby totally ill-prepared teachers are charged with directing these vital and fundamental interest[sic] of our children, along paths which lead to indifference, carelessness and neglect – which must eventually take its toll."[7]

School Physical Education across the Provinces

Was Lamb correct in his assessment? What was the situation in the provinces at this time with regard to school-based physical education?[8] In 1934, the McGill School of Physical Education contacted each provincial Department of Education asking them to provide information about the status and qualification of physical education teachers, in addition to the requirements and programs for physical education, in their public elementary and high schools. A comprehensive report of the findings was compiled by one of Lamb's students.[9] The study took place around the same time as the *Syllabus of Physical Training for Schools 1933*, published by the British Board of Education, was being adopted throughout Canada, replacing the older 1919 version, although neither of these texts was revised by the Strathcona Trust to fit Canadian needs. The 1933 *Syllabus*, designed primarily for students up to eleven or twelve years of age, relied more on a system of Danish gymnastics developed by Niels Bukh, which focused on flexibility, suppleness, and rhythm. Bukh was familiar to Canadians because along with a troupe of twenty-five young Danish gymnasts, he toured several Canadian cities in the fall of 1931 presenting a program of athletic exercises, tumbling, folk dances, and songs. It was so popular in Calgary, for example, that at least 7,000 came to the evening performance with many turned away from an earlier school matinee.[10] The 1933 *Syllabus* was much longer than its predecessors, reaching 350 pages, with more attention to organizing and teaching games, swimming, and dance. It too was quickly adopted, even if teachers had to buy their own copies.

There was remarkable curricular consistency throughout the country with all but one province utilizing the Strathcona *Syllabus* for elementary schools, and some also for secondary schools. In Quebec, Cécile Grenier (see box 4.1), the assistant director of physical education at the Commission des écoles catholiques de Montréal, translated some of the *Syllabus* into French for use in Catholic schools. In Saskatchewan, however, the influence of Ethel Mary Cartwright, previously at McGill and now a professor of physical education at the University of Saskatchewan, was clearly in evidence. Replacing the *Syllabus* in Saskatchewan schools was a "modern" program including play, organized games, gymnastics, athletics, calisthenics, dancing, and other rhythmic movements. Outdoor recreation such as hiking, field excursions, and picnics were also part of the elementary curriculum. By way of explanation, Cartwright wrote: "In common with all other forms of true education, the process is one of growth and liberation of capacity from within. It is not a system of formal drill imposed by external authority and requiring automatic response to the word of command; but rather a rich and varied program of opportunities for children to express themselves in wholesome, purposeful forms of play and other types of physical exercises."[11] The difference between the elementary and secondary physical education programs was that most public schools followed the *Syllabus* to the letter, whereas high schools incorporated a more varied program of indoor and outdoor games especially if they had access to a playground. Schools with a proper gymnasium offered more apparatus gymnastics and calisthenics.

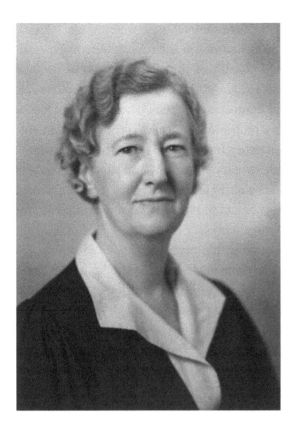

Figure 4.1. Ethel Mary Cartwright, 1942 (University of Saskatchewan, University Archives and Special Collections, Photograph Collection, A-3222)

The main challenge in the 1930s and 1940s for physical education in Quebec was to modify people's attitudes towards the subject. One of the first steps was to change the name from "physical training" to physical education, which also included broadening the subject beyond military drill and calisthenics. Jack Lang, who in 1930 was appointed Supervisor of Physical Training and Fire Drill for the Montreal Protestant School Board, worked hard (together with Dr. Lamb) throughout the Depression years to change these perceptions. Lang's philosophy was that physical education (specifically, education through the physical) should merit the same amount of attention as any other subject in the curriculum at both the elementary and secondary level. He was also responsible for creating the Montreal and District Athletic Association, which eventually brought the Protestant and Catholic schools together into one body.[12] As for the Commission des écoles catholiques de Montréal, René Bélisle for the boys and Cécile Grenier (see box 4.1) for the girls were pioneers in the development of physical education during this era.[13]

Almost all teachers of physical education also taught one or more academic subjects, and there were very few "specialists" anywhere except in some of the larger cities. In the Maritime provinces, for example, there were no specialists at all. At this time, there were only four institutions in the country offering specialist training in physical education – McGill University, the University of Toronto, the Margaret Eaton School (see chapter 3), and the University of Saskatchewan. Graduates of these programs (except graduates of McGill who taught in Quebec Protestant schools) also had to obtain a professional teacher's certificate from a normal school before they could teach in either an elementary or a secondary school. The most common qualification of elementary school physical education teachers was still the Strathcona "B" Certificate obtained at a normal school, although some provinces were also offering specialist courses in physical education, primarily for secondary school teachers, at summer schools.

The time devoted to physical education within the total curriculum varied considerably throughout the country. For elementary schools, the hours per week ranged widely with Saskatchewan the highest at one hundred minutes and Prince Edward Island the lowest at twenty minutes, although in British Columbia there were no definite time periods set aside. In secondary schools, British Columbia, Manitoba, and Ontario all required ninety minutes or more per week, and with most other provinces it was eighty minutes, although again Prince Edward Island required only twenty minutes or less.

As time went on, there were increasing concerns about the role played by the Department of Militia and Defense in the training of physical education teachers for elementary schools. Between 1933 and 1940, for example, approximately 10,000 students in the Ontario normal schools had received the Strathcona "B" Certificate through the forty-five-hour course, which was usually taught by a military officer loaned to the school for six to eight weeks by the Militia Department. In 1936, the Ontario Committee of the Strathcona Trust summed up their dissatisfaction succinctly: "However well the Strathcona Drill may be adapted for the training of men it is quite unsuited for the culture of children."[14] There were further complaints that military officers were not up to date with the 1933 *Syllabus*, and more importantly, they had no understanding of how to teach children. Nonetheless, the "B" certificate examination was retained, although in 1939 the Department of Education established its own physical education course and exam in normal schools, which also qualified teachers.

Secondary school teachers in Ontario were never subjected to the rigours of obtaining the Strathcona Certificate because the Department of Education certified them in "physical culture" through its own diploma course.[15] However, as the Ontario secondary curriculum evolved, including compulsory courses in health and physical education, there was clearly a need for university-trained teachers in these

BOX 4.1. CÉCILE G. GRENIER (1907-2003)

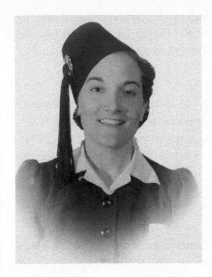

Figure 4.2. Cécile G. Grenier, 1939 (Archives UQÀM, Fonds d'archives Cécile-G. Grenier, 71P:020:F3/7)

One of seven children whose father, a medical doctor, believed wholeheartedly in the importance of sporting activity, Grenier grew up in an environment of healthy exercise, both at home and in the boarding schools she attended. She trained as a teacher, and in 1927 was hired by the Commission des écoles catholiques de Montréal (CECM), where she taught at the elementary and high school levels for the next ten years. Although not trained specifically in physical education, she educated herself through taking lessons in various sports, attending short courses (she acquired the Strathcona "B" certificate), and trying out her ideas with the students she taught. Her reputation grew, and in 1938 she was appointed the assistant director of physical education for the CECM. She soon travelled to Sweden to learn more about Ling gymnastics at the college in Stockholm that Per Henrik Ling had established many years before. Here, Grenier found the basis for her developing philosophy of physical education, especially for girls and women: "Physical culture or hygienic gymnastics is based on the repetition of movements aimed at the development of musculature, range of joint movements and major organic functions. When the movements are well known, they can be advantageously punctuated by musical phrases and thus we obtain *rhythmic gymnastics* ... which prevent stiffness and are very suitable for young girls and women."* Above all, physical education was a form of bodily expression that allowed females to express their feelings through movement. Thus, all forms of dance played a major role in Greiner's teaching despite the disapproval of the nuns who ran the schools, and the Catholic ban on dancing.

Realizing there was nowhere at this time for francophones in Quebec, especially women, to gain training in the teaching of physical education, Grenier founded the private, non-profit Institut d'éducation physique (IEP) in Montreal in 1939. Here, she offered courses in the evenings and during the summers, and also formed an elite group of female gymnasts (of good demeanour, excellent character, and good health) who performed publicly in Montreal and elsewhere to illustrate the work of the institute.

> Grenier went on to have a very long career in physical education, retiring in 1971. Fluently bilingual, she was well known throughout Canada especially through her work in the early days of the Canadian Association of Health, Physical Education, and Recreation (CAHPER), and with other organizations. However, her heart and soul were with the multitude of girls and women she trained through her institute.
>
> For more information, see Detellier, *Mises au jeu*, 89–105, and Leduc and Girard, "Le statut professionnel," as well as an interview (in English) conducted by Stuart Davidson in 1978 (Stewart Davidson fonds, Library and Archives Canada, Item number 435312). The quotation followed by an asterisk (*) is from Detellier, *Mises au jeu*, 103; translated by M. Ann Hall.

subjects. For many years, the University of Toronto had offered a diploma course in physical training but only for men. Although there were several attempts to offer a course for women, one did not become permanent until 1928, and by 1931 it was changed to a three-year arts course with the fourth year devoted to physical education, after which a diploma was granted. As we discussed in the previous chapter, a three-year Bachelor of Health and Physical Education degree program was approved in 1940 – the first in Canada – along with the formation of the School of Physical and Health Education. The 1940 class consisted of six men and eleven women, which by 1945 had expanded to an enrolment of one hundred men and 121 women.[16]

Physical Education in the Indian Residential Schools

In 1932, with now eighty residential schools under its jurisdiction, Indian Affairs reported that the "health of Indian children studying in boarding schools continues to receive special attention. Good medical supervision has been arranged and much thought has been given to physical education, proper diet, and sanitation."[17] By 1938, Indian Affairs claimed that "residential schools are now equipped to provide worth-while instruction in agriculture, gardening, carpentry work, boat-building, tailoring, dressmaking, cooking, handloom weaving, and physical culture."[18] These studies were combined with the regular courses of study supplied by provincial departments of education, although for Indigenous students, the tendency was to provide a practical course of study with less emphasis on academic subjects. However, to what extent were students at the residential schools receiving instruction in physical culture or education?

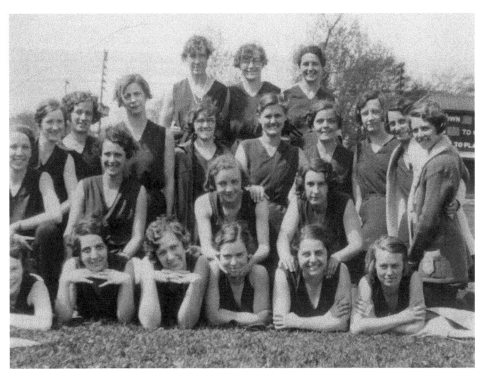

Figure 4.3. Specialists in Physical Education, Ontario College of Education, 1930–1 (University of Toronto Archives, 2006-29-3MS)

We examine one institution in particular, namely, the Pelican Lake Indian Residential School (also called the Sioux Lookout School), which tells a rather different story.[19] Located in northern Ontario, some 350 kilometres northwest of Thunder Bay near Sioux Lookout, it was established by the Anglican Church and drew students from the relatively close Lac Seul First Nation, but also from the widely scattered bands making up today's Nishnawbe-Aski Nation. Many of the students came from communities and families in remote areas, where they experienced a traditional lifestyle. The heavily forested property comprised 287 acres, bordered by Pelican Lake to the north and the main CNR transcontinental line to the south. Land was cleared and levelled near the school for farming operations, mainly by male student labour. The main school building was a three-storey structure including classrooms, two basement playrooms, medical dispensary, chapel, and girls' and boys' dormitories. Although opened in 1926, the school was not fully operational until 1929 with 103 students, and when running at capacity it could accommodate 125 students.

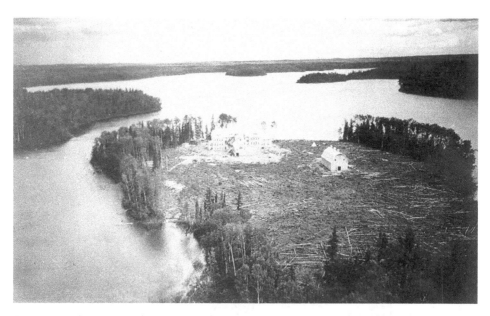

Figure 4.4. Pelican Lake Indian Residential School, c. 1927 (The General Synod Archives, Anglican Church of Canada, P75-103-S7-130)

Poor drainage meant that the area surrounding the school was less than ideal for sports and recreation. Snow covering the fields in winter, and muddy conditions in spring and fall made outdoor activities difficult if not impossible. An assessor undertaking the school's first official inspection commented on the lack of recreation space: "Goodness! Where do the children play?"[20] Nonetheless, local school administrators worked to provide facilities and equipment for physical activities under difficult conditions. Although there were designated play and recreation rooms in the basement of the main building, seeping rainwater curtailed indoor physical activities for long periods of time. The lake was always important to the school's recreation program with swimming in summer and skating or hockey in winter. Like all other residential schools of this era, recreational activities and sport, aside from providing some fun, had the broader purpose of eliminating "Indianness." A 1940 pamphlet advertising the Pelican Lake school stated: "Unlike their playmates of civilization, the Indian children's recreation must be cultivated and developed, as they lack the knowledge of creating their own amusements. Strange as it may seem, the average Indian cannot swim, so that their recreation becomes an education. Once taught, they become keen, and display good sportsmanship and courage."[21]

Like all industrial schools of this era, the labour required to keep Pelican Lake running was supplied mostly by the students through the half-day system. The boys

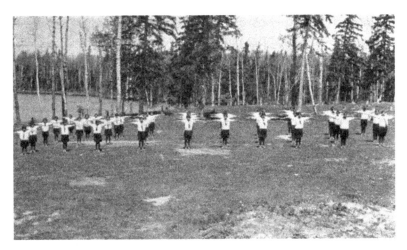

Figure 4.5. Girls' physical training class at Pelican Lake Indian Residential School, 1941
(The General Synod Archives, Anglican Church of Canada, GS75-103-B131-F4)

worked the farm by seeding, cultivating, harvesting, and caring for the animals. They also continued to clear brush and stumps from the land. The girls worked in the laundry, kitchen, dairy, sewing room, and helped to keep the dormitories clean and tidy. This left little time for recreation, and to make matters worse, Indian Affairs was reluctant to provide funds for athletic and recreational equipment, so that the school was mostly dependent on donations from local church groups for sporting equipment (e.g., skates) and uniforms. By 1945, the lack of recreational opportunities was still very noticeable at Pelican Lake School. The Indian agent responsible pointed this out, also noting that under proper supervision, such activities "would go a long way toward developing character and physique."[22]

How typical was Pelican Lake among the residential schools in general? In his report to the 1996 Royal Commission on Aboriginal Peoples concerning the history of residential schools, historian John S. Milloy wrote the following: "As that story unfolds, one conclusion becomes unavoidable: despite the discourse of civil and spiritual duty that framed the school system, there never was invested in this project the financial or human resources required to ensure that the system achieved its 'civilizing' ends or that children were cared for properly. Nor was there ever brought to bear the moral resources necessary to respond to systemic neglect or to the many instances of stark physical abuse that were known to be occurring." He went on to point out that throughout the history of the system, "the church-state partners were aware of these sorrowful circumstances and, moreover, that they came to understand the detrimental repercussions for all Aboriginal children of their residential school experience."[23] In his highly respected history of residential schools, *Shingwauk's Vision,* J.R. Miller called them "instruments of attempted cultural genocide" primarily because former students "bitterly recalled enforced attendance, non-Indian staff who denigrated Aboriginal culture and mistreated them, inadequate food and excessive chores, runaways and beatings, and, perhaps most persistently, the way in which their residential schooling experience at Shingwauk had failed to prepare them to be successful after they left the school."[24] In her book about Indigenous health and healing in British Columbia, historian Mary-Ellen Kelm notes that the "goal of residential schooling was to 're-form' Aboriginal bodies, and this they did. But the results were not the strong, robust bodies of the schools' propaganda, well-trained for agriculture and domestic labour, but weakened ones, which, through no fault of their own, brought disease and death to their communities."[25]

In these major studies of residential school history, in addition to the now numerous first-hand accounts of residential school survivors, there is rarely any reference to "physical education" as opposed to sports, games, and recreation, which are infrequently mentioned. As we have seen in chapters 1 and 2, calisthenics and physical drill were sometimes encouraged and taught as a form of physical education. Yet, as a curricular subject or program, physical education was next to impossible to organize or teach mainly because most residential and day schools had no facilities for such activities. Some had basement areas, obviously designed for play activities, but they were totally inadequate for rigorous and varied physical education. Besides, they were often only used for storage or assembly purposes. In addition, most schools never had a properly cleared or graded playing field with many still overgrown with shrubs, thistles, grasses, and weeds, rendering them unusable for sports and games.[26] The exceptions were rare.

In chapter 5, we continue the story of the Pelican Lake Residential School with regard to physical education, sport, and recreation throughout the remainder of its history.

Dominion–Provincial Physical Training Programs

As the Great Depression of the 1930s brought about mass unemployment, hunger, and homelessness, governments sought ways to raise the general level of health and morale, especially among youth. British Columbia, for example, with its favourable climate and general attractiveness became a mecca for drifters riding the rails and looking for work, especially in Vancouver. As the city's Superintendent of Playgrounds, Jan (also known as Ian) Eisenhardt struggled to provide some sort of organized activity for the swelling number of "hobos" congregating in the city parks and playgrounds looking for something to do. A recent immigrant from Denmark, Eisenhardt was familiar with the folk high school movement, popular in Nordic countries, where gymnastics and sports training played a major role. He began to introduce this concept into the Vancouver playgrounds, but soon realized there were far more who wanted to take part than there were leaders and facilities available.

In 1934, backed by the province's Minister of Education George Weir, Eisenhardt proposed a scheme of free, volunteer-run games and recreation classes that became known collectively as the Pro-Rec (provincial recreation) program.[27] His plan would not have reached government level in the first place had it not been for Weir, a strong advocate for physical education, whose support was crucial in the first year of the program. Free classes were offered, initially to unemployed men, and later to all those aged fifteen and over who were no longer in school. In what was arguably the most successful community sport and recreation program of any national fitness initiative of this era, the Recreation and Physical Education Branch of the Department of Education provided instructors for the various Pro-Rec activities as well as basic gymnastics apparatus and athletic equipment, while local communities were expected to offer the facilities.

Membership grew rapidly through participation in a wide range of activities, including dance, gymnastics, keep-fit, swimming, boxing, wrestling, weightlifting, and various team sports. In the first season, 1934–5, nineteen Pro-Rec centres in six different cities were established with an enrolment of just under 3,000.[28] By 1938–9, there were nearly 27,000 registered participants in Pro-Rec, with over sixty per cent female. Mass demonstrations of young women's fitness classes – many of them wearing a light-blue one-piece gymnastic suit and special shoes made from canvas – were held occasionally in Vancouver's Stanley Park, where there could be as many as 2,000 participants and thousands of spectators.

The fact that Pro-Rec attracted more women than men was unusual for sport and physical recreation programs in this era. The success of the keep-fit classes and the mass displays were partially responsible. Also, Pro-Rec's slogan, "Health, Beauty, Diet and Sports" was similar to "Movement for Life" of the Women's League of Health and Beauty, since both emphasized the "glamour, goodness and modernity of health and fitness."[29] Created in 1930 by Mary Bagot Stack in England, the League's purpose was to promote healthy motherhood and universal peace by encouraging women to incorporate fitness into their daily lives: good health, it was argued, led to peace, not war. Mary died unexpectedly in 1935 at which time her daughter, Prunella, took over leadership of the League. Touted as the "most

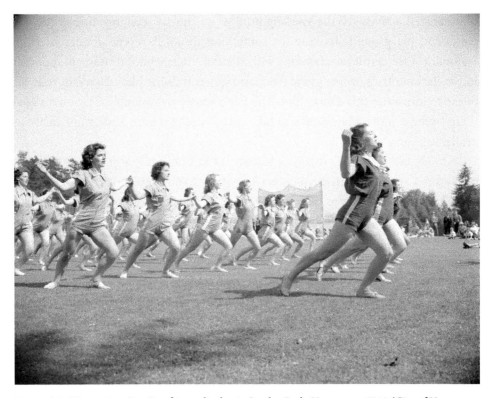

Figure 4.6. Women in a Pro-Rec fitness display in Stanley Park, Vancouver, 1940 (City of Vancouver Archives, 1184-2355, Jack Lindsay photographer)

physically perfect girl in the world," Prunella came to Toronto in September 1935 for the official launch of the League in Canada. An enthusiastic audience packed Toronto's Eaton Auditorium, where 130 new Canadian League members, dressed in uniforms of black shorts and white tops, gave a demonstration of rhythmic exercises. "Our system is for women and planned for women," stated Stack. "We don't want to develop the muscles of ball players; such a system would be wrong for us."[30] By 1936, the League had attracted over 1,000 members in Toronto; two years later this had grown to over 5,000, with branches in other Ontario centres as well as Montreal. In Britain, under the leadership of Prunella, who had observed and admired the mass movement spectacles in Germany, there was little concern in the League about the growing association between fitness, fascism, and duty to the state.[31] The war itself severely curtailed the activities of the League; many of its branches closed, and it never recovered to the level of its heyday in the 1930s.[32]

In 1937, the federal government passed the Unemployment and Agricultural Assistance Act, which provided funds for approved training and development

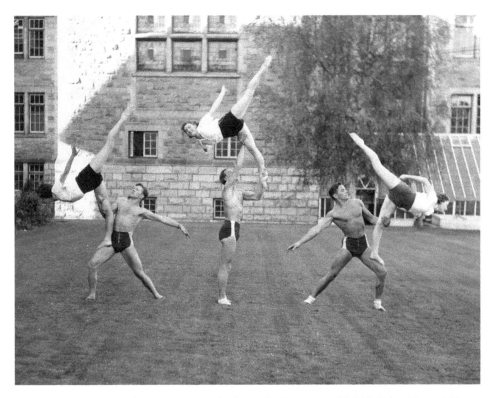

Figure 4.7. Pro-Rec members putting on a display at the University of British Columbia, c. 1940 (City of Vancouver Archives, Sp P46.4)

projects for unemployed young people, male or female from the ages of eighteen to thirty, through equal cost-sharing arrangements with cooperating provincial governments. Physical training projects to maintain health and morale were included as an acceptable category, in large part due to Eisenhardt's work, and the favourable, nation-wide reputation of his Pro-Rec program. The Dominion–Provincial Youth Training Programme subsequently provided grants to enable Pro-Rec to establish more centres, hire more instructors, and purchase more equipment. The 1939 Youth Training Act continued this support, with its provisions for the training of young people to prepare them for gainful employment.

The availability of funds prompted other provinces to look more closely at BC's Pro-Rec to determine if they should initiate a similar program. Quebec, for example, signed an agreement in 1937 whereby activities and instruction would be provided in the larger, urban centres in cooperation with private organizations. Officials in Alberta had been observing Pro-Rec for some time, prompting the province's premier, William Aberhart, early in 1938, to contact George Weir inquiring if

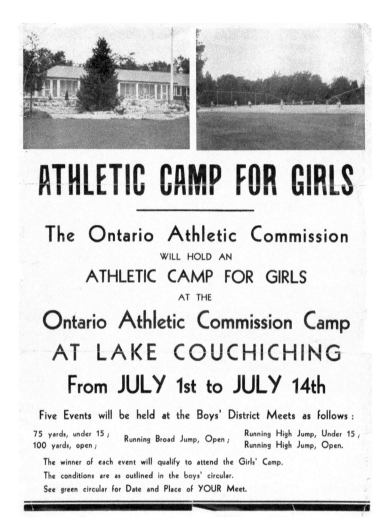

Figure 4.8. Poster announcing a camp for girl athletes at the Ontario Athletic Commission Camp, c. 1938 (University of Toronto Archives)

Eisenhardt could consult with public agencies and private organizations interested in recreation. After much planning and consultation between the two provinces, classes began in Alberta in the fall of 1938. During the first year of operation, thirty-one centres opened with a registration of almost 8,000 members, almost three-quarters of whom were unemployed. By 1940–1, there were 107 centres handling a registration of 6,000 trainees for a five-week course.[33] There was, however, a considerable difference in the Alberta program in that communities were given more responsibility for the establishment of centres, programs differed from centre to centre, and mass displays of fitness were not an important feature. In the summer of 1939, Saskatchewan also initiated a physical training project by making use of Pro-Rec instructors from British Columbia; their program ran in much the same manner as in Alberta. Manitoba also established a leadership training program with experimental centres established in twelve towns.[34] Overall, about $1.5 million a year was provided to support these various provincial schemes.

In 1929, to commemorate its tenth anniversary, the Ontario Athletic Commission (OAC) purchased seventeen acres of farmland along the shores of Lake Couchiching, near Orillia, Ontario (using tax money from professional sports teams). During the next two years, they landscaped playing fields, laid a 440-yard cinder track, built a swimming dock, erected and furnished cabins, a dining hall, and other buildings necessary to accommodate at least sixty athletes plus staff. They began operating two three-week summer training camps for high school athletes (males only) from around the province, mostly in track and swimming.

Women benefited from the camp for the first time in 1934, when the Department of Education began holding an annual week-long workshop for female physical education teachers from across the province. After several refusals, the leaders of the Women's Amateur Athletic Federation of Ontario persuaded OAC Commissioner Lionel Conacher to let them use the camp for their own leadership development program, and then to subsidize the participation of outstanding female athletes across the province. The Margaret Eaton School held its September camp counsellor course for their students at OAC in 1936, 1938, and 1940 (see chapter 3). It was also made available to the Department of Education for the upgrading of physical education teachers during the Second World War.[35]

Wartime National Physical Fitness Act

A small but vocal lobby considered these provincial programs inadequate, and they would settle for nothing less than a national, federally funded initiative in the area of fitness and physical activity directed especially at the youth of the nation. For example, in 1938 Arthur Lamb and others created the National Physical Fitness League, which "publicized the costs and benefits of improved fitness in a number of imaginative special events, radio broadcasts, and publicity campaigns that prefigured today's familiar campaigns of ParticipACTION."[36] The position of the federal government, still focused on the lingering effects of the Depression, was that recreation, fitness, and preventive health were the responsibility of local and provincial governments, which was certainly the case for physical education within the school systems.

What drew the federal government into the crusade was the high percentage of rejections among those entering military service during the Second World War. Near the beginning of the war, it was estimated that one-third of those recruited would be rejected because they could not walk five miles. The number of males who were actually rejected continued to climb and reached the level of 40 per cent of those who volunteered for active duty and 50 per cent of those who were conscripted.[37] Certainly the question remained as to whether a man declared unfit for military service was indeed physically unfit. Although it was a military problem, it was also a much broader issue: "War teaches valuable lessons but it should not be necessary to have a war to make people realize that the health and fitness of children and of young people are of paramount importance to the country" stated an editorial in the *Canadian Public Health Journal*. It went on to suggest that health education, including healthy habits and fitness, should be part of the school curricula because physical education was still confused with health training: "Teaching children to play games is considerably different from training them to live in health."[38] Soon, and for the first time, physical fitness came under the purview of the federal Department of Pensions and Health (later renamed Health and Welfare). The long-term plan was to integrate physical fitness with future health insurance schemes.

The National Physical Fitness Act was proclaimed on 1 October 1943 and by February of the following year a National Council on Physical Fitness had been appointed. Ian Eisenhardt of Pro-Rec fame and now a major in the Canadian military, was selected as the council's paid, full-time director, and its membership consisted of nine individuals (all male), each representing one of the provinces. The Council's purpose was straightforward – to promote the physical fitness of the people of Canada. It was to do this by "promoting the extension of physical education and coordinating and encouraging those people and activities that were associated with this objective."[39] More specifically it was to "assist in the extension of physical education in all educational and other establishments; encourage, develop and correlate all activities relating to physical development of the people through sports, athletics and other similar pursuits; train teachers, lecturers and instructors in the principles of physical education and physical fitness; organize activities designed to promote physical fitness and to provide facilities therefor; and cooperate with organizations ... engaged in the development of physical fitness in the amelioration of physical defects through exercise."[40] To accomplish these ambitious goals, a small fund of $225,000 (about $3.5 million today) was to be distributed to the provinces through a cost-sharing program. With his usual irony, Lamb supported the funding: "We no longer raise an eyebrow at the eleven million dollars we spend every day for death and destruction. Are we going to question an annual expenditure towards

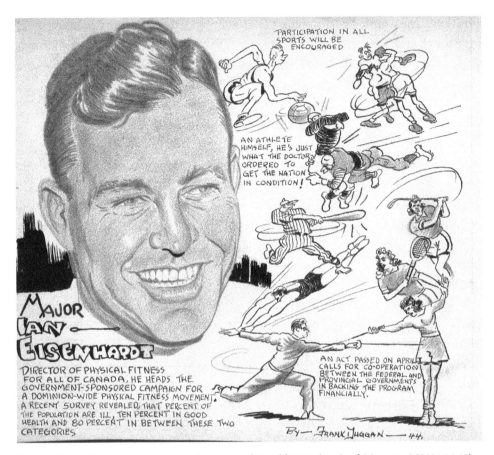

Figure 4.9. Ian Eisenhardt cartoon in the *Montreal Herald*, 1944 (McCord Museum, M2001.74.12)

safeguarding the health and fitness of generations to come, which would only last our fighting forces approximately thirty minutes?"[41] For his part, Eisenhardt was as optimistic as always about what could be achieved: "We must bring the lessons taught in the playing fields, in the gymnasiums, and in our health courses into the daily life of the children; we must persuade our people that one can never 'retire' from active participation in physical training – that life is activity."[42]

At the first meeting of the Council in May 1944, its members approved a series of resolutions, which, as we will see in the next chapter about the postwar era, were overly ambitious and difficult to implement. All communities were urged to set up their own physical fitness programs in cooperation with Provincial and Dominion Councils; universities should conduct a physical fitness program for all students and establish degree courses in physical and health education; and the many excellent military leaders of physical fitness and recreation should be hired for postwar positions. The Council also ambitiously recommended one month's camping every year for all children ages five to fourteen (there being over two million children of this age in Canada at the time).[43] We continue the postwar story of the National Council on Fitness in the next chapter.

Youth Movements in the Depression and Wartime

The devasting impact of the Depression prompted the formation of several new youth organizations among which the Canadian Youth Congress, founded in 1935, was one of the best known. It acted as the coordinating body for local "youth councils" formed in several large Canadian cities, and at its peak represented the major youth organizations, including the YMCA, with a total constituent membership of over 400,000. It held annual conferences, sent delegates to the World Youth Congress, and lobbied the federal government for youth-oriented legislation that would reverse the effects the Depression. In 1936, it issued the Declaration of the Rights of Canadian Youth calling for youth employment programs, social security, improved health, recreation, and educational facilities, and world peace. Sadly, it had a brief and stormy history, and as one historian noted, it was "beset by conflicts between communists and non-communists, and by harassment from the RCMP."[44] It survived until 1942, when it was declared an illegal organization under the Defence of Canada Regulations.

By 1936, many of the youth organizations founded before the First World War (e.g., the Y's, Boy Scouts, and Girl Guides), and those established in the postwar years (e.g., Trail Rangers, Tuxis Boys, and CGIT) had enrolled over two million adolescents across the country. In fact, the Depression likely helped boost their membership.[45] The Girl Guides, for example, doubled their membership between 1933 and 1937, suggesting that Guiding provided a "wonderful opportunity for interesting and wholesome recreation in those lean days, when other forms of amusement [were] more costly."[46] Several of these youth groups also played a vital role in the war effort. With their quasi-military structure, the Girl Guides saw a stepped-up emphasis on emergency preparedness, physical fitness, homecraft, nursing, and first aid. They also participated in traditional female home-front activities – knitting, sewing, making bandages, acting as messengers, typists, chauffeurs, and whatever else might be helpful. Similarly, the Boy Scouts collected salvage, promoted and grew Victory gardens, served as messengers, telegraph operators, and first-aid attendants, and took part in Victory Loan Campaigns.[47]

In 1942, Indian Affairs reported that a large number of senior pupils were displaying a keen interest in organized movements such as the Girl Guides, Boy

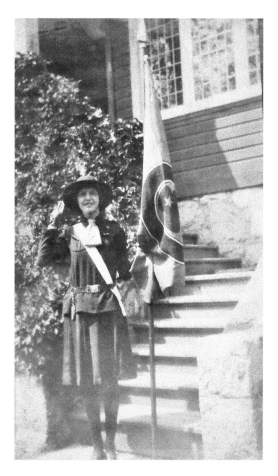

Figure 4.10. Kathlyn Hall (Ann's mother) as a Girl Guide, 1930 (courtesy of Nancy Mitchell)

Scouts, and Cadet Corps. At this point across Canada, there were seventy-eight residential schools, 275 day schools, and ten combined white and Indian day schools, with a total enrolment of just over 17,000 students. However, that "large" number turned out to be quite small with only two residential schools (both in Alberta) and five day schools (in Ontario, New Brunswick, and British Columbia) reporting a youth group. These statistics were followed by a gratuitous and confusing statement: "These organizations provide the Indian Youth with valuable lessons in the art of self-government. They encourage him, too, to assume responsibility for the accomplishment of tasks that he can complete better and more economically for himself than any other agency that might be designed to help him."[48] Unfortunately, we know little about the role of these and other youth organizations within the Indian residential and day school system during the Depression years and wartime, except to say that they were probably the exception rather than the rule. Following the war and into the 1950s, there was considerably more interest in creating positive experiences for Indigenous youth within the traditional youth organizations.

To ensure that youthful voices were heard, especially during postwar reconstruction, a Canadian Youth Commission (CYC) was established in 1940 largely through the initiative of the national YMCA.[49] It was an independent body created to study the problems facing youth aged fifteen to twenty-four; to draft reports and recommendations based on these studies; and to promote the acceptance of these recommendations by governments and private youth-serving agencies. There were fifty-four commissioners representing all regions of Canada; the Protestant, Catholic, and Jewish religions; the major political parties; various sectors of industry, labour, and agriculture; and both genders. Through surveys, interviews, and briefs about jobs, health, recreation, clubs, marriage, family, and citizenship, the commission heard from youths – although none were Indigenous – across the land. Overall, they were scholars and school dropouts, workers in industry and agriculture, civilians and armed services personnel, churched and non-churched, urban and rural, male and female, married and single, French and English.[50] The CYC also held provincial youth conferences, usually over a weekend with a youth keynote speaker. Those attending were split into discussion groups around the major topics of employment, education, family, health, religion, recreation, and citizenship.

Nonetheless, it is worth examining some of the ideas and recommendations regarding physical education in two of the reports published by the CYC, namely about health and recreation, because they provide an indication of what young people of this generation considered important and necessary in these areas.[51] The CYC committee on recreation, for example, constructed a questionnaire, in both English and French, and sent out 5,000 copies to selected volunteer workers, many attached to youth agencies, throughout the country. Volunteers placed them in the hands of young people, fifteen to twenty-four years, chosen in accordance with instructions prepared by the committee. Of these, about half of the surveys were completed and returned, and the committee chose 1,600 to meet the requirements of a national sample of Canadian youth culture (although there were fewer returns from French Canadian youth).

Questions ranged from the type and amount of recreation equipment that young people owned or could borrow; leisure-time activities in which they spent more than an hour a day; how frequently they dated or had friends of the opposite sex; what sport and games they played or would like to play; memberships in clubs or teams; participation in cultural activities like painting, drawing, music, and drama; attendance at movies; and finally, how and where they spent their vacations. Most importantly, they asked youth to give their opinions about recreation in their communities and to suggest improvements.

One recurring theme addressed the unrealized opportunities for recreation within schools, which according to youth, could make better use of school property and equipment, especially out of school hours. Also addressed was the place of recreation (including physical education) within the school curriculum, which brought forth some insightful recommendations:

> We recommend ... that the school curriculum from the primary grade to matriculation, include adequate instruction in and supervision of leisure-time recreational activities – athletics, sports, physical education; music, art, reading, etc. – in order that youth may develop vigorous and healthy minds and bodies and live a healthier, happier life. (CYC Youth Hearing, Vancouver, BC)
>
> ... That there be instituted in the school curriculum, beginning with grade one, and continuing throughout the entire period of a student's time at school, a programme for developing the human body and giving health education covering all phases of it. This programme is to be made compulsory to all people, unless they are medically unfit. A government certified instructor is to take charge of this programme. (CYC Conference, Calgary, Alberta)
>
> ... Training for recreation should begin in public schools with a broader system of recreational activities such as: athletics, games, dancing, hikes, crafts, art, music, dramatics. (Hamilton and District CYC Conference)[52]

Taking aim at the rationale behind the National Fitness Act of 1943, the recreation report also emphasized that health is not just a matter of physical fitness, and that the "mental hygiene" aspects of recreation were also worth considering. Activities should not be seen as ends in themselves, but as a means to the social development of individuals. Small groups were more conducive to individual growth than mass activities, and a varied program appealing to different people was better. "In the physical education field itself," continued the report, "we must see to it that our aim is the all-round development of participants. Our goal must not be to develop 'muscle men,' nor a few champions, nor to crush individuality through the pressures of a mass discipline." Instead, what was needed was a broad programme "rich in content, free of ideas of mass displays, and focussed on the full cultural development of all our Canadian young people."[53] This criticism was clearly aimed at the relatively narrow focus of the National Council on Physical Fitness, and perhaps unfairly at the highly popular mass demonstrations of Pro-Rec, especially in British Columbia. Moreover, setting up yet another Council for the purpose of promoting other recreational activities not within the realm of fitness was impractical. Alternatively, it was suggested that the Department of Health and Welfare recognize the need for a broader definition of physical fitness and adjust the act accordingly. This, of course, never happened (see chapter 5 as to the fate of the National Fitness Act).

On the other hand, the CYC's Committee on Health took a broad view of this topic, although it was never clearly defined, at least not in their report. The chair of the committee was the Deputy Minister of Health in the Dominion Government, who previously had been Director of Medical Services for the Canadian Army. The committee members came mostly from the army, government, or medical professions. In order to guide youth groups studying the problem of "health" and ultimately preparing briefs, the committee developed a brief guide with useful statistical information as well as a series of questions related to prevention, treatment, and health services.[54] Sixty-seven briefs were received from various youth groups across the country.[55] One recommendation, mentioned in twenty-six briefs, was that "physical fitness programmes be promoted in and out of schools as a preventative health measure." More specifically, it was suggested that a "well-balanced, organized programme for physical education in the schools should be checked up closely by school inspectors," and that there be less emphasis on "championship sports." [56]

Unfortunately, despite all the information and discussion it generated about youth during 1940s, the Canadian Youth Council was not made permanent, and little in the way of policy ensued from its many recommendations.[57] Also, as far as we can tell, the CYC made no effort to survey Indigenous youth, nor to ask for their views about any of the issues they considered important to non-Indigenous youth.

The late 1920s through to the early 1940s were challenging times in Canada, as was true for most industrialized countries, culminating in the devastating loss of life among the soldiers, airmen, sailors, and civilians who fought in the Second World War. The war brought some relief from the Depression years, however, as the country ramped up its munition factories, aircraft plants, shipyards, and other manufacturing in the overall war effort. Women, who often stayed at home following marriage, were also mobilized – some joined the army, navy, or air force, while others were employed in non-traditional trades required by the war industry.

The war, argued one Canadian politician, "brought to light that a large number of our young people were not physically fit; it showed the need of a national movement to promote physical fitness among men, women and children, and our whole system of education from elementary schools to the universities seemed to have been lacking and deficient."[58] Hence, in 1943 the National Physical Fitness Act was proclaimed followed by appointments to the National Council on Physical Fitness. The various youth movements were reinvigorated through their war efforts and asked to voice their opinions about postwar reconstruction. Regarding the recognition and importance of physical education, there was some progress through the creation of a national association; a re-evaluation of school-based physical education curricula; and the growing recognition of the need for specialists in the field through university-based degree programs. Sadly, most Indian residential and day schools still lacked the necessary facilities and teachers to be able to include physical education as a regular, instructed school subject.

CHAPTER FIVE

Setting a Heroic Agenda – Realizing the Possibilities

For far too long educators have paid *lip service* to the value of physical education. But lip service alone will not make a nation physically fit. If the schools are to be held responsible for the state of fitness of the youth then drastic alterations in the programs, facilities, and equipment of our schools are essential. Lip service must be changed into practical service, and there must be a complete re-evaluation of the curriculum.

Robert Jarman, 1945
(italics in original)

This call to action came from Robert Jarman of Winnipeg, who at the time was president of the Canadian Physical Education Association.[1] He also pointed out that "one of the greatest lessons the war has brought home to us on this continent is that we were living in a fool's paradise regarding the fitness of our youth." Peace fitness, he argued, is as vitally important as war fitness. Physical education can no longer be looked on as a frill, and it must be given a much higher priority than in the past. "The school of the future must be judged not merely by its powers to equip academically, but by its ability to provide and maintain a program which will create a morally and mentally fit and sturdy citizenry."[2]

We have called it a "heroic agenda" because so much was promised over a relatively short space of time – basically over a little more than two decades – and much of it was indeed accomplished.

Promoting Fitness for the Masses

As discussed in chapter 4, the National Physical Fitness Act (1943) was largely a response to a military problem, especially the shortage of physically fit recruits during wartime. Major Ian Eisenhardt, director of the National Council on Physical Fitness, through his statements and articles, maintained the military aura that had prompted the federal action in the first place. "There is a revival in Canada today in the interest in keeping fit," he wrote, "and our boys and girls in the Navy, Army, and the Air Force are setting a good example for the whole country." He also argued that national fitness was the result of individual fitness: "The war has taught us a lesson; the present drives for blood, money, salvage, and many other joint efforts, have only been successful because of teamwork."[3] Eisenhardt was an eloquent champion for those who hoped that a fitness program would complement a national health insurance program. However, the federal government shelved health insurance after the war and cut back on many other social programs, including physical fitness. There were also issues with the National Council, the principal one being that its purpose – "to promote the physical fitness of the people of Canada" – was not clear.[4] Was it to take a leadership, executive, or advisory role, or all three? There were also severe limits on the amount of funding it had at its disposal: $225,000 to be distributed to the provinces through federal–provincial agreements, and an additional $25,000 for administrative purposes. Most provinces joined the program, but several were reluctant. Ontario, for example, decided to develop its own plan with an emphasis on improved school physical education, adult education, and community physical fitness. The latter, argued the Ontario Director of Education Dr. J.G. Althouse, must also be accompanied by the development of character and citizenship to achieve the "spiritual fitness for living in a democracy."[5] Eventually, after much hesitation and delay, Ontario entered the program in 1949 as did New Brunswick, unlike Quebec, which never did.

In 1945, the program was transferred to the Welfare Branch of the Department of Health and Welfare, and it was no longer confined to the narrow and concrete terms of physical fitness. The committee structure of the National Council was eventually expanded to include leadership training, industrial recreation, athletics and the Olympics, cultural and rural activities, swimming and lifesaving, and also health and medical gymnastics. Eisenhardt resigned as director in October 1946 to take up a position with the United Nations in New York. He was primarily responsible for the recreational activities of the staff appointees to the United Nations, who came from all over the world. Doris Plewes, a teacher from London, Ontario, who had been the volunteer executive secretary to Eisenhardt, moved to Ottawa to become the assistant director of national fitness, but was never appointed director. It was not until October 1949 that the position was filled by Ernest Lee, the British Columbia director of physical education and recreation. A prominent athlete and active coach, he had a bachelor's degree in physical education from the University of Oregon and was past president of the British Columbia CAHPER branch.[6] However, he lasted less than a year because of the many difficulties in implementing the National Council's multi-faceted program with limited resources. It was also clear that the federal minister responsible, the Honourable Paul Martin, was less than supportive, arguing that there were "greater priorities for Government to consider in Canada and that there were many things in a free society that people should do for themselves ... The question of jurisdiction in the sports field was provincial and municipal."[7] After Lee's resignation, a new national director was never appointed primarily because no one wanted the job.

After the war there was a re-evaluation of provincial fitness programs. Pro-Rec, for example, was perceived by many as a Depression-based project that had served its purpose in the postwar era. There was also criticism and a lack of support from various sectors. The YMCA had always been concerned about Pro-Rec's emphasis on gymnastic activities, which they saw as a publicly financed infringement on their territory. Physical educators were critical of Pro-Rec's program, centralization, and educational background of its instructors. A committee investigating the policies and programs of the Recreational and Physical Education Branch was critical of Pro-Rec's emphasis on physical fitness to the exclusion of other forms of recreation. In 1953, the newly elected Social Credit government of British Columbia decreed that all government-operated recreation classes be discontinued, effectively bringing an end to Pro-Rec.[8]

The National Council on Physical Fitness met for the last time in December 1952, lacking the funds to continue with its programs, and the National Physical Fitness Act was quietly repealed by the government in June 1954. As for Doris Plewes, she remained in Ottawa for many years as a consultant in fitness and recreation with the federal government, frequently travelling the country to promote physical education and fitness. In many ways, she was ahead of her time.[9] At the 1954 British Empire and Commonwealth Conference on Physical Education in Vancouver, she talked about "physical illiteracy," likening it to the academic variety: "Clumsiness is a kind of muscle-stuttering, commonly found in a large number of cases in varying degrees of intensity. If a youngster stutters, something is done for him. If he's clumsy, he receives contempt."[10] Prompted by the dismal results in the United States, where the Kraus-Weber fitness test measuring minimum muscular strength and flexibility showed that 60 per cent of American children were out of shape compared with only 9 per cent of their European counterparts, Plewes coordinated the testing of over 60,000 Canadian children and adults from coast to coast using the Canadian Physical Efficiency Tests.[11] This battery of seven tests, and the subsequent standards, were based on a person's age, body weight, and height. She was also responsible for initiating a series of short (ten-minute) ice hockey instructional films completed in 1956. Initially, she envisaged a series of booklets put together by a team of writers, including Bill L'Heureux at the University of Western Ontario. He eventually took over the project, and the eight-part series (in English and French), sponsored by General Mills, was produced through Crawley Films.[12] By this time, Plewes was almost sixty, yet she remained a valuable role model: "Her own hair is white, but her youthful enthusiasm and trim figure are proof that she practices what she preaches about being fit – not fat."[13] In a paper circulated at the Second British Empire and Commonwealth Conference on Physical Education in Wales in 1958, Plewes argued that Canadian children lack the "sturdiness and staying powers of our pioneers," reiterating the importance of testing the fitness of the population for the purposes of reference, motivating interest, and assessing progress.[14]

With the loss of the National Council on Physical Fitness as well as most provincial fitness programs, governments demonstrated a continued disinterest in funding fitness initiatives. Into this void jumped a homegrown and highly vocal expert, namely, Lloyd Percival, who was quickly gaining a reputation as a successful coach. Early in 1944, Percival tried to convince the National Council on Physical Fitness to include his "Sports College," a weekly radio program airing on CKOC in Hamilton, within its mandate, but his request was summarily dismissed. Instead, Percival persuaded the CBC, in cooperation with the YMCA, to broadcast his "Sports College of the Air," which became an immediate success.[15] Each half-hour program was jam-packed with sports and fitness related information. Initially directed only at young males, it was never dull and often included interviews with sport celebrities. Each episode ended fittingly with the motto: "Keep fit, work hard, play fair and live clean."[16] By 1946, it had attracted between 750,000 and one million listeners per episode. Percival also began to explore other venues to promote his message, which brought about the "Play Better" publications – initially small booklets on how to play better hockey, football, basketball, and other sports as well as how to build a better body or how to be a better coach. Many of these were expanded in later editions, each of which could be ordered at very little cost.

Percival also began conducting his own fitness surveys, often receiving national attention through magazine and newspaper articles. "Our Flabby Muscles Are a National Disgrace," for example, was published in *MacLean's* magazine. In 1953, some 1,800 Canadians – supposedly a representative sample based on urban or rural, age, sex, and economic status – were assessed using fifteen simple fitness tests with "appalling" results. In the age twelve to sixteen group, for instance, only 50 per cent passed the tests, with a rapid decline from then on in terms of increasing age. Most subjects failed all tests demanding endurance. "We place no value on physical fitness," ranted Percival, claiming that our sedentary lifestyles, poor food habits, and lack of facilities and organizations for mass participation in sports explained the results.[17] Another example was the *Don Mills Mass Fitness Test*, where Percival tested 300 children (age six to twelve) in the Toronto suburb in 1957 using the Kraus-Weber fitness tests and found a 59 per cent failure rate.[18]

Percival's surveys and publications, and indeed the Sports College itself, were mostly ignored by the growing number of fitness experts in Canadian universities, many of whom had completed graduate study in the United States. During the late 1950s, the *CAHPER Journal* published an increasing number of articles by young Canadian physical educators who were soon to become leaders in fitness research. One physical educator who reached out to Percival was Earle Zeigler at the University of Western Ontario (now Western University). Zeigler's primary concerns were that people trained in "tests and measurements" were not engaged in the Sports College research, and that products recommended by the college were not properly tested. In a lengthy response, Percival defended his research and products, and at the same time pointed out that "we are desirous of cooperation with those at work in this field in Canada but so far practically all our attempts to develop any such cooperation has met with dismal failure."[19]

In 1959, Prince Philip, the Duke of Edinburgh, was invited to become the president of the Canadian Medical Association.[20] In a hard-hitting and much-publicized speech at his installation, he pointed to several indicators, such as an increase in admissions to public and mental hospitals and the high level of disability among children, that indicated a phenomenal increase in what he called "sub-health" within the Canadian population. At the individual level, this produced mental tension, emotional instability, delinquency, as well as lower stamina and resistance to disease and poverty. He also pointed out that Canada's achievements in sport were hardly in keeping with a country that had one of the highest standards of living in the world. All this affluence, he argued, has

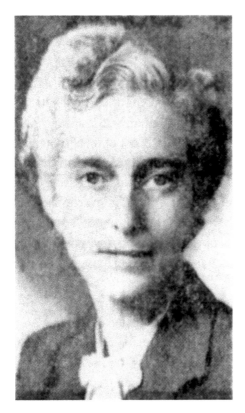

Figure 5.1. Dr. Doris W. Plewes, 1948 (*Vancouver Sun*, 24 July 1948, 6)

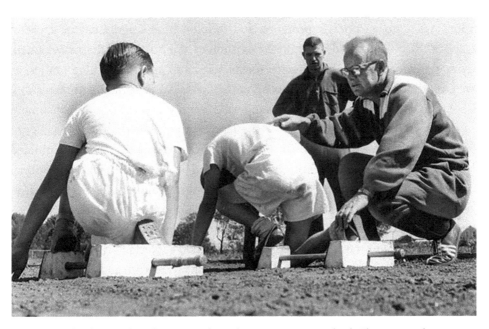

Figure 5.2. Lloyd Percival teaching young boys the sprint start, 1966 (Erik Christensen photographer, courtesy of Judith Scott)

the "same effect upon the community as a plaster cast has on the muscles of the body."[21] Doctors, he contended, not only fight disease and disability, but they should also take responsibility for the effects of sub-health, especially the lack of physical fitness among the Canadian population. He also quoted directly from Doris Plewes's 1958 conference paper, pointing out the startling inadequacies regarding the provision for physical education in Canadian schools (discussed in the next section). Therefore, argued Prince Philip, the "root of this problem of sub-health lies in the state of the physical fitness of the younger generations and therefore in the physical education of the children."[22] As a solution, he suggested four immediate and essential actions: proper physical education in schools; adequate recreational facilities for all ages and sections of the community; extension of the work of youth organizations both in scope and age; and finally, an organization to publicize sports and recreational activities and to encourage people to take part in them.

To add insult to injury, Canada's performance at the 1960 Summer Olympics was, according to a *Globe and Mail* editorial, a national and international disgrace. Only *one* medal (a silver in men's rowing) had been won, and Canada ranked thirty-two out of forty-four competing countries. "We are becoming a nation of flabby, overweight weaklings," proclaimed the editorial, and "we are bringing our children up to be the same."[23] The resulting panic contributed to the federal government's decision in 1961 to introduce new legislation (Bill C-131) – the Fitness and Amateur Sport Act – "to encourage, promote, and develop fitness and amateur sport in Canada."[24] The act provided for the establishment of a National Advisory Council, federal/provincial cost-sharing agreements, grants to sport governing bodies, as well as scholarships and research programs in physical education and recreation. Research into physical fitness was supported mainly through the establishment of four research institutes, located at the University of Alberta, the University of Saskatchewan, the University of Toronto, and the Université de Montréal. Initiated by the CAHPER Research Committee, one funded project was to establish national norms of physical performance for Canadian children and youth (from seven to seventeen years of age). Initiated in the fall of 1964, the study involved a representative sample of 500 boys and 500 girls in each age group among 135 randomly selected schools in the ten provinces, totally 11,000 subjects.[25] The six tests – sit-ups, broad jump, shuttle run, flexed arm hang, fifty-yard run, and 300-yard run – measuring strength, speed, and endurance provided a set of comparative norms. Teachers were encouraged to test their students each year. As a follow-up study, and to evaluate fitness in a more "objective and refined" manner, the CAHPER

Research Committee undertook to test the physical work capacity of over 2,000 children and youth using a bicycle ergometer. Not surprisingly, they found that males were superior to females as well as being overall higher in body weight.[26]

In 1968 during a federal election, Prime Minister Pierre Trudeau promised to investigate amateur sport in Canada, which is why the Task Force on Sport for Canadians was created.[27] Although the resulting report was focused mostly on professional hockey, its primary recommendations were about enhancing federal government involvement in amateur sport generally, resulting in the creation of Sport Canada. In 1970, the federal government eliminated most of the program supports for fitness, deciding instead to concentrate on high-performance sport as a more prominent and explicit strategy to strengthen the spirit of nationalism and pan-Canadian unity.

Sad State of Physical Education in Canadian Schools

As the Canadian Physical Education Association (CPEA) expanded, local and provincial branches were being established, with some more active than others. The Edmonton branch for example, examined school physical education in the province of Alberta in 1948 through a high-powered committee that included a teacher, the superintendent of schools, the curriculum director for Alberta, and several faculty members from the department of physical education at the University of Alberta. The problems they uncovered were numerous: a lack of facilities, unqualified instructors, extremely low budgets, and no provincial supervisor of physical education, to name just a few. Especially in rural schools with often no facilities or space, it was difficult to do anything more than calisthenics. Physical education was compulsory for grades one to ten, but only optional in grades eleven and twelve, where just a handful of students opted to take the class. In some areas of the province, religion actually forbade sports, although some of the younger students were allowed to play softball. The committee made a series of recommendations aimed at alleviating some of these problems.[28] In Manitoba, the provincial government established a committee in 1957 to study physical education (and recreation) in the province. Chaired by Frank Kennedy, from the athletic department at the University of Manitoba, it was composed of men (and one woman) involved in the leadership of physical education and recreation. They travelled throughout the province seeking information through formal hearings, written submissions, interviews, and correspondence on how to improve Manitoba's physical education and recreation programs, and they published their findings in an extensive report.[29]

After the National Fitness Act of 1943 was passed, Nova Scotia was among the first provinces to sign the agreement. It received only $11,300, augmented by an equal amount from the province; its top priority was to develop physical education in the schools.[30] In 1944, when Hugh Noble arrived in Halifax as the first supervisor of physical education for Nova Scotia, he found that secondary schools were still following the militaristic Strathcona Trust program with little if any physical education in the elementary schools. He travelled the province for a year, meeting with school principals, teachers, home and school associations, health authorities, and others asking what they thought should happen with regard to school physical education. After gaining a sense of what people wanted, he again travelled the province laying out his ideas about how they could implement these programs. The postwar expansion of secondary schools, both urban and rural, brought intensive lobbying to ensure the inclusion of gymnasium facilities. By 1946, Noble had been joined by Dorothy Walker, a graduate of the Margaret Eaton School, who had taught for several years at a private school in Toronto. Noble and his staff conducted "teacher institutes" by bringing together teachers from small schools to introduce them to the "new" physical education. They also instituted summer schools to train already qualified teachers in physical education, and they began working with universities in the Atlantic provinces hoping to interest them in creating physical education degree programs.[31]

Even in Ontario, where school physical education was more established, there were serious issues in the rural areas. Winnifred Prendergast at the Normal School in London, Ontario, conducted a survey of physical education in the rural schools of western Ontario in 1945. She found that one-quarter of the 168 schools surveyed made no provision whatsoever for even recess supervision, instruction, or direction; another 27 per cent supplied some equipment such as a ball or bat, but no supervision; 22 per cent had supervision for "play periods" two or three times a week; 22 per cent had daily supervision; but only 2 per cent of the schools had an acceptable playground program.[32]

Ten years later, in a paper circulated at the Second British Empire and Commonwealth Conference on Physical Education and quoted extensively by Prince Philip in his 1959 speech to the Canadian Medical Association, Doris Plewes laid out the ongoing, stark reality of physical education in Canada. She began by pointing out that each of the ten provinces had complete jurisdiction over public (tax-supported) education within their province, and that the federal government provided for "Indians, Eskimos, and persons living in the Yukon and North-West Territories." Consequently, at that time there were twelve different programs of education within Canada. Furthermore, extensive immigration, coupled with an extremely high birth rate after the war had "multiplied educational inadequacies in spite of the fact that hundreds of new schools are being built each year, and teacher recruitment is at all times high."[33] The result, she argued, was that the inadequacies for the provision of physical education in Canadian schools were startling.

The lack of gymnasium space meant that some students in large schools had no physical education whatsoever, where others were limited to one brief period a week. Some provinces permitted the conversion of gymnasia into classrooms as well as the construction of new schools without a gymnasium, and limited outdoor facilities discouraged general participation in sports and games. While all provinces included physical education in their courses of study, it was frequently on a voluntary basis only, and several provinces still made no provision beyond grade ten in secondary schools. "These two factors," Plewes argued, "added to the lack of grants for capital construction, make it difficult to secure either adequate facilities for *all* the pupils or sufficient time allotment to achieve limited minimum goals with even average success."[34]

Another problem identified by Plewes was the lack of trained teachers of physical education, especially in the elementary schools, and specifically female. In 1953–4, for example, there were just over 40,000 teachers employed in the elementary schools of eight provinces (no information was available for Ontario and Quebec), and of these, only 187 held any kind of certification to teach physical education. Assuming the situation in Ontario and Quebec was comparable, this meant that only 0.5 per cent of elementary school teachers in Canada held a physical education certificate, many of which were obtained in a four- to six-week summer course. The issue of teacher shortage was certainly recognized by the physical education profession, but what to do about it was unclear. Ella Sexton, an inspector with the Physical and Health Education Branch of the Ontario government, laid out her ideas in an extensive, two-part article in the *Journal of CAHPER*.[35] The causes for the shortage, she argued, were the "high marriage mortality" rate especially among young women teachers; heavy teaching loads and responsibilities; inadequate school gymnasium facilities; the low prestige of physical education compared with other subjects in the curriculum; and physical education teachers' unwillingness to sell their profession as a vocation to their students, or to challenge the interests and capabilities of their senior students. Among her solutions were recognizing the importance of pupil–teacher relationships, educating the public about the benefits of physical education, and creating bursaries and scholarships for students wishing to study physical education at universities.

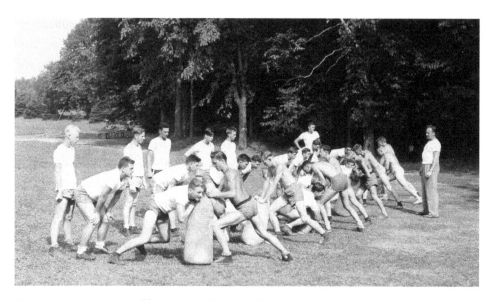

Figure 5.3. First Ontario Athletic Leadership Camp for boys, Lake Couchiching, Ontario, 1948 (University of Toronto Archives)

One program that seemed to be working was the opportunity for senior secondary school students to attend the Ontario Athletic Leadership Camp, on the shores of Lake Couchiching, for a two-week summer program designed to develop leadership and organizing skills through athletics and sport-related activities. Every secondary school in the province was permitted to select a girl and a boy based on high academic standing, leadership qualities, and active membership on at least one school team. One hundred and twenty leaders were accommodated on each course – two for the girls in July and two for the boys in August – with all expenses (travel, living costs, tuition) paid for by the Department of Education. The camp's staff were chosen from the best secondary school physical education teachers; the camp program was planned for the purpose of establishing goals, introducing skills of recreational games and sports, and providing opportunities for the staff to study the abilities of each individual camper. Students were also given the opportunity to practice-teach some phase of a sport activity to their cabin mates, who in turn assessed the effectiveness of the teaching. Identifying teacher potential specifically in physical education was also a purpose of the camp. Records indicated that a substantial percentage of these leaders had entered the teaching profession.[36]

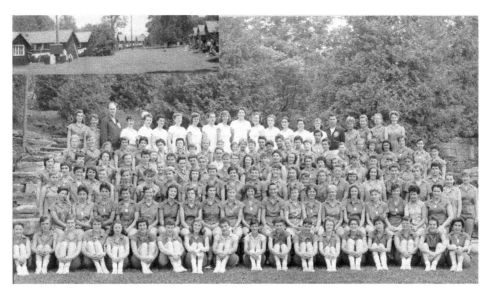

Figure 5.4. Ontario Athletic Leadership Camp for girls, Lake Couchiching, Ontario, 1958 (courtesy of Ann Hall)

Doris Plewes continued to argue that physical education programs should not only develop children's potential physical powers to a greater extent, but also encourage their maintenance at a reasonably high level throughout adulthood. It is the responsibility of physical educators, she contended, to assist and reinforce the developing physical powers of children and youth during the school years by making them less accident prone, enhancing their emotional stability, improving their "organic vigor," and, at the same time, recognizing and appreciating individual differences in physical capabilities.[37] This was certainly a tall order given the precarious state of physical education in general and the lack of qualified teachers, especially in the elementary schools.

Contested Terrain of Movement Education

In the years following the Second World War, Canada's approach to physical education in schools continued to be affected by transatlantic influences, and especially through waves of émigré physical educators from Britain. These newcomers played a significant role in the transfer and exchange of new professional practices. Notable among them were women trained at Britain's female physical education colleges, who brought with them novel and progressive methods of student-centred teaching for use in schools and post-secondary institutions. Their understanding and promotion of movement education, as the initiative was called, gradually gained traction in schools, colleges, and universities across Canada, but at the same time it provoked considerable controversy and debate.

Movement education first appeared in British primary schools. It focused on learning and expression by offering young children a variety of creative movement experiences. The 1933 *Syllabus of Physical Training for Schools* (discussed in chapter 4), based upon Ling's Swedish gymnastics, began to give way to tentative experiments that encouraged the exploratory use of large climbing apparatus and a variety of improvised equipment. During the war, British children at play "borrowed" apparatus that had been installed in many parts of the country primarily for commando training, and without instruction invented activities of their own making, which prompted physical educators to experiment with scrambling nets, frames, ropes, poles, etc., using them to guide children through discovery and practice.[38] As well, creative approaches to teaching gymnastics and dance were fostered by enthusiastic followers of modern dance exponent Rudolf Laban. All were facilitated through a growing interest in progressive child-centred approaches to teaching and learning, especially in elementary schools.

The movement education philosophy was most clearly laid out in two books about physical education in the primary (elementary) school, which replaced the older *Syllabus* handbook. *Moving and Growing* discussed how children develop as they grow; their powers of movement and agility; how the school day can be planned to take account of their needs and limitations at different ages; and how different forms of physical education can be used to develop versatility and skill.[39] *Planning the Programme* was much more of an instructional manual through the discussion of facilities and equipment, planning the lessons for physical training, games, dance, and swimming, complete with helpful instructions and drawings.[40] Both volumes were beautifully and generously illustrated with photos of children enjoying uninhibited movement. "This new and particularly sound approach to the problem of developing a child's physical powers through movement is timely and greatly needed," wrote the influential Doris Plewes, asserting how the new approach was a move away from the drill master towards the educator. "A careful study of these two books," she continued, "will prove most helpful to teachers in elementary schools who are sincerely concerned with the all-round education of boys and girls and who see opportunities to assist them to develop strong bodies in and through physical education in schools."[41] Marking a significant departure from the former military emphasis on drill, posture, and Swedish gymnastics, the

BOX 5.1. RUDOLF LABAN (1879–1958)

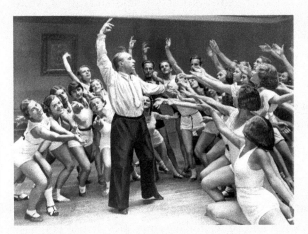

Figure 5.5. Rudolf Laban with dancers of the Berlin State Opera, 1934 (Sueddeutsche Zeitung Photo/Alamy Stock Photo)

During the 1930s in Germany, the Austro-Hungarian Rudolf Laban worked with the Nazi regime by directing major dance and music festivals, all funded through the propaganda ministry, until 1936 when his production designed for the Berlin Olympics was banned as unsuitable. No longer able to work, Laban fled to Paris and then in 1938 to England, where he found refuge at Dartington Hall, a large country estate in Devon that housed a progressive school and flourishing centre for the arts. Over the years, visiting performers included modern dancers such as Ruth St. Denis, Ted Shawn, Anna Pavlova, and Martha Graham. Dance teaching at Dartington was thus eclectic and included Dalcroze eurythmics, Isadora Duncan's "barefoot dancing," folk dance, dance-mime, ballet, Uday Shankar's Indian dancing, and various forms of central European modern dance. Laban's arrival, however, encouraged a version of modern dance known as "Ausdruckstanz" (expressionist dance). For him, dance evolved out of gymnastics and an awakening of spatial and rhythmic sensibilities. Every movement, he claimed, whether spontaneous or planned, has an "effort quality" expressed in the rhythm of bodily movement such as floating, dabbing, wringing, thrusting, pressing, flicking, slashing, and gliding. In this sense he held similar views to Émile Jaques-Dalcroze (see chapter 3) in that beyond the body there was something only dance could reach.

Laban was assisted in his dance research and teaching by his close associate Lisa Ullmann, a German dance and movement teacher who came to Dartington in 1933. Together, they founded the Laban Art of Movement Guild in 1945 and the Art of Movement Studio in Manchester in 1946; some years later the studio moved to Addlestone in Surrey. Ullmann translated Laban's work, organized teaching workshops, ran modern dance holiday courses, and provided most of the teaching. The studio's one-year course for qualified physical education teachers was recognized by the Ministry of Education in 1948, the same year that Laban's textbook for teachers, *Modern Educational Dance*, was published

> and distributed widely. He developed a system of movement notation, called Labanotation, involving the essential elements of space, time, and weight, which were combined with the overall characteristic of flow. Laban himself was not particularly interested in schools or children, and it was primarily others who adapted his movement theory for use in working with children especially within the school setting.
>
> For more about Laban and his work, see Nicholas, *Dancing in Utopia*; Preston-Dunlop, *Rudolf Laban*; Maletic, *Body-Space-Expression*; and Vertinsky, "Schooling the Dance."

new movement education curriculum consisted of activities such as dance and dramatic movement as well as games and educational gymnastics. It also emphasized the pedagogy of child-centred exploration, self-expression, and open-ended tasks rather than formalized responses to commands.

The introduction of movement education into Canada during the 1950s came some years after it developed in Great Britain and only slowly found its way into the physical education curriculum of Canadian schools. A lack of clarity about what exactly movement education was, and how it should be taught, as well as resistance from mostly male physical education teachers who tended to favour a motor skills and games-based approach, all contributed to this hesitancy. The idea, explained movement education supporters, was not to teach children directly, but to provide them with the best conditions to learn. At first, they admitted, learning may seem like a rather roundabout and slow process, but that was because it was achieved through the child's guided exploration rather than a follow-the-leader pattern. As well it was noted that the learning that took place might well become more readily transferable to other situations.

Among the relatively few studies examining the effects of these transatlantic exchanges in movement education in Canada are those that focus on the Ontario experience.[42] First of all, it was important for Canadian physical educators to see and to learn what was happening in British physical education. "Watch Britain!" announced CAHPER representative Joyce Plumptre Tyrrell in 1953 after visiting several women's physical education training colleges in England. "These were not faddists," she enthusiastically reported about the British teachers she met, "but well-balanced, widely educated women who were bringing to their jobs humour, understanding and vision."[43] After McGill University physical educator Ruth Duncan spent six weeks in England visiting primary schools and observing movement education classes, she reported: "Not only does it improve children's ability to move freely and with control ... Knowing this, we can't ignore it nor can we be content to say that what we have been doing is good enough."[44]

At the same time, British-trained physical educators visited Canada to demonstrate the principles of movement education and to help train Canadian teachers. Indeed, some were already in Canada, having immigrated following the war.[45] Nora Chatwin, for instance, was not a physical educator but an experienced primary schoolteacher from Liverpool when she came to Canada in 1946 as an exchange teacher. Nonetheless, physical education had been an important part of her general teaching experience with young children, which she sought to replicate in her first job in Timmins, Ontario, despite the lack of indoor facilities and outdoor playing fields.[46] Chatwin decided to stay in Canada and went on to teach briefly in Ottawa. In 1952 she was appointed by Gordon Wright, then director of the newly established Physical Education Branch in the Ontario government, as the first elementary school consultant for the province. Spearheaded by Chatwin's influence, a number of British–Canadian teacher exchanges were facilitated through conferences, workshops, and summer schools. The latter were especially valuable in supplementing the training of Canadian physical education teachers at a time when the rapidly growing population had led to a critical shortage of teachers (see previous section). Those hosted in Ontario (held eventually in Toronto, Guelph, Hamilton, North Bay, and Sudbury) started up in 1947 and were initially designed to update teachers in the field and offer certification in physical and health education. Often lasting up to six weeks, summer schools provided opportunities for physical education teachers to both instruct and take courses in the same location, to share ideas, and establish lifelong friendships. One summer school course was held in England with fifty-one Canadian teachers visiting schools for a week followed by instructional classes for two weeks at the Chelsea College of Physical Education in Eastbourne.[47] Between 1947 until the last Ontario summer school in 1970, Chatwin invited more than fifty British education specialists to come and teach workshops, introducing some 1,600 Canadian teachers to movement education sessions as well as attracting British teachers to job opportunities in Ontario and elsewhere in Canada.

Chatwin was also instrumental in the development of teaching manuals; the first one, *Physical Education for Primary Grades* was written by Chatwin herself. It was followed by *Junior Division Physical Education*, compiled by a committee drawn from teachers and supervisors of physical education in Ontario, although again Chatwin did the writing.[48] Together these manuals provided teachers with appropriate school physical education content from grades one to six, which included introductory activities, activities with small apparatus, cooperative group games, sport-type activities, as well as folk and creative dance. It was the first time that the term "creative dance" had appeared in the physical education curriculum. The rights to these manuals were bought by CAHPER, and they were distributed and made popular from coast to coast. Somewhat later, Sheila Stanley published her influential text, *Physical Education: A Movement Orientation*, which was more directly based on the philosophy and principles of movement developed by Rudolf Laban.[49] Similarly, Glenn Kirchner and his colleagues Jean Cunningham and Eileen Warrell at Simon Fraser University published their book *Introduction to Movement Education* in 1970 along with a series of instructional films.[50]

When the English-trained teachers arrived in Canada, they expected schools to be equipped with apparatus similar to the type found in Britain, which was clearly not the case. Mary Liddell, who immigrated in 1952, successfully lobbied for funding to import expensive climbing apparatus from England. Gordon Wright, then president of CAHPER, was aware that other provinces were interested in purchasing climbing apparatus and a committee was struck to investigate the possibilities. At the same time the Assistant Commissioner of Penitentiaries was exploring the possibility of using the industrial shops at the Joyceville Institution near Kingston, Ontario, to manufacture gymnasium and physical education equipment. The task of designing the Canadian Climber fell primarily to Mary Liddell, Nora Chatwin, and other members of the CAHPER equipment committee. In 1961, the first prototype was installed and tested in Mary Liddell's Toronto school. The Canadian Fold-Away Climber, including frames, beam-ladder, ropes, and metal ladder cost half the price of an imported unit and became one of the major products of the Joyceville shop. By 1969, they were producing about 200 units annually, distributed throughout the country with some even exported to the United States. Production ended in 1980 because the apparatus failed to remain financially competitive. By 2000, the Climber and other similar units were scarce in Ontario schools, and no doubt across the country, having either been removed for safety reasons or fallen into disuse by teachers not trained in their use.[51]

Thus, it was primarily due to Nora Chatwin's efforts and her associates, that the British movement education philosophies and methods obtained traction in Canada. The content, and the ways in which they were received and supported, however, inevitably differed from province to province, where each had specific educational policies and structures in relation to curriculum development and implementation. Nevertheless, when CAHPER honoured Chatwin for her efforts in 1971, the citation noted that not only had her influence transcended Ontario

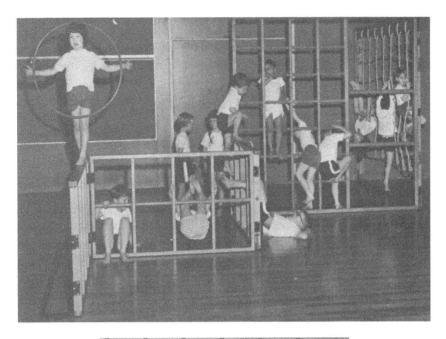

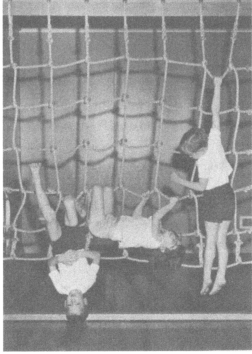

Figure 5.6. Movement education in elementary school (Sheila Stanley, *Physical Education: A Movement Orientation*. Toronto: McGraw-Hill, 1969, 105 and 207)

but that there were few elementary school teachers in Canada who had failed to be influenced in some way by her "Chatwinian" philosophy and guidance in physical education.

Movement education philosophies and teaching approaches spread slowly across Canada through visiting experts, summer school programs, and new arrivals from England in response to Canadian advertisements in the 1950s for teachers. Valerie Proyer and Lois Pye, for example, saw such an ad and took the opportunity to emigrate to Nova Scotia, immediately obtaining teaching positions.[52] Personnel in the Nova Scotia government's physical education division were impressed with these women and in 1953 invited them to teach in their summer school program. Pye taught a course on movement utilizing an educational gymnastics and developmental games approach. In 1954, Ruth Foster, the influential director of physical education for girls and women in the British Ministry of Education, toured Nova Scotia (also Quebec and Ontario) giving workshops on movement education. This prompted Canadians Hugh Noble and Dorothy Walker to spend time in England studying this new approach to physical education. Walker, for example, spent a year in 1958–9 at the I.M. Marsh College of Physical Education, and subsequently encouraged further visits from English specialists to teach movement education courses at summer schools.[53]

From its early foothold in Ontario and Nova Scotia, movement education spread westward into other provinces. News items in the *Journal of CAHPER* were often about female physical educators from the Prairie provinces who visited the British women's physical education colleges for movement education and modern dance instruction or who attended workshops and international conferences before returning to their home institutions to share their ideas. In Alberta, for example, Marion Irwin, supervisor of girls' physical education in Edmonton, invited Margaret Caudwell, a graduate of Anstey College in Birmingham, to teach in a summer recreation leadership program in 1963. She in turn convinced Margaret Ellis, who had trained at Chelsea College in the early 1950s, to take a position in the Faculty of Education at the University of Alberta. Joyce Boorman, a graduate of St. Gabriel's College in London and the Laban Art of Movement Studio emigrated in 1968 to teach at the University of Alberta, where she became an international authority on children's creative dance.

In British Columbia, Helen Goodwin came to UBC from Derbyshire, England, in 1955, having trained at the Laban Art of Movement Studio. She taught movement education to students in the School of Physical Education as well as choreography in the theatre department, where she developed a dance company; she also conducted dance workshops in the university's extension department. Extraordinarily talented, she was considered one of the prime forces in new and experimental performance art in Vancouver during the 1960s and 1970s. Anne Tilley was another British physical education teacher who came to Vancouver in 1957 to complete her degree at UBC's summer school. Trained at the Dartford College of Physical Education in Kent, Tilley had answered advertisements for teaching opportunities in Canada and begun to teach physical education at Hamilton Teachers' College in Ontario. During that time, she twice joined Nora Chatwin's summer schools at McMaster to gain degree credentials before deciding to move to British Columbia and complete her credentials at UBC's summer school. "It was all a bit of hit and miss in Vancouver," she said, "contrary to the more organized system in Ontario, for we were at the end of the railway line in a province growing and developing."[54] While there she was hired by the School of Physical Education to teach a variety of physical activity courses, including educational gymnastics, to first- and second-year students. A year later she was invited to join the Faculty of Education to teach movement education along with a growing cluster of other well-trained movement specialists, including Evelyn Wiseman, an early childhood education specialist who had worked with A.D. (Dave) Munrow and colleagues at the University of Birmingham's Department of Physical Education.

Indeed, many of the British émigrés, who came to Canada to teach in schools and universities, had earned diplomas from colleges of physical education in Britain, which were not considered the equivalent of a university degree. Subsequently, most were required to attain post-graduate degrees through programs mostly in the United States, where especially in the 1960s there was far more choice in physical education graduate study than was available in Canada. Many completed these requirements through summer schools and others took a leave of absence from their home university. Those who attended American universities were often exposed to the developing programs of "modern dance." The initial impetus for dance education in the United States had been established by physical educator Margaret H'Doubler, who in 1927 created the first university degree program for physical educators in dance education at the University of Wisconsin.[55] Through her efforts, she had opened the gym door for dance studies to enter higher education. In 1931, the American Physical Education Association established a National Dance Section to promote the constructive development of all types of dance education leading to the inauguration of summer schools for dance at Bennington College in Vermont led by Martha Hill, a former student of H'Doubler. It was Hill and her associates, strongly influenced by the theatrical modern dance performances of Martha Graham and company, who took dance education in a new and more professional direction. This paved the way for the conservatory model of dance at the Julliard School in

New York City but caused diminishing enthusiasm for movement education and modern dance in American schools, which were less akin to the Laban and British connection evident in Canada. Beyond the mid-twentieth century, movement education in American schools became increasingly marginalized in favour of the growing focus on skill training and fitness. Nonetheless, the initial Anglo-American summer courses on movement education held in Britain, which Canadians also attended, were an important venue for learning and exchange.[56] There was, however, a growing feeling among the Canadians that the Americans were slower and more hesitant to articulate pedagogical approaches to movement education.

By the mid-1960s in Canada, among the universities across the country offering a degree program in physical education, twelve of the women's departments offered some type of modern dance course.[57] However, dance pioneer Rose Hill of McMaster University questioned why it did not form a more integral part of the physical education training curricular at all levels. Why were students more deficient in this area than any other? And why was it largely taught and pioneered only by women? She offered a number of potential solutions: teach modern dance much earlier in school programs; offer in-service training for teachers willing to teach the subject but who lack the confidence and skill; form a group of professional physical educators with a special interest in modern dance; and create a specialization within physical education degree programs. At the same time, Hill touched upon one of the central issues related to similar programs – whether they be called movement education, modern dance, creative dance, educational gymnastics, or by some other term – the increasing resistance, mostly by male physical educators.

The basis of this resistance can best be summed up as follows: "With an emphasis on games, gymnastics, and dance, the movement approach was largely resisted by male specialists who feared that the acquisition of specific sports skills and the development of the desired behavioural attributes would be compromised."[58] This became clear as articles began to appear in the *Journal of CAHPER* questioning the movement education approach. For example, the head of physical education at a collegiate in Scarborough, Ontario, agreed that although movement training for young children was an excellent program, he worried this would become the only method for teaching of sports skills. He also warned that the young British teachers arriving in Canada would "displace more experienced, skillful Canadian teachers in our Training Colleges" and concluded that unfortunately "this field has now been invaded by some well-meaning egotists who wish to achieve a 'short cut' to an administrative post."[59] Another commentator worried that rhythmic exercises now formed the basis for many physical activity lessons, noting that "it is very difficult to decide exactly what is their purpose. Too many explanations begin with the words 'I think,' and are not based upon fact or research."[60] Some years later, a male professor at the University of Saskatchewan, in an article entitled "Movement Educators – Beware!," argued that although movement education had many virtues, it should not be taught to children older than nine or ten years because by then the "material needs to be intensified and expanded towards teaching specialized skills and complex sports techniques."[61]

The tenor of the debate around the concept and teaching of movement education, as well as the gender division that it evoked, echoed the same increasingly bitter movement/anti-movement debates that took place in England.[62] A.D. (Dave) Munrow, for example, famously argued that the teaching of generalized movement skills advocated by movement educators was not as good training for developing specific skills as the old-fashioned way of simply practising them. He reflected a dominant, male physical education view that advocated a biomechanical approach to movement. It also praised the merits of exercise physiology, which sought to measure rather than evaluate, and which was more linked historically with fitness training than were the insights of modern dancer Rudolf Laban.[63] It set the stage for a debate over the nature of gymnastics, which became, in effect, a debate over the definition of physical education writ large and by extension, its degree worthiness. Indeed, the debate prefigured a fight for survival among the female physical education colleges in England, which were slowly being absorbed into the institutional fabric of the polytechnics or colleges of further education.[64] The fate of movement education in the elementary schools followed a similar path.

Resistance to the movement education curriculum in Canada paralleled the British experience albeit more slowly and with less vitriol. The growing demand for teachers with a university degree directly affected the nature and substance of school physical education across the provinces, including the role of movement education. By 1971, summer school programs were absorbed into the colleges of education. It was primarily the summer schools that had exposed teachers to movement education as it developed in England, while teachers also travelled south to study somewhat different American approaches. Movement education in Canada thus lost its unique promotional resource network. The philosophy of child-centred learning in elementary schools would persist in a variety of ways in the future despite the outspoken opinions of Canadian historian Hilda Neatby and what she called "My Small War with the Educators." "The present preoccupations with bodybuilding and character moulding," she complained, "are useless and may even be dangerous so long as we neglect and starve the mind." Her claim that progressive education's fascination with process at the expense of content had done children a terrible disservice by depriving them of a full and rich curriculum resonated with male physical educators, who demanded a more direct teaching approach to sports skills and gymnastics training. They did flinch, however, at Neatby's critique of Canada's universities and those working in them in non-traditional areas such as physical education: "They are costing more than society can or is willing to afford … we have too many of them … and too many of the wrong people and we are keeping them happy by letting them do the wrong thing."[65]

Similarly, there was growing resistance to movement education in the United States, which was summed up by a female teacher who concluded that criticisms stemmed from an emotional and narrow focus upon physical education orchestrated by male physical educators invested in promoting specific skill development for sport.[66] One noted sarcastically that "some of the movement education postures on movement may be useful in some types of dance but have little use elsewhere."[67] Some years later, influential physical educator Earle Zeigler observed that "so-called modern dance still seems unacceptable to the majority of male physical education teachers and coaches and their attitude is conveyed to the boys and young men in their classes as well."[68] Such critiques spoke to the broad gender-related divisions within the profession of physical education that had developed first in England and later diffused to North America, largely through female physical educators deeply invested in the methods and educational benefits of movement education and modern dance. They also prefigured ongoing debates and quarrels about the most effective ways to physically educate Canadian youth as fitness regimes gained increasing popularity, and the popular male teaching style of a sport skill-based form of physical education retained its dominance.

Physical Education in the Indian Residential and Day Schools

By 1950, responsibility for Indian Affairs was transferred to the Department of Citizenship and Immigration, nicely dovetailing the assimilationist goals of the former with the mandate of the latter, which was to educate, train, and integrate newcomers into full citizenship. Along with this came the decision that "Euro-Canadian physical activities would be used to address the government's concern about physical fitness and health among Indigenous people while simultaneously facilitating their assimilation into mainstream society."[69] To meet these goals, Indian Affairs advertised for a Supervisor of Physical Education and Recreation whose responsibilities included carrying out a program of physical education and recreation on Indian reserves and in schools (day and residential);

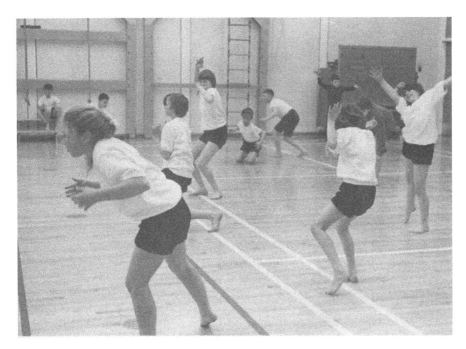

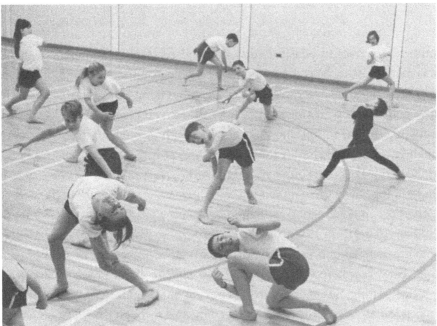

Figure 5.7. Creative dance in elementary school (Joyce Boorman, *Creative Dance in Grades Four to Six*. Don Mills: Longman, 1971, 5 and 27)

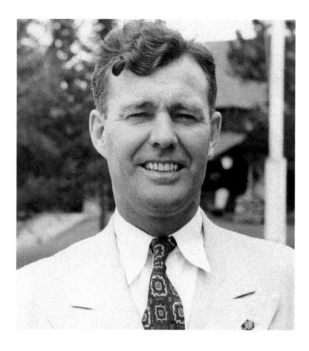

Figure 5.8. Ian Eisenhardt, 1950 (Canada's Sports Hall of Fame / SPORTSHALL.CA)

conducting courses in physical education and recreation for Indian agents and teachers of the schools; cooperating with provincial authorities in joint programs of physical education and recreation; and finally, taking care of the usual administrative duties such as writing reports and making recommendations.[70] At the time, Ian Eisenhardt was in Europe working with youth through a UNESCO program; nonetheless, he applied for the job, and given his previous experience with Pro-Rec and the National Council on Physical Fitness, he was appointed in February 1949.[71] Almost immediately there was a noticeable increase in articles about physical education, sport, and recreation in the *Indian School Bulletin*, a newsletter published by Indian Affairs from 1946 to 1957, whose purpose was to bring "some assistance to our teachers and an indication of Departmental policy in the field of education."[72] However, there was still little in the *Bulletin* about physical education in the school setting; rather, most articles were about organized sport, and therefore primarily about boys. "The expectation confirmed through the *Bulletin*'s narrative was that boys and men would lead public and active lives, while girls and women would lead private and domestic lives, engaging in physical activities for decorum and health, not for character building and certainly not for reward. This also implied that the majority of programme resources, especially for organised sports, would be directed towards boys and men."[73]

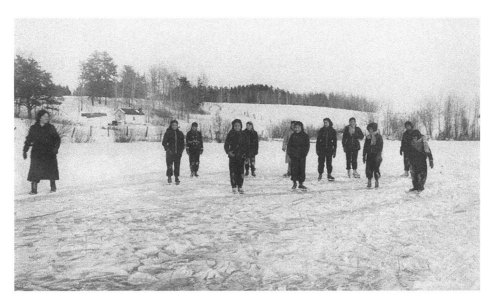

Figure 5.9. Skating on Round Lake at Celia Jeffrey Indian Residential School, Kenora, Ontario, c. 1951 (The Presbyterian Church in Canada Archives, G-5475-FC-21)

One of Eisenhardt's first tasks, between April and October 1950, was to visit a number of residential and day schools to survey their sport and physical education facilities and programs. At this point, there were sixty-nine residential, 329 day, and five combined schools across Canada with a total of just over 23,000 students. The majority (fifty) of residential schools were located in the Prairie provinces and British Columbia, as were more than half the day schools.[74] In all, Eisenhardt visited thirty-two residential schools, twenty-one day schools, and twenty reserves in Quebec, Ontario, Saskatchewan, Alberta, and British Columbia. His subsequent reports were comprehensive in that they itemized indoor and outdoor facilities, sports equipment, games and sports played (ice hockey was the most popular for boys, followed by soccer), social activities, general health and hygiene, and frequency of medical inspections. However, when it came to physical education, it was clear that few schools were following the provincial curriculum mandated in the public schools. Sadly, it was mostly absent due primarily to the lack of a gymnasium or even an adequate playroom, any sort of equipment, or a qualified teacher. Comments from the school principals such as "will be started, when gym is ready"; "trying to follow curriculum in spite of great difficulties"; or "not yet organized" spoke to the difficulties.[75]

Eisenhardt tried to push Indian Affairs into providing more funding to enhance the physical education and sport programs in the schools under their

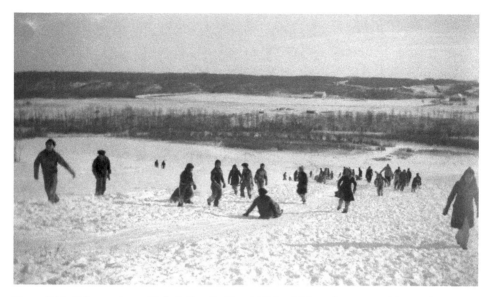

Figure 5.10. Tobogganing at Birtle Indian Residential School, Manitoba, c. 1950 (The Presbyterian Church in Canada Archives, G-3253-FC-12)

jurisdiction and on the reserves. In an article entitled "The *Canadian Red Man* of Today," he claimed that Indian Affairs would aim at "a higher degree of social organization" through which a program of health and recreation for all "Indians" in schools, on reserves, and in hospitals would "in addition to improving hygiene habits, and building better health – bring joy and health to the Indians."[76] He also made reference to a greater investment in physical education in the residential and day schools through better playing fields, gymnasia, and equipment; the training of young "Indian" men and women in physical education; and the appointment of trained physical education teachers to the residential schools. He sought publicity for his cause, which generated several newspaper articles and columns, not all of which were positive. One in particular rankled Eisenhardt for the rest of his life. It was written by Charlotte Whitton, a syndicated columnist before she became the mayor of Ottawa, whose basic argument was summed up accordingly: "If the Indians of Canada need stimulated syncopation, songs and games for their health – and culture – are there none of their own blood and traditions who could be found in this country or this continent, to be put in charge of such a plan?"[77] The negative publicity and the unwillingness of Indian Affairs to provide additional funding for "sports and games" helped to marginalize Eisenhardt within the department such that in December 1951, after serving less than two years, he resigned.[78]

In 1951, the Indian Act, the federal statute defining the government responsibilities for Indigenous peoples, underwent major revisions that aimed "to make possible the gradual transition of Indians from wardship to citizenship and to help them advance themselves."[79] One important revision called for the dismantling of the school system and included provisions that authorized the Minister of Indian Affairs to enter into agreements with provincial governments and municipal school boards to educate Indigenous children. These schools were to follow provincial curricula, including programs of physical education and extra-curricular involvement in sports.[80] Back in 1945, just before he resigned as director of the National Council on Physical Fitness, Eisenhardt recommended that the federal government treat "Indians and Eskimos as the 10th Province under the *National Fitness Act*" in order to improve their sport and recreational opportunities.[81]

The position of supervisor of Physical Education and Recreation at Indian Affairs remained vacant after Eisenhardt's resignation, and lacking an advocate, the area continued to be underfunded. A national survey of both residential and day schools in 1956 concluded: "In most of the schools there appeared to be little or no physical education program. A number of schools had no facilities for such activities. Basement areas were obviously designed for playing areas, but they were very inadequate and were utilized for storage or for assembly purposes. A large number of school sites were not properly cleared, graded, and prepared for playing purposes. Many were still in a wild state; others were overgrown with shrubs, thistles, grasses and weeds presenting a very unkempt and neglected appearance."[82] A new supervisor was appointed in 1957, namely Findlay Barnes, who previously had been principal of the Edmonton Indian Residential School, just northwest of the city and near St. Albert.[83] In an article in the *Indian School Bulletin*, Barnes outlined the requirements of a "well-planned, well-organized, and well-integrated physical education program" as an integral part of the school curriculum.[84] The program he suggested was traditional physical training: mainly calisthenics, games and sports, track and field meets, and gymnastic stunts such as club swinging and pyramid building. There was no evidence that Indian Affairs was paying any attention to new curricular developments such as movement education.

In chapter 4, we discussed one residential school in particular with regard to physical education and sport, namely, the Pelican Lake Indian Residential School (also known as the Sioux Lookout School), which existed from 1926 until it was shut down in 1969. What we saw previously was that there were no appropriate facilities at the school for curricular physical education, although some recreational activities took place such as skating, hockey, and swimming primarily because the school was situated beside a large lake. For the boys at least, their physical activity was primarily work as they laboured in the fields surrounding the school.

By the late 1940s, the school's capacity had increased to about 150 pupils with a much larger staff; as well, the half-day system had been replaced by full-day classroom instruction. A proper ice rink was built outside on the playing field behind the school, which allowed for the further development of boys' hockey. The Black Hawks club was formed, and even though many boys had not skated before, the team was entered into the bantam division of the local hockey league. Therefore, hockey for boys and skating for both sexes were the basis of the "physical culture" program at the school at least during the winter.[85] During his 1950 tour of residential schools, Ian Eisenhardt visited Pelican Lake and recommended that the substandard condition of the fields be improved, which did happen. A boys' playground for younger students was created with swings and teeter-totters, but the girls needed to wait longer for theirs. Another outdoor rink was added a few years later, this time with outdoor lights so that winter evenings could be spent skating or playing hockey.

As early as 1952, there was discussion with Indian Affairs about the need for a proper, indoor gymnasium at the school, and possibly the reconstruction of an old barn. These negotiations dragged on for ten years before a gymnasium was finally built and ready for student use by the fall of 1962. By then, the majority of older students travelled to Sioux Lookout to a public school for their education with only the younger, elementary school students staying at Pelican Lake. In 1969, the school, which by then was mostly a residence, was taken over by the federal government, and therefore no longer run by the Anglican church. It operated solely as a hostel until 1978 when it was torn down.

The photographs we have included in this chapter, and in chapter 4, of smiling, carefree residential schoolchildren at play should not be taken as representative of their experiences at these schools. Although they depict a sense of physical well-being and general happiness, this was not true for most children who generally were forced to attend a residential school. Put bluntly, these images also help to obscure the realities of the abuse, both physical and sexual, within the residential school system.[86] Within the archival record, there are many photographs of smiling sports teams, almost all male, and usually of hockey, football, or basketball. One study has shown that less than 5 per cent of sport and recreational photos featured girls.[87] It is worth remembering that whatever physical education, sport, or recreation was available in the residential school system during this era it was directed mostly at males, and not females. On the other hand, studies of similar photos are

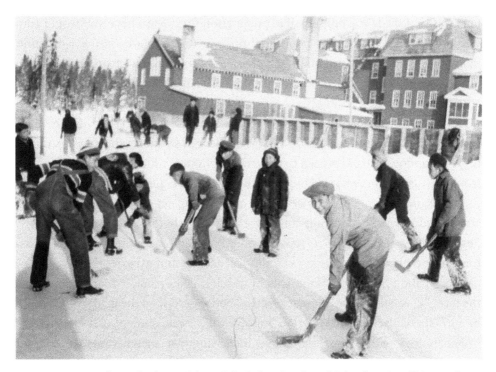

Figure 5.11. Boys playing hockey at Pelican Lake Indian Residential School, c. 1951 (Shingwauk Residential Schools Centre, Algoma University)

being used to elicit memories from the participants, and at the same time repatriate these images to their source for reinterpretation, thus returning the power to tell stories firmly back in the survivors' hands. One such study involved photos and former students from the Pelican Lake Indian Residential School, especially related to boys' hockey.[88]

The National Physical Fitness Act (1943), which we discussed at the beginning of this chapter, was an important catalyst in promoting teacher training in physical education at universities across Canada. These university programs began almost immediately: the first at the University of Toronto, which had been established in 1940; then followed by McGill (1945), British Columbia and Queen's (1946), Western Ontario (1947), Ottawa (1949), Alberta (1950), Saskatchewan and Laval (1954), Montreal (1955), McMaster (1956), and New Brunswick (1957).

By 1960, there were thirteen schools or departments of physical education (or physical education and health) within Canadian universities. The purpose of the degree programs was to train teachers and specialists in "physical education." The idea was to provide the best possible preparation for the teachers who would educate the children of the baby boom and postwar immigration. At the same time, many universities were still offering a physical education service program to first- (and sometimes second-) year students, as well as intramurals and inter-collegiate athletics.

Yet it was not long before the vision of research-based, progressive teacher preparation and physical education for all was challenged by those who advocated for a more discipline-based approach to university "physical education," as we have seen from the disparagements of Hilda Neatby in *So Little for the Mind*. Throughout the 1960s, more Canadian universities began offering degree programs, but not all considered "physical education" an appropriate name because it did not adequately describe the study of "man-in-movement" which "embraces the mechanical, anatomical and physiological aspects of physical activity and explores the psychological, social and physical environments in which it takes place."[89] Many argued that the term "kinesiology" or "human kinetics" better described the field. For example, in 1967 the University of Waterloo approved the establishment of a Department of Kinesiology with a new orientation. Increasingly, science became the core for many degree programs in an ever-increasing recognition that universities were training "movement scientists" rather than physical educators. *Kinesiology* was the label being used more frequently to describe this area of study. Between 1960 and 1969, twelve more Canadian universities began offering a variety of degrees (the most popular were a BSc or B.P.E.) in the field, bringing the total to thirty-five. We further examine these significant and continuing changes to university-based programs in the next chapter.

CHAPTER SIX

Changing Times and New Initiatives

Physical Education in the elementary schools is fast becoming one of the biggest success stories in Canada.

Fred L. Martens, 1982

By 1970, the paradigm of uniform, compulsory physical education was rapidly eroding. Within the schools, the idea of required instruction in any subject was under attack from progressive educators, students, and their parents in favour of "choice" and "child-centred" instruction. The bellwether for this change was a much-publicized Ontario study, *Living and Learning* (also known as the Hall-Dennis report after the co-chairs, Emmett Hall and Lloyd Dennis,) published in 1968.[1] Its recommendations to put students' needs and dignity at the centre of public education reflected widespread sentiments, especially among the young. In an increasingly freedom-seeking, even hedonistic, youth culture, the once admired example of the physical education teacher calling out prescribed drills to a regimented class was strikingly out of place. In most provinces and school boards, uniform physical education (K–12) gave way to a variety of optional approaches. The same pressures eliminated compulsory physical education for undergraduates in Canadian universities.

Changing Context

Outside the schools, several important supports for physical education disappeared, while innovative competitors emerged. The federal government ended its financial support for the training of physical educators in universities, preferring to spend that money on high-performance sport. Canadian universities, most of which had established faculties of physical education during or immediately after the Second World War, began to shift their focus away from teacher preparation to the disciplinary study of human movement with an emphasis upon exercise physiology, a trend variously called human kinetics, kinanthropology, exercise sciences, and eventually, kinesiology. The new community colleges that sprang up in several provinces began to prepare students for careers in public and private recreation, exercise therapy, and commercial fitness that in many ways provided alternatives to school-based physical education. Parents who could afford private sports camps, clubs, and gyms wondered out loud why their children still had to take physical education in the schools.

The landscape was changing in other significant ways as well. Three decades of unprecedented economic growth had enabled activist governments to build new roads and sewers, schools, hospitals, and medical care for an increasing population. But in the 1970s, the economy began to sputter in the face of a bewildering combination of recession and super-inflation ("stagflation") and international changes such as the end of the gold standard and the OPEC-led rise in oil prices. As governments struggled, many citizens began to doubt the central place of the state in Canadian society, arguing for a much greater role for corporations, entrepreneurs, and non-governmental organizations. By the 1980s, the now-familiar cutbacks to public education began to bite.

It was a fractious time in other ways as well. The hegemony of British ideas and the Protestant ethic that once characterized most of Canada, even in francophone Montreal, was under assault from many sides. After acrimonious public debates, "God Save the Queen" and the Union Jack–emblazoned red ensign were replaced by "O Canada" and the red-and white maple leaf flag as the national anthem and flag of Canada. In Quebec, an ascendant nationalism sought to be "maîtres chez nous" (masters in our own household), using the provincial state to reform every major institution in the interests of the francophone majority. Quebec nationalists challenged the right of the federal government to speak, tax, and spend for Quebeckers and some even called for complete autonomy. In English-speaking Canada, a strong nationalist movement in the arts led to an outpouring of new forms of cultural expression in theatre, film, painting, literature, and music. Canadians from non-English or non-French backgrounds sought to distance themselves from the tensions between Quebec and English-speaking Canada, successfully arguing for an official policy of multiculturalism to affirm the broad diversity of citizens' backgrounds. Italian, Ukrainian, Chinese, and Portuguese Canadians gradually turned "ethnicity" from a marker of second-class immigrant status to a proud source of community richness. Other strong popular movements in labour and the environment pushed for further transformations.

In 1972, the National Indian Brotherhood (the forerunner of the Assembly of First Nations) produced a policy statement, "Indian Control of Indian Education," marking a watershed moment in Indigenous education.[2] It was a clear and unequivocal call for local control of education by First Nations communities and parents. The federal government's response was a slow, devolution approach whereby residential schools were gradually phased out, federal day schools were reduced in number, and schools under Indigenous administration grew proportionally. By the end of the 1970s, only fifteen federally controlled residential schools were still operating, yet the marginalization, cultural loss, and abuse of Indigenous children would continue for several decades more in forced adoptions and day schools.

First Nations activists, led by the Indian Association of Alberta, the Union of British Columbia Indian Chiefs, and the National Indian Brotherhood, forced the federal government of Pierre Trudeau to withdraw a major policy initiative (known as a *white paper*) intent upon completely assimilating the Indigenous population, eliminating all treaties, and converting all land on reserves to private property. Indigenous peoples across Canada were shocked, and their rejection of the white paper's proposals in 1969 inspired a renewed Indigenous resurgence and resistance. In 1982, Prime Minister Trudeau initiated the patriation of the Canadian Constitution, but without any protections for or consultations with Indigenous peoples. Indigenous associations and activists quickly responded with a series of demonstrations and appeals, including the Constitution Express, a chartered train that staged protests in cities and towns between Vancouver and Ottawa, and legal presentations to the United Nations and European governments. In 1982, the government relented, introducing what became Section 35 of the Constitution Act, which states that "the existing Aboriginal and treaty rights of the Aboriginal peoples of Canada are hereby recognized and affirmed."[3]

Towards the end of the period covered by this chapter, the 1996 Royal Commission on Aboriginal Peoples in Canada, a five-year investigation into Indigenous life, on- and off-reserve, published its five-volume, 4,000-page report, with over 400 recommendations. It covered a vast range of issues including the sports and recreational needs of Indigenous people, and the necessity for health and healing especially among Indigenous youth. One section of the report, entitled "A Healthy Body: Physical Fitness, Sport and Recreation," pointed out that young people appearing before the commission emphasized the need for physical activity, leadership training, coaching, recreation program training, and participation in cultural activities like music and drama. Boredom was a major problem in Indigenous communities with few resources. The need to provide sports and recreation rooted in Indigenous traditional culture was also emphasized. A series of recommendations addressed these concerns, but none had anything to do with physical education, such as incorporating traditional, Indigenous physical activities and games in school physical education classes and programs.[4]

A boisterous feminist movement also pushed for legal and social changes, demanding equal opportunities for girls and women and social transformation in every sphere of society. The 1970 Royal Commission on the Status of Women recommended that "the provinces and territories ... ensure that school programmes provide girls with equal opportunities with boys to participate in athletic and sports activities, and ... encourage girls and women to participate in athletic and sports activities."[5]

Did compulsory physical education as moral and physical preparation for nation-building have a future in this rapidly changing context? Many wondered whether it was still relevant. Donald Macintosh, the respected director of physical and health education at Queen's University, wrote that unless physical educators "look carefully and intelligently at the shortcomings within the profession and at the changing society and take the steps necessary to ensure that physical education programs will meet the future needs and interests of Canadians," the profession could become extinct.[6]

Many physical educators took up the challenge. The seventies, eighties, and nineties witnessed significant growth, innovation, and public support, with renewed emphasis upon physical fitness and competitive sports. But it was always a patchwork of policy and practice. The Canadian Association for Health, Physical Education and Recreation (CAHPER) tried in vain to resurrect the idea of a coordinated, pan-Canadian curriculum focused on compulsory, daily physical education. As a result, intention and practice varied enormously from province to province, board to board, school to school, and even classroom to classroom. Inspirational programs could flourish alongside resistance and lethargy, and fitness and sports were often taught in isolation from each other. The subject was always contested, which is the story of this chapter.

Making Physical Education Relevant

Some students and their parents sought the complete abolition of physical education, but most just wanted it improved. In 1970, one of the co-authors of this book conducted a survey and engaged focus groups with Toronto-based youth.

BOX 6.1. DONALD MACINTOSH (1931–1994)

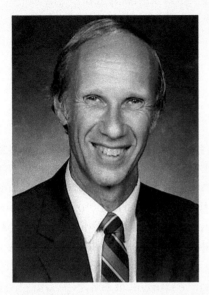

Figure 6.1. Donald Macintosh (courtesy of Susan Lederman, Queen's University)

"Dr Mac," as his students called him, arrived at Queen's University in 1965 as the new director of the School of Physical and Health Education. He followed pioneer physical educator, Fred Bartlett, who retired after seventeen years at Queen's. In announcing Don's arrival, a *Queen's Journal* article briefly outlined his background, but also provided his height (6'3") and weight (about 200 pounds), as if these statistics were some sort of qualification for his new job. Indeed, Don was a superb all-round athlete having been an all-star junior football player, a provincial (Alberta) tennis champion, a university basketball player, and the captain of the Canadian men's Olympic basketball team that competed at the 1956 Summer Olympics in Melbourne, Australia.

He also had a strong academic background: a BEd in Physical Education from the University of Alberta (1954), an MSc from the University of Washington (1960), and a PhD from the University of Oregon (1964). Still in his early thirties when he arrived at Queen's, Don had gained teaching and coaching experience mostly in Edmonton at Victoria Composite High School and at the University of Alberta. In every sense, he was a well-trained physical educator with the academic qualifications to gain the respect of his colleagues in an institution of higher learning.

As we have outlined in this chapter, he was also a leading, sometimes pleading voice for university physical education departments to return to what he called the heart of the profession: sport, dance, and physical activity. In his R. Tait McKenzie Address to CAHPER in 1992, two years before his untimely death from cancer, Don made it clear that the move away from this centrality had negatively impacted the profession. Specialization and the preoccupation with academic respectability within physical education, he argued, meant that the field no longer had a central focus. During the latter years of his career, Don co-authored three important texts related to Canadian sport policy: *Sport and Politics in Canada* (1987), *The Game Planners* (1990), and *Sport and Canadian Diplomacy* (1994).

Principal David Smith of Queen's University, speaking at a memorial service for Don, said that "Canada has lost one of its finest sports policy leaders." He also

> called him "a person of great warmth and caring who touched many lives in the athletic community on this campus and in Canadian university sport."* The Donald Macintosh Memorial Visiting Scholar Fund brings prominent scholars in the sociology of sport or sport policy to Queen's for a one-day conference each year.
>
> * *Queen's Journal*, 28 June 1994, 3.

While respondents complained that physical education classes were repetitive, regimented, and redundant, most went out of their way to say how much they enjoyed sports and physical activity, especially informal activities like frisbee, swimming, and camping. They expressed the hope that they could learn and pursue the ones they wanted in a more supportive environment.[7] Leaders like Donald Macintosh accepted the critique and sought ways to restore the subject's relevance. "There is little question that there will be an increasing demand for opportunities to participate and gain instruction in many sports, creative movement activities, and physical recreation endeavours," he wrote. "The key ... is for the physical educator to be expert in creating a successful and satisfying environment for the learning of movement skills. Movement skills are vehicles by which people realise the outcomes espoused by our profession – physical development and health, social opportunities and competencies, and opportunities for expression and self-realization."[8]

While games and team sports continued to dominate the curricula in many schools, students were given more choice in the activities they could take, and teachers were encouraged to offer a broader variety of skills and activities, with an emphasis upon "carry-over" or "life-time" activities. Many school boards made agreements with local recreation departments and even private clubs so that students could learn to ski, golf, sail, figure skate, or play tennis, while some constructed or rented outdoor education facilities to enable students to learn to canoe, camp, rope climb, and snowshoe.[9] Many of these classes were co-educational, ending the strict segregation that characterized much of physical education in the decades immediately following the Second World War. There were experiments with timetabling to enable more instruction-appropriate blocks of time. Some boards even tried to group students by ability and experience to enable teachers to engage students at their own level. In a pilot project in Toronto's Northern Secondary School, for example, two teachers who would subsequently become Olympic coaches (Andy Higgins and Tom Watt) took two classes of young men, one selected based on chronic inactivity or complete inexperience, the other for their athletic accomplishment, and showed that both could learn more effectively when grouped with others at the same level. The beginners showed the greatest improvement. By the end of the class, they had overcome their fear and developed the confidence to seek more opportunities for themselves. Unfortunately, when Higgins and Watt left the board to coach at the University of Toronto, the experiment was discontinued. While some physical educators continued to call for students to be grouped according to need, ability, and interest, rather than age, academic grade, and sex, very few boards could make it work.[10]

Max Fourestier and the Vanves Experiment

The most influential new approach came from France. It had a long fuse. In 1950, Dr. Max Fourestier, the doctor for the Gambetta Elementary School in Vanves, a suburb southwest of Paris, rekindled an experiment begun in Lyon in the 1930s to realize a better balance between intellectual and physical development. Instead of the traditionally heavy French schedule of academic courses, the school day was divided into two, with academic instruction in the morning, and physical education, art, music, and supervised instruction in the afternoon. The time devoted to academic subjects was reduced to four hours a day, while that for physical education expanded to eight hours a week. It came to be known as the "1/3 system" because approximately one-third of the weekly curriculum was devoted to physical education.[11] Fourestier then reintroduced another bold idea from the 1930s, which was universal instruction in winter sports. The school took pupils to the Alps for one month each winter, all expenses paid, to teach skiing and other forms of outdoor winter activity. Eventually, the "snow classes" evolved into a comprehensive, interdisciplinary embodied pedagogy about the mountains, their environment, and cultures, as well as winter sports.[12]

The Vanves experiment was carefully monitored, evaluated, and replicated in other French cities (although it never became widespread), and in Belgium and Japan with the same results. Despite the fears of parents that their children would fall behind academically and catch colds and other illnesses during the "snow classes," the exact opposite turned out to be the case. Those taking the program had better results academically and experienced less stress. They exhibited better health, motor development, and balance. They were also judged to have matured faster, and to interact more constructively with their peers.[13]

Fourestier was a brilliant publicist and networker. He began presenting the details of these results to the media and major conferences, including the Fédération Internationale d'Éducation Physique, which in 1958 held their congress as part of

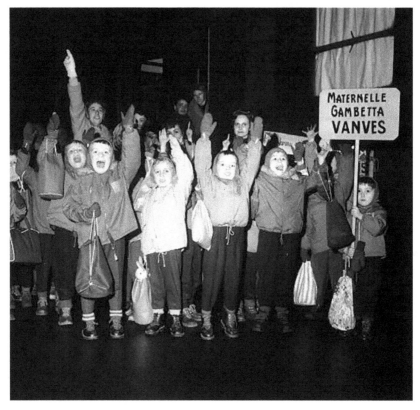

Figure 6.2. Children from the Gambetta School Kindergarten in Vanves, France, leaving for their first ski class trip, February 1959 (Keystone-France/Gamma-Keystone via Getty Images)

the World's Fair in Brussels. He also invited colleagues from around the world to see the Gambetta School first-hand, and soon drew the attention of physicians, educators, and the media in Quebec. In 1954, *La Presse*, the most popular French daily newspaper in Canada at the time, applauded the Vanves experiment in an editorial. After Fourestier spoke at a conference in Montreal in 1963 and met with senior Quebec educational officials, the first "snow classes" were introduced in the Laurentians.[14] Within a few years, there was a steady stream of Quebec educators to the Paris school. They included senior government officials, influential university faculty and their doctoral students, teachers, trade unionists, and prominent youth and sports leaders. It was a propitious time for progressive new ideas in Quebec. The "Quiet Revolution" was well underway. The government was in the throes of transforming the once decentralized, elitist, patriarchal network of Catholic and Protestant schools into a highly centralized, secular, universal, and gender-equitable system, following the recommendations of the Royal Commission of Inquiry on Education in the Province of Quebec, known as the Parent Commission after its chair, Alphonse-Marie Parent. The commission commented favourably about the Vanves experiment. The integral role of physical education and physical activity became a permanent feature of Quebec public education, from kindergarten to Cégep (Collège d'enseignement général et professionnel), the publicly funded first step in post-secondary education in Quebec. Some urban and rural school boards, notably Trois-Rivières and Pont Rouge, replicated the Vanves model exactly.[15]

Excitement about the Vanves experiment soon found its way into English-speaking Canada. In 1968, Jack Mackenzie, supervisor of physical education in Regina, visited the Gambetta School. Upon his return, he persuaded several Regina principals to implement the "1/3 system" and publicized the promising results to colleagues in university faculties of education and physical education. Within a few years, schools in Victoria, Nanaimo, Coquitlam, and Abbotsford in British Columbia as well as North York and Renfrew County in Ontario, introduced the model. In 1976, a CBC television crew visited both Regina and Vanves and the resulting documentary encouraged still others to adopt it.[16]

Several Canadian schools added innovations of their own. The Blanshard Elementary School in Victoria, for example, made running the primary vehicle for physical fitness, requiring every student to run every day as a complement to the physical education classes. Depending upon age and ability, the daily requirement was between 400 and 1500 metres. It soon became a source of pleasure and accomplishment for many students, with intrinsic motivation replacing compulsion. Blanshard built the program to teach students to monitor their own fitness by recording pulse rates, test results, and nutrition in a daily diary, and used this information to teach the basics of physiology, anatomy, and nutrition. It became an exemplar of "student-centred learning," helping students learn about their own bodies and the effects of different habits and interventions, and ultimately take responsibility for their own health. Teachers across the country soon made the daily exercise regime a pedagogy of self-awareness, physiology, and health. It showcased the benefits of "self-directed" learning.[17]

As in France, the new programs were carefully monitored to convince sceptics. At the Blanshard school, cognitive skills were measured by the standardized Canadian Test of Basic Skills in eleven subjects; psychological tests and surveys of parents and teachers for attitudinal changes; and three fitness tests, one strength and two aerobic, used for psychomotor changes. Not surprisingly, the greatest improvement occurred in children's cardiovascular fitness. Children's attitudes towards physical education, the school, and themselves became much more positive.

Despite the reduced time for academic classes, children's scholastic levels remained the same or slightly improved. Similar results were found in other boards. For example, in North York in Toronto: "a majority of teachers ... feel that time given to physical activities is *not* done at the expense of other subject areas"; "more teachers are involved more frequently in personal physical activities outside of school"; and "nearly all pupils (95%) reportedly enjoy physical education."[18] Two follow-up studies of the Trois-Rivières experiment twenty-six and thirty-four years later confirmed the earlier results, namely that a significant program of daily physical activity enhanced aerobic function, muscle strength, and physical performance, and most importantly did not detract from academic accomplishment.[19]

These efforts also led to new ways to improve teaching. Most provinces and territories relied upon generalist teachers with little or no training and experience in physical education to teach in the elementary schools. It was one of the reasons why physical education was so frequently cancelled – many teachers were afraid to teach it. The gold standard was a physical educator with a specialist degree in every school who could conduct much of the teaching and serve as a resource for other teachers. But in his 1977 survey, Stewart Davidson found that only Prince Edward Island, as well as the Catholic and Protestant schools in Montreal, employed specialists for all schools.[20] Few school boards could afford them, and even then, principals who did not value physical education often assigned these specialists to general classroom duties.

The "1/3 system" helped strengthen non-specialist teaching. It necessitated a much more engaged classroom generalist, which in turn led boards to implement extensive in-service training. Another response was an itinerant system, with teams of specialists travelling to a circle of schools on a regular basis, providing top-notch instruction to students and raising the level of instruction in all classes.[21] Still another approach was to focus on teachers' fitness, on the grounds that teachers who exercised regularly would be more comfortable teaching physical education themselves and would serve as effective role models. In Manitoba, a provincial task force made the generalist teacher's fitness a priority, recommending fitness testing, counselling, subsidized fitness classes, workout gear, and equipment for teachers, and dressing rooms with showers for every elementary school.[22]

Children and Physical Activity

A growing body of research on children and the consequences of physical inactivity also gave impetus to the renewal of physical education. In the early 1960s, the Fitness and Amateur Sport Directorate (FAS) in the federal Department of National

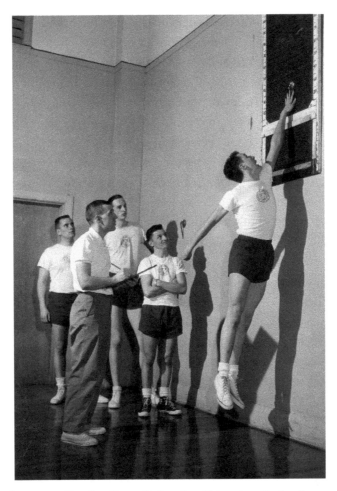

Figure 6.3. Professor Donald Bailey, Physical Education, University of Saskatchewan, measuring vertical jumps, 1960 (University of Saskatchewan, University Archives and Special Collections, Photograph Collection, A-1611, photographer: Gibson)

Health and Welfare helped establish four university-based exercise physiology labs to study Canadian fitness. In one of them, Donald Bailey of the University of Saskatchewan conducted a nine-year study on the relationship between children's physical activity and their growth and development. Bailey's team took more than 100 physical and biological measures, including nutrition, on 150 boys and 100 girls annually. Arguing that the capacity of adults was a function of activity during a child's period of growth, they focused on aerobic capacity as the most sensitive metric of overall physical condition. The results were alarming. Bailey's conclusion was: "*For the ordinary Canadian child (not the athlete or the exceptionally skilled, but the ordinary boy) physical fitness as expressed by aerobic power factoring out size, seems to be a decreasing function of age from the time we put him behind a desk in our schools.*"[23] In other words, just at the time when Canadian children needed exercise and movement for healthy growth and development, they were imprisoned behind a desk by their schools. Bailey delivered his indictment at a national conference on fitness and health in Ottawa in December 1972, and it quickly became a widely shared concern. He called upon the medical profession to contribute to a campaign for adequate physical education: "There are thousands of competent, hardworking physical educators in schools across this country whose efforts are being frustrated by a system of education that gives so little priority to physical education for *all* children. What a great thing it would be for them if each provincial medical association would say, 'Physical activity is an important factor in good health, we urge each and every school board in the country to ensure that every child in every grade gets at least one period of organized physical education per day.'"[24] Bailey also promoted the benefits of the "1/3 system" discussed earlier.

Another recipient of FAS funding, Roy J. Shephard of the University of Toronto, published a stream of research studies from his own lab; comparative analyses from countries around the world; and elaborate estimates of the social and economic costs of physical inactivity. In *Endurance Fitness*, first published in 1969, Shephard estimated that the health costs, loss of productivity, and social disruption caused by physical inactivity had cost the Canadian economy $1.78 billion in 1965, about $300 per wage earner. In the 1977 edition, he estimated that if increased physical activity reduced cardiovascular disease in the Canadian population by only 25 per cent, the savings would approximate $750 million.[25]

ParticipACTION

In 1971, the findings of Bailey, Shephard, and other scientists provided fodder for a new agency the federal government helped establish to keep the imperative of physical fitness front and centre in the Canadian imagination. Initially called Sport Participation Canada, it was quickly rebranded as ParticipACTION to make the name bilingual and position it as non-governmental. While it received a subsidy from the federal government, it needed to finance its various advertising campaigns with corporate donations and sponsorships, an early example of public–private partnership. The new agency sought to change Canadian attitudes and behaviour towards fitness through social marketing. The initial idea was to guilt Canadians about their low levels of fitness, encourage them to adopt regular exercise, and improve their nutrition. In its most famous advertisement, ParticipACTION took a

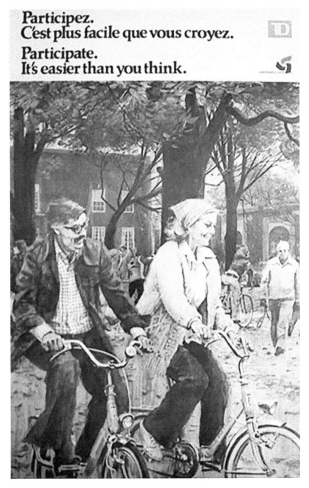

Figure 6.4. ParticipACTION poster from the early years of the fitness campaign, 1973–9 (courtesy of the ParticipACTION Archive Project)

draft statement by Roy Shephard that "*some* Swedish men at age sixty had the same fitness level as *some* Canadian men at age thirty" and turned it into a categorial claim that "the average 30-year-old Canadian is at about the same physical shape as the average 60-year-old Swede."[26] The ad was illustrated by a film of a young man in a red and white track suit struggling to keep up to a white-haired, bearded man in a blue and yellow outfit jogging comfortably. In subsequent years, ParticipACTION's ads became more encouraging, with a focus on the joys of physical activity as well as the health benefits. But the strategy remained much the same: promoting fitness through social marketing. The messages were also heavily loaded with appeals to Canadian unity.

ParticipACTION's social marketing was a poor substitute for a comprehensive strategy and substantive policy with clear, widely agreed-upon goals and timelines; coordinated investments in facilities, programs, and skilled leaders; and monitoring and evaluation. Whether eliciting guilt or inspiration, social marketing is not enough. People need genuine opportunities to change their behaviour, and public programs to eliminate or at least reduce the economic and social barriers to participation. Scholars found that even where there were concentrated marketing campaigns, as in a ten-year pilot project in Saskatoon, there was little actual improvement in overall fitness levels. The ads emphasized individual responsibility for personal change, completely ignoring the growing literature on the social determinants of health, including the cost, work, transportation, gender stereotypes, and other social barriers to participation. Advertisements were highly dependent upon the sponsoring corporations, which meant that they were often focused on affluent urban consumers, with very little effort to reach out to those who had least opportunity to participate in physical activity and sports – the urban and rural poor, Indigenous peoples, working women, immigrants, and persons with disabilities. Some campaigns even partnered with unhealthy products, such as the ads stamped on refined sugar packages and matches distributed in coffee shops and restaurants.

Although scholars have been critical of ParticipACTION and its actual contribution to population health and fitness, they all agree that it was highly successful in selling its brand, creating awareness about the low overall levels of fitness in Canada, and linking the idea of fitness to a sense of Canadian nationalism. Where the marketing industry standard for success is considered 70 per cent brand recognition, and a rating above 70 per cent is considered unsustainable, ParticipACTION repeatedly achieved recognition at or above 90 per cent.[27] The problem is that after quickly agreeing that physical activity is important for health, most people point out with regret that it's very difficult, if not impossible, for them to achieve or sustain. Sadly, neither ParticipACTION nor the federal government ever sought to tackle the obvious barriers with significant, coordinated investments in the actual facilities, programs, and services that would enable more Canadians to become active.

ParticipACTION is important to our story (see also chapter 7) because it broadened public awareness about the costs of physical inactivity at a time when physical educators sought to create a coordinated national strategy for physical education. Its messaging helped give visibility to a series of regional, provincial, and territorial conferences as well as published reports about elementary school physical education. Each recommended daily instruction in physical activity for every elementary schoolchild in Canada.

Quality Daily Physical Education

The ideal for Quality Daily Physical Education, or QDPE as it is widely known, was set out by CAHPER in a national consensus statement prepared by a representative committee of educational leaders and university researchers chaired by Stuart Robbins of York University. *The National Report on New Perspectives for Elementary School Physical Education Programs in Canada*, published in 1976, called for a minimum of thirty minutes of daily, quality instruction, with the principles of child growth and development as its base; a wide range of movement experiences with appropriate competition; and qualified, competent teachers with adequate and appropriate facilities and equipment. The report put a heavy emphasis upon fitness, arguing that "a good physical education program contributes to the total fitness of each child. It includes physique, organic, motor components and psychological and social elements as well. Physical fitness is of such importance that every part of the program must include vigorous physical activity."[28] CAHPER sought to recruit the federal government to QDPE, recommending that it provide incentive grants to provincial governments and school boards for implementation, in addition to a range of programs and resources to upgrade the skill levels of teachers. It also asked the federal government to ensure that "minimum standards for physical education facilities and equipment are established and met" and to appoint a "Royal Commission on Sport Competition for Young Children."[29] Despite its concerns about Canadian fitness and high levels of polling support for QDPE, the federal government rejected these recommendations. In addition to its preoccupation with high-performance sport, it was reluctant to take the lead on a matter so clearly within provincial and territorial jurisdiction. No province or territory mandated QDPE either. It meant that at the governmental level, there was neither leadership nor money for a coordinated Canadian strategy.

Undaunted, CAHPER and its provincial and territorial counterparts encouraged individual boards, schools, and teachers to institute QDPE. They distributed model policies and curricula and set out guiding principles and minimum standards. The standards included a focus on the acquisition of self-knowledge and the habits of fitness, a wide range of activities, qualified and enthusiastic teachers, and a high rate of active student participation in every class. The overarching idea was to encourage a lifetime of fitness. The resource materials distributed by CAHPER gave teachers tips on how to select activities for a balanced program, how to administer the activities, and how to evaluate the results.[30] Some provinces developed their own resources. In British Columbia, for example, the Health Activity Program (HAP) was created to supplement and enrich health, science, and physical education programs for children four to eight years old. It included modules designed

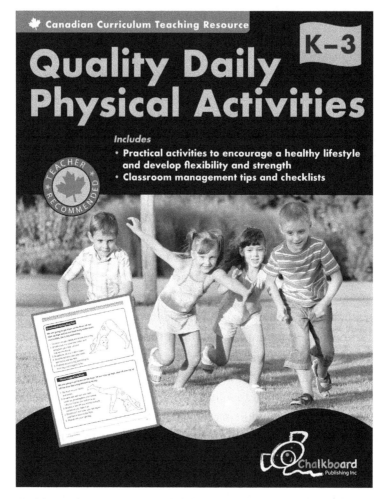

Figure 6.5. Useful Canadian resource on quality daily physical activities (courtesy of Chalkboard Publishing)

to help students understand and appreciate how the body works in terms of heart fitness, sight and sound, breathing fitness, and action/reaction.[31]

While the exact number of participating schools cannot be determined with precision, several knowledgeable observers concluded that there was widespread take-up.[32] In 1982, Fred Martens of the University of Victoria wrote that "physical education in the elementary schools is fast becoming one of the biggest success stories in Canada."[33] In 1995, Henry Janzen of the University of Manitoba observed that the "1970s were the Golden Years for physical education."[34] In 2003, CAHPER recognized 784 schools as meeting its principles and standards for QDPE. That number, which represented only about 8 per cent of the 10,000 elementary schools in Canada at the time, no doubt underestimates the spread of QDPE, because the CAHPER certification required a time-consuming formal application and adjudication.[35] Many schools and teachers simply taught or conducted fitness classes on their own. They could draw upon a growing number of instructional resources, including curricular materials produced and distributed by individual school boards, and packaged programs such as the Heart and Stroke Foundation's Jump Rope for Heart and the Canadian Fitness Award. The latter encouraged teachers to impart physiological knowledge and experience around six performance tests – a 50-metre run, a 300-metre run, flexed arm hangs, short speed run, sit-ups, and a standing long jump.[36]

How effective was QDPE in developing lifelong habits of fitness? The longitudinal studies of the "1/3" experiment in Trois-Rivières suggest small but significant benefits. When the students in the experimental group became middle-aged, they expressed more positive attitudes towards physical activity than their counterparts in the control group and had fond memories of the program and their physical educators. But the researchers found only a slightly higher determination to practise physical activity. They suggested that major economic and social changes – which included the closure of paper mills, the north-shore railway, and the port; the growth of the retail trade and several new industries; and significant out-migration to the larger cities of Quebec and Montreal – may have disrupted participants' life patterns to the point that they found it difficult to continue regular physical activity no matter what the intention.[37] Their speculation supports a long-standing concern about the decentralized and disconnected nature of QDPE. No matter how effective and influential physical educators are in imparting self-knowledge about the determinants of fitness for health, the experience and skills of appropriate activity, and an abiding appetite to stay fit, the system ultimately left students on their own after they left school. There was no guidance to the programs, facilities, and services they could access after graduation, let alone a coordinated public strategy to help them sustain regular physical activity while navigating the challenges of higher education, employment, and establishing a household. At a time when "health" mostly meant the treatment of disease and not prevention, when public recreation was increasingly cut back or forced to implement user fees, and when an increasingly privatized fitness industry made "pay for play" even more expensive, it is no wonder that the effects of QDPE gradually wore off.

Establishing Dance within Physical Education

Dance is a complicated artistic and movement phenomenon that has never fit easily into the school curriculum. "Housed within the physical education curriculum and the arts curriculum," suggest historians, "dance has been used to convey an array of educational objectives including moral and social development, social etiquette, physical skill, creative self-expression, health and fitness."[38] In the early 1900s, "dancing steps" were taught within physical training lessons as a means of promoting a graceful carriage, considered more important for girls than for boys.[39] The revised 1933 *Syllabus* suggested that dancing, which meant folk and national dances, be taught for one period a week during physical training.[40] However, as we have seen in chapter 5, it was not until the postwar period of child-centred education that creative dance became popular, especially in elementary schools, primarily through the efforts of British-trained movement education specialists.

By the mid-1960s, there was sufficient interest and professional expertise in dance education across Canada to create the CAHPER Dance Committee, initially chaired by Rose Hill at McMaster University. One of their first tasks was to survey the state of dance in schools. It found that the majority of provincial elementary and high schools taught folk dance as part of their physical education curriculum, but very few included creative or modern dance. For the next three decades, a relatively small group of dedicated dance educators worked hard to promote "expressive" dance (as opposed to folk, tap, or ballet) by creating a national communication network, offering dance workshops, organizing dance conferences, establishing provincial dance committees, and encouraging research about dance. They also worked hard to convince deans of education and physical education to improve the dearth of university-level dance courses.[41] Others published influential texts primarily on movement education for elementary schoolchildren which also featured a section on "dance" as a viable subject area.[42]

In 1994, after years of lobbying their professional association to include "dance" as a legitimate and distinct area of study within physical education, CAHPER became CAHPERD.[43] While dance in higher education flourished, the renewed emphasis on health and fitness in school physical education meant that whatever dance was taught in schools became part of general exercise programs.

Sport in Schools

Another powerful influence upon physical education in the 1970s and 1980s was sport. A popular element of school culture from the late nineteenth century, sport grew steadily in importance during the interwar years. Sports were taught as part of physical education, and students played them in both intramural and interscholastic competitions organized by the school. There were few opportunities for children and youth outside the school and municipal playgrounds, and most were limited to basketball, hockey, volleyball, and track and field. Up until the 1950s, most community clubs catered only to adults. In most parts of Canada, both girls and boys participated in school sports, although boys' opportunities dwarfed those available for girls, who had inferior facilities and fewer resources. To be sure, there were regional differences in how opportunities were organized. Interscholastic competition for girls was strongest in western Canada. In southern Ontario, the maternal feminism of the girls' rules movement and the woeful inequality of resources discouraged vigorous competition between schools, but intramural sports were well organized and focused on developing girls' leadership. The sister-led Catholic schools in Quebec took a similar approach for similar reasons. Despite their challenges, schools introduced many girls and young women to sports. Among immigrant families where respect for education was high, sports in the schools legitimized their daughters' interest.

With the postwar baby boom, sports grew rapidly as a popular form of social and skill development and recreation for children and youth. The number of community opportunities for them increased and adults gave up their own participation to direct, coach, fund-raise, and transport their children's teams and leagues. Schools continued to play a leading role, adding sports like badminton, field hockey, gymnastics, rugby, soccer, and tennis, and also hiring physical educators based on their ability to teach and coach in specific sports. Schools gave many students their first formal instruction and experience in sports, and the new schools built to accommodate the rising student cohorts included spacious, well-equipped facilities.

In many schools, sports became the dominant form of student culture, engaging the most students, elevating student leaders, setting the rhythms for "school spirit," and creating reputations for the local area. Sports also reinforced male privilege, conferring status and opportunity disproportionately to boys and men, and advantaged male and marginalized female teachers. But both students, and courageous and creative physical educators, insisted upon opportunities for girls and young women too. In 1976, Donald Macintosh and Alan King reported on a comprehensive study of high school sport they had conducted the previous year in Ontario.[44] They found that in schools of 800 or fewer students, 52 per cent of the student body participated in interscholastic sports that academic year, and another 10 per cent had participated at some point during their time in the school. In larger schools, 35 per cent of the school population competed that year, while another 10 per cent had some interscholastic experience. The ratio of male to female student athletes was 59:41. Sixty-four per cent of the student athletes took part in two or more sports. Similar percentages of the student body participated in intramural sports, and those opportunities drew still other students. High school students of both sexes participated in intramurals in roughly equal numbers. Finally, 85 per cent of the students surveyed attended at least one interscholastic contest as spectators and 9 per cent volunteered as administrators, officials, or trainers. The investigators also found that virtually all surveyed coaches were teachers in their respective schools – it was a requirement in many boards – and that a significantly higher percentage of students involved in interscholastic sports achieved above-average grades than students who did not play sports for the school, suggesting that both coaches and students were effectively engaged in the academic programs of the school as well. Clearly, in the year and schools surveyed, sport played an integral, even galvanizing role in secondary education.

The synergies between school sports, classroom physical education, and physical fitness were less clear, especially as many high schools eliminated the compulsory requirement for physical education in grades 11 and 12. Curricular physical education did benefit from new and improved athletic facilities, and the popularity of successful coaches who also served as physical education teachers. Macintosh and King found that only 42 per cent of the teacher-coaches (but 62 per cent of women teacher-coaches) had qualifications in physical education and were likely to teach that subject. They also found that enjoyment, health and fitness, and a liking for physical activity were the most prominent reasons students gave for their participation in school sports.[45]

Sports greatly complicated physical educators' responsibilities in integrated classrooms because it forced them to address the thorny gender issues embedded in the culture of sports that were rarely addressed in society. It was an almost impossible task. How does a teacher encourage girls in the classroom when they had far fewer and poorer sporting opportunities outside the classroom, and women's sports were virtually banished from the mass media and thus the public discourse? Teachers had to struggle against the deeply entrenched but unspoken pedagogy of sports that was designed to strengthen masculinity at the expense of girls and women, which made them comfortable and familiar for most boys and men, but unfamiliar, even alien, to some girls and women. An earlier generation of feminist physical educators had sought to address this issue by developing a distinctly women's culture of sports, with a focus on women's empowerment, health, well-being, and friendships, supported by women's leadership and distinctly women's organizations, events, and communications. But they faced many obstacles and were rarely able to provide opportunities comparable to those enjoyed by boys and men. By the 1960s, they had little to offer a younger generation of sports-interested young women who wanted the same undifferentiated opportunities of men's sports.[46]

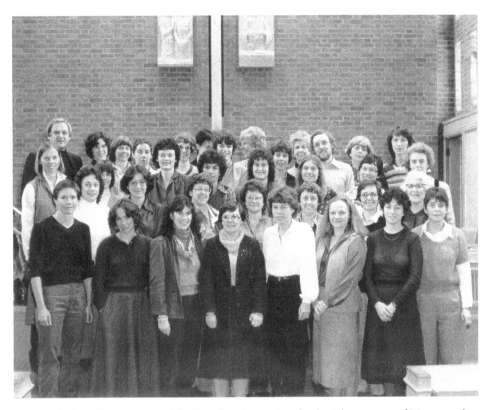

Figure 6.6. Founding members of the Canadian Association for the Advancement of Women and Sport, 1981 (courtesy of CAAWS, now called Canadian Women & Sport)

In the integrated class, most boys entered the gym with prior sport experience, so that they monopolized the teacher's attention and received the best marks. While athletically gifted or ambitious girls jumped at the opportunity to play or learn sports, others found them difficult to learn, especially when they were constantly being compared with more experienced boys. The task required sensitive deconstruction and refashioning, as sports feminists argued when they called their new organization the Canadian Association for the Advancement of Women *and* Sport (CAAWS) to signal that to fully accommodate girls and women they had to change the character and meaning of sports, as well as the number of opportunities. But it was very difficult to achieve in a single classroom. "Equal access did not ensure equal participation. The practice of ignoring gender and letting boys and girls mix in a curriculum that had previously been strongly gendered and differentiated ... exacerbate[d] rather than dissipate[d] differences between them, creating hostility and attenuating students' and teachers' stereotypical attitudes."[47]

The federal government's turn to high-performance sport in the early 1970s intensified the pressure on schools and other institutions to emphasize competitive sports according to the traditional male model at the expense of other approaches to education for the body. The new federal agency, Sport Canada, and the provincial/territorial sports ministries which it inspired, rapidly transformed the once amateur, volunteer-led, and highly decentralized community-based sports governing bodies into the integrated network of state-directed, -financed, and -monitored Ottawa-based, non-governmental bodies now known as "the Canadian sport system." Governments created a whole new layer of competitions, including the Winter and Summer Canada Games and various provincial regional multi-sport games, and they also encouraged the hosting of international mega-events such as the Olympics, Commonwealth, Pan-American, and World Student Games. Sport Canada and its provincial/territorial counterparts gradually professionalized the Olympic sports, creating full-time jobs for administrators and coaches in addition to living grants for the best athletes. The mass media gave tremendous new visibility to these activities through increased coverage, especially on television. In 1976, the Canadian Broadcasting Corporation telecast the Montreal Olympics in colour sixteen hours every day. Yet while the Canadian teams competing in international events like the Olympics demonstrated that women as well as men could excel, the rapid growth of the male-exclusive, capitalist sports cartels in Canada – the Canadian Football League, the National Hockey League, and Major League Baseball – and the spillover coverage of the US-based National Basketball Association and National Football League, intensified the dominance of masculine sports. Increased revenues and the unionization of players doubled and trebled salaries, making them much more attractive to middle-class boys and their families.

These developments provided powerful incentives for coaches to recruit and athletes to specialize. They encouraged the ambitious athlete and their families to seek better opportunities outside the school and accelerated the creation of for-profit and community-based sport camps and training programs for that purpose. In the snapshot taken by Macintosh and King in 1975, small but significant differences were already evident in the motivations of those who played for school teams and those who sought out-of-school opportunities, the latter expressing "the desire to develop a high level of sport" much more frequently.[48] These and other changes created tensions that only grew, undermining the role of the school as the provider of all. They also contributed to the elevation of the class base of Canadian sport because, increasingly, only the middle and upper classes could afford "pay for play" for their children. Even state schools gradually turned the focus from sport as education to sport for sport's sake. Several observers raised the concern that those physical educators who coached spent much more time preparing for practices and games and mentoring student athletes than instructing the students enrolled in their classes who did not play for their teams.

The women's movement of the 1960s and the dramatic performances and uncompromising advocacy of Olympic athletes like Abby Hoffman, Marion Lay, Nancy Greene, and others inspired many girls and young women to take up sports. They faced pushback in a variety of time-worn forms, from the fear mongering of moral physiologists that sports were unladylike and dangerous to the refusals of decision makers to grant them access to facilities. Such was the culture of entitlement for boys and men that even those schools that supported girls and women struggled to provide them with teams, competitions, coaches, facilities, and funds. Macintosh and King found that the boys' programs surveyed in Ontario in the 1970s enjoyed from 63.5 to 66.8 per cent of the available funds.[49] It was not only budgets and the number and quality of playing opportunities. A wave of integrations of once separate men's and women's physical education departments took place in schools, colleges, and universities in the 1970s, giving men most of the resulting jobs, enabling them to stall the movement towards equality. The entire period was a long struggle for legitimacy, opportunities, and resources, in both schools and communities. Athletes and advocates employed a variety of strategies, often resorting to human rights tribunals and the courts to win access to better opportunities. It helped that Sport Canada quickly realized that Canadian women excelled in international sports, often outperforming their male counterparts. It began to fund their training and living expenses on an equal basis and publicize their achievements through the Athlete Information Bureau. Through the persistent lobbying of advocates, Sport Canada established a women's program, which more systematically funded women's opportunities. The establishment of CAAWS in 1981 brought another strong voice to the advocacy.[50] The number of women participants would slowly grow in all sectors of Canadian sports, especially in schools, colleges, and universities. But it was a long struggle.

Physical Education and Sport in the Universities

Physical education was rapidly changing in higher education, too. Ever since the beginning of the twentieth century, Canadian universities required every undergraduate to take some form of physical education, while offering extra-curricular athletics on an optional basis. Some universities granted diplomas in physical training for teachers, fitness instructors, and camp counsellors, and after the Second World War turned them into degree programs. As institutions struggled to respond to the radically different circumstances of the 1970s, all three of these program offerings would be transformed.

Compulsory physical education for undergraduates was an early casualty. It had been one of the great achievements of the field, ensuring that every student had an opportunity to learn and play sports as a healthy balance to academic responsibilities. But by the early 1970s, most requirements were dropped. In part, it was a response to the liberalization of the undergraduate curriculum. Even if they wanted to, the rapid increase in enrolment meant that most universities no longer had the facilities to conduct such programs for everyone. Gradually, they pivoted, offering an increasingly wide and innovative variety of fitness, body awareness, dance, and instructional classes, financing them with student fees and pay-for-play. But such optional programs have never been able to reach more than a small fraction of the student population. The low rates of participation reflected the inequalities of income, gender, and Indigenous, racial, and religious backgrounds, as much as student interest and the increasingly frantic pace of everyday life. Universities also offered opportunities to faculty, staff, alumni, and alumnae, as well as members of the community on a membership or pay-for-play basis.

Up until the 1960s, most universities conducted extensive intramural programs for men and women, organized by separate and unequally funded men's and women's departments, often using completely different facilities. Both programs relied heavily upon student leadership for their direction and operation. In addition, most universities fielded teams in intercollegiate sports, increasingly with professional coaches, again organized separately for men and women, often with different facilities and unequal financial support. Given the time required for ground transportation – train, bus, and car travel being the most convenient and affordable means until the 1960s – most competitions were regional.

In men's team sports like basketball, Canadian football, and hockey, intercollegiate games attracted large audiences and mass media coverage, providing a steady stream of revenue to finance programs and facilities. At the University of Toronto, for example, men's football regularly filled the 27,000-seat Varsity Stadium and men's hockey the 4,500-seat Varsity Arena. Going to the game, cheering for your alma mater, and belting out the school song were a bonding staple of student life. Prominent male student athletes were celebrated throughout the student body, extolled by faculty and administration as exemplars of student excellence.

During the 1960s, many familiar, long-cherished aspects of athletics lost support or even came under attack, while new universities and innovative approaches changed the narrative. At the big-city universities like Alberta, British Columbia, McGill, and Toronto, the crowds for men's team sports gradually evaporated,

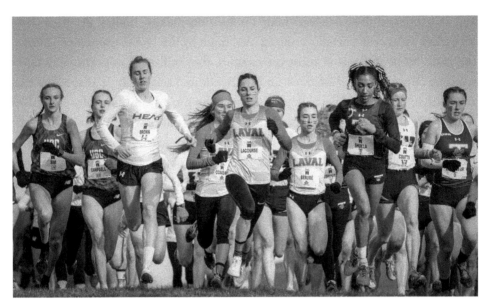

Figure 6.7. Canadian university women athletes in action (Mathieu Belanger, www.mathieubelanger.com)

costing athletic departments a major source of revenue and on-campus support. Intercollegiate sports faced competition from a growing variety of entertainments, including live music and theatre, and licensed restaurants. Students competing for marks felt that they had less time for sports, and the increasingly radicalized youth culture turned away from them, dismissing sports as "bastions of the establishment." As the focus of the established universities shifted to research and graduate studies, some male athletic directors worried about the future of sports on their campuses. On the other hand, many of the new universities, created to accommodate the children of postwar immigration and the baby boom, made athletics a point of identity and student life. They invested significantly in facilities and intramural and intercollegiate programs, and they sought to establish their reputations by beating the established universities in their chosen sports. With the democratization of air travel, a new coalition of athletic directors strengthened regional conferences and created a fully Canadian network for competition, the Canadian Intercollegiate Athletic Union (now U SPORTS).

Women's activism forced significant changes in university sports. As female enrolments grew, university women demanded equal opportunities in intramural and intercollegiate sports. Gradually they changed the public face of Canadian intercollegiate sports with dramatic performances in a growing range of sports and events, and also thoughtful, visible leadership on decision-making bodies. But their drive for equality was only partially realized. Although by the 1990s, women constituted the majority of students at most universities, they still had proportionally fewer sporting opportunities, resources, and well-endowed scholarships, disparities that continue to this day. Male coaches benefited the most from new jobs created by the growth in women's sports, as did male administrators when the once separate women's and men's athletic departments were integrated in the 1970s and 1980s. During the period of most rapid growth, men's coaching positions in women's sports more than doubled, while women's positions decreased. It has not improved significantly in the years since.[51]

The post-1960s growth of Canadian intercollegiate sports was punctuated by frequent debates between universities and regions over the conditions of student athlete eligibility (now limited to five years). However, the most bitter debate concerned "athletic scholarships" to keep our athletes at Canadian universities rather than encourage the "brawn drain" to well-endowed institutions in the United States that were willing to provide living stipends, tuition, and training expenses for high-performance athletes.

The further professionalization of coaching, the intensification of training and competition, and the stalling of gender equity pushed Canadian university sports much closer to the international model of high-performance sports. Student athletes continued to do well in their courses, generally achieving grades higher than the university average, but they became less and less involved in the traditional undergraduate experience. As the training and travel demands of their sports intensified, they found they had significantly fewer opportunities to engage with other students, pursue their intellectual curiosity in open-ended ways, and contribute to political and cultural life. Most of them were willing to pay that price, but the disconnect raises the question of whether intercollegiate sports still belong in Canadian universities and colleges.

The Rise of Kinesiology

By 1976, thirty-five Canadian universities offered full degree programs to prepare physical education teachers.[52] Students took courses in anatomy, biology, physiology, psychology, sociology, and an arts and science minor they could teach; skill development in a variety of sports and activities; and lesson planning and class organization. As was the case in other professional programs (e.g., forestry and nursing), many programs were essentially shared operations, governed and coordinated by schools or departments of physical education, with teaching cobbled together from a small faculty of their own as well as other academic divisions like arts, science, and medicine. In some universities, students graduated with two degrees – one in physical education and the second in arts or science. Others earned three degrees: physical education, arts/science, and education. In the 1960s, many provinces offered scholarships to students in physical education through a shared-cost agreement with Fitness and Amateur Sport. Graduates greatly strengthened the quality of physical education across the country, and many went on to important roles in public education and other fields.

By the early 1970s, these creative arrangements began to unravel, stretched by both appetite and fear. Ambitious faculty with graduate degrees from research universities began to imagine a field much broader than teacher preparation, with a vision to study and teach about every aspect of human movement. Some sought to pursue this through the structure of an established discipline such as physiology, history, philosophy, or sociology, joining with colleagues at other universities, including mainstream scientists and scholars without formal ties to physical education, in order to gain support and stake out the intellectual territory through conferences, and scientific or scholarly journals. For example, in 1967, the Canadian Society for Exercise Physiology and the North American Society for the Psychology of Sport and Physical Activity were established; and in 1972 the North American Society for Sport History was formed. CAHPER played the role of midwife in several of these initiatives, convening sessions under these frameworks at its annual conferences, and, where journals did not exist, publishing the emerging scholarship. In 1970, for example, the CAHPER history committee initiated a series of academic symposia on the history of sport and physical activity, with a Canadian focus. In 1978, the sociology committee published twelve monographs on various aspects of contemporary sports, and the North American Society for the Sociology of Sport was established later that year.

Another approach was to create an entirely new discipline focused on the study of the human body in motion. The person most associated with this vision was University of California, Berkeley, psychologist Franklin Henry. He called for the transformation of physical education in the university from a program of professional preparation into a new, interdisciplinary field of inquiry. It would draw upon the already established disciplines of anatomy, physiology, cultural anthropology, history, sociology, and psychology, and integrate their insights and methodologies into an entirely new way of studying physical activity.[53] According to Henry's colleague and biographer, Roberta Park,

> Henry was convinced of the great, but barely tapped, potential within the field that until recently was almost universally known as "physical education." He was dedicated

to enhancing its status and took pains to show faculty of other departments its possibilities. At the same time, he insisted that physical educators must become more fully engaged in *producing* the knowledge upon which the claims of their field were based ... This would require that some substantial portion of the profession (but certainly not all) must devote sustained attention to basic research ... Henry was concerned that too much of what presumed to pass for "science" and "theory" was little more than unfounded opinion. No field could gain respect, indeed survive, in such circumstances.[54]

Henry's approach found the greatest favour with experienced physical educators who began graduate studies and research after they had established their careers as teachers and coaches. They well understood that physical activity comprised multiple dynamics, and thus required investigation and explanation from an interdisciplinary perspective, and not that of a single discipline. As such, men (they were almost all male) assumed the leadership of academic physical education and tried to reconstitute their units on an interdisciplinary basis, giving them such names as "exercise sciences," "human kinetics," "kinanthropology," and eventually "kinesiology." One such leader was Earle Zeigler, the founding dean of the Faculty of Physical Education at the University of Western Ontario. In the early 1990s, he observed that there were more than 200 different names for the units once associated with physical education across North America. His preference was for "developmental physical activity."[55]

These new ways of thinking were also driven by fear. With the abolition of compulsory physical education and the levelling of the school-age population, the demand for teachers was drying up. It became harder to recruit new faculty with research degrees because they wanted nothing to do with teaching physical activity. As universities became preoccupied with research, they became less and less interested in supporting financially challenged professional faculties with little academic distinction of their own. Already low on the academic totem pole, faculties and departments of physical education worried about fragmentation, even elimination. As long as applications remained strong, physical education had a chance, because enrolment drove revenue at most universities, but the long-term forecast predicted decline. Increasingly, students sought careers in the health sciences. Academic physical education quickly needed to reinvent itself.

There was little consensus about the road ahead. Faculty members, students, alumnae and alumni fiercely debated "whose knowledge counts" through curriculum meetings, hiring and promotion, and research. If the academic culture encouraged scholars and scientists to battle for their own theoretical frameworks and methodologies, those habits made it difficult for them to agree upon a shared, multi-disciplinary approach. Meetings opened deep divides between interdisciplinary and disciplinary approaches, and the critical social sciences and humanities against the instrumental sciences of physiology and human performance. It also divided those who continued to support a place for instruction in physical activity, and the traditional link to athletics, against those who sought to abolish both of these.[56]

Out of the plethora of names, a consensus slowly emerged around "kinesiology." By the 1990s, two very different definitions emerged. The most widely accepted meaning was a broad, holistic approach that encouraged the study of human movement from a range of disciplinary perspectives. While faculty research and teaching increasingly focused on a single discipline like physiology or sociology, or sub-disciplines like exercise biochemistry, many deans and chairs forged undergraduate curricula that required students to take courses in several disciplines, with the option to specialize in the upper years. The best programs became exemplary liberal arts programs, with students acquiring knowledge and research skills in all the main avenues of academic inquiry, from the humanities and social sciences to the biological and physical sciences. It was a challenge for programs to integrate these various components into a relevant whole, and sometimes students complained that there was little connection between courses in different disciplines. Gradually programs introduced explicit courses and experiences to help faculty and students gain an interdisciplinary understanding.

These debates and initiatives had the effect of marginalizing instruction in physical activity, including dance and outdoor education, in many institutions. They also led departments to sever their organizational links to athletics. When faculty at McMaster University voted to abolish the physical activity component of the curriculum and separate from athletics, for example, they celebrated it as a major victory. But there was also a counter trend. In those programs that retained a physical activity component, teaching physical education enjoyed something of a revival. At the University of Toronto, students successfully lobbied for an enlarged physical activity component to their degrees, so that they could explore embodiment and acquire the knowledge and skills required for teaching a range of activities to various populations.

Programs gradually gave students the opportunity to take their degrees in either kinesiology or physical education. When the Canadian Council of University Physical Education and Kinesiology Administrators (CCUPEKA) established an accreditation system in the late 1990s to establish standards for undergraduate education, it did so within two-degree pathways – kinesiology broadly defined and

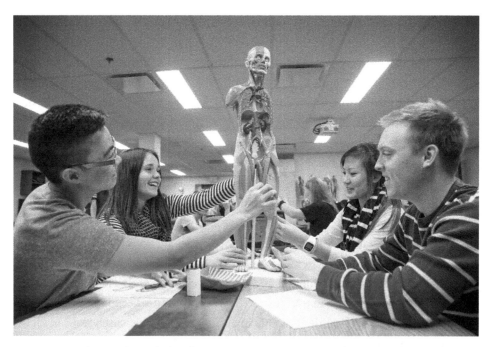

Figure 6.8. Students in the Bachelor of Kinesiology program, Faculty of Kinesiology, Sport, and Recreation, University of Alberta (courtesy of the University of Alberta)

physical education teacher preparation. At the time of writing, twenty programs across Canada enjoy accreditation in kinesiology, and ten in physical education, with nine universities recognized with accreditation in both fields.[57] A much narrower meaning of kinesiology that focuses on physical activity therapy has also emerged with the establishment of the Canadian Kinesiology Alliance/Alliance Canadienne de Kinésiologie in 2001, which we discuss further in the next chapter. Kinesiology advocates increasingly seek recognition as a regulated health profession.[58]

By the 1990s, participation rates in sport and physical activity across the Canadian population were in sharp decline. Adult participation in sport fell from 45 per cent in 1992 to 34 per cent in 1998, and physical activity as a broader category including non-competitive activities like hiking levelled off at 38 per cent of the population. Children were 40 per cent less active than thirty years earlier, and the prevalence of overweight children sharply increased from 15 per cent of the age cohort among boys in 1981 to 25.4 per cent in 1996 and 15 per cent among girls to 29.2 per cent.[59] The determinations were complex, to be sure. Some of the contributors were unintended consequences of decisions that in other ways improved the educational experience for many children and youth. For example, the consolidation of small schools into large, comprehensive schools in rural areas gave students specialist teachers and much better facilities, but the associated transportation meant that they spent as many as two hours a day sitting on a bus rather than playing after-school sports or walking or riding to school. The same occurred in large urban areas with the decision to allow students to attend any school they chose, even if it meant they had to take transport to do so.

At the same time, it was hard not to draw the conclusion that some of the decline was linked to the deliberate abolition of compulsory physical education, cuts to programs, and the renewal, in provinces like Ontario, of the idea that physical education, school sports, and the arts were "frills" that should not be funded within the basic school envelope. After-school sports were also hurt by teachers' strikes; since coaching was usually volunteered in most boards and contracts, it was the easiest labour to withdraw. The costs of sports soared, as schools were required to purchase safer, better equipment to reduce injury, and mitigate travel risks by replacing student carpooling with chauffeured buses. Higher costs often meant user fees for students and fund-raising for their parents, practices that created new economic barriers and inequalities for participation.[60] The continuing super-valorization of high-performance sports for children and youth reduced the importance of school sports in the public schools, and more wealthy parents preferred to put their sports-loving children in private schools with better facilities and programs. Teachers, provincial associations, and boards worked creatively to improve the quality of opportunities, but they faced a perfect storm of battering winds.

CHAPTER SEVEN

Seeking Optimism in a Contested Field

A rich education for the whole child necessarily requires physical education to be afforded the time that is afforded to other core subjects. The greater the time spent in physical education, the greater the opportunities for the development of students' learning, health, and fitness.

Robinson et al., 2019

Well into the twenty-first century, it seems unnecessary to express the sentiment that children in school require quality time in physical education, not just to learn new skills, but also for health, fitness, and embodied respect for social diversity. Presumably physical education is well and truly established within the provincial and territorial school systems, and no longer marginalized or viewed on a different, even lower, level than other core subjects. Canadian universities, specifically faculties, schools, or departments of physical education and/or kinesiology are uniquely preparing students for the demands of teaching the subject in our schools. Perhaps most important of all, today's physical education as taught in schools, colleges, and universities is culturally relevant in its recognition and affirmation of the diverse cultural identities of students.

If only all this and more were true. Writing about physical education as it has changed and evolved over almost twenty-five years into the twenty-first century has been an enormously difficult project, and we have struggled with what to include and exclude. Also, all aspects of the Canadian school system were thrown into disarray when the COVID-19 pandemic appeared and became deadly early in

2020. We discuss the effects and resulting implications of the pandemic for physical education in the next chapter, the Afterword, because we will likely still be dealing with them when this book is published.

For this chapter, several useful Canadian books published in the last twenty years have been enormously helpful. The first is *Stones in the Sneaker*, edited by Ellen Singleton and Aniko Varpalotai, an eclectic compilation of important issues in health and physical education with chapters ranging from understanding student experiences in physical education to issues of race, gender, disability, and the law. Also edited by Singleton and Varpalotai is the more recent sequel *Pedagogy in Motion*, another interesting collection of essays that challenged all "physical and health education professionals to renegotiate and interrogate the theories, practices, methods, and future innovations of their shared 'community of inquiry.'"[1]

The work of Daniel Robinson and Lynn Randall, and specifically their edited book *Teaching Physical Education Today: Canadian Perspectives*, has also been inspiring. Twenty-four professors from sixteen different Canadian universities in the nine provinces with physical education teacher education (PETE) programs contributed chapters to the book, while an additional sixteen professors from other universities in Canada also contributed as reviewers. The scope of the book is broad and divided into three sections – introduction, pedagogy, and content – whose purpose is to help and inspire an emerging generation of health and physical educators. From the perspective of the three co-authors of *Educating the Body*, we have learned a great deal and it has helped us decide upon the focus and content of this chapter.

What needs to be remembered, however, is that *Teaching Physical Education Today* represents the ideal – what physical education within our elementary and secondary school systems could and should look like – and not necessarily what actually happens in reality. In 2018, for example, only 35 per cent of five- to seventeen-year-olds reached their recommended physical activity levels as outlined in the Canadian 24-Hour Movement Guidelines for Children and Youth.[2] Given that all students in Canada are required to take physical education throughout elementary school and part of secondary school, the subject can be expected to have a positive impact on the health of Canadian children and teenagers, and encourage their lifelong participation in physical activity. The central question we ask in this chapter is whether that is actually happening.

Physical and Health Education Curricula across Canada: A Snapshot

Comparing physical and health education curricula today across a vast country like Canada can be a futile and sometimes perilous exercise. Each province and territory controls its own curricula, which are often (or not) undergoing change or renewal. Since they are produced by governments in concert with teachers, they are not exempt from political influence.[3] In sum, they are inherently political documents. Nonetheless, one recent study attempted to provide "a greater understanding of the landscape of grades 1 to 9 Canadian physical and health education curriculum by analysing curricular aim statements, organizers, and learning outcomes," as well as examining the instructional time allocated to physical education.[4] The study (conducted in January 2014) was limited to grades one to nine because in subsequent grades there is often more than one physical education course offering per grade, and physical education requirements for graduation vary. Also, there are considerable variations within the provinces and territories. Manitoba, Ontario, and Quebec offered a combined health and physical education program, whereas the remaining seven provinces offered physical education (as separate from health education). The three territories adopted the curricula of neighbouring provinces: the Yukon utilized British Columbia curricula, and the Northwest Territories used Alberta's, whereas curriculum and resources developed in Nunavut (in both English and Inuktitut) are adapted from other Canadian jurisdictions. Finally, in provinces with separate francophone curricula, only the anglophone curricula were studied.

The analysis showed that the state of physical and health education in Canada was very similar to that reported in Europe and other countries around the world. The primary stated aim was the acquisition of knowledge, skills, and attitudes for healthy active living (or lifestyle, or for life) through physical activity. For all provinces and territories, the gaining of movement skills was dominant, with healthy living taking second place, and fitness activities having a more tertiary role. However, as grades progress, there was a shift in emphasis from movement skills to healthy living and fitness skills. Learning outcomes were best achieved through involvement in physical activity and movement skills, or in some cases "kinesthetically," a broader term that includes the physical activity and movement in physical education settings such as gymnasiums, open spaces, or outdoors using different types of equipment and learning activities.[5]

The recommended instructional time allocated for physical education varied considerably within the provinces, as shown in figure 7.1. In Canada, the idealized standard of 150 minutes per week has been followed in only some provinces and territories (e.g., British Columbia, Alberta, Saskatchewan, Manitoba, and Nova Scotia). It is also recognized by Physical and Health Education Canada (PHE Canada) as the minimum standard for both elementary and secondary schools applying for their Quality Daily Physical Education (QDPE) award.[6] Moreover, although some insist that Quality Physical Education is much more important than

Province	Grade 1	Grade 2	Grade 3	Grade 4	Grade 5	Grade 6	Grade 7	Grade 8	Grade 9
BC	10% (90–100 hr/year)							10% (90–100 hr/yr)	
AB	10% (PE & Health)						10% (PE & Health)		
SK	150 min./wk					150 min./wk			
MB	11% (75% PE, 25% HE)						9% (75% PE, 25% HE)		
ON	At discretion of individual schools – no government guidelines								110 hr/yr
QC	120 min./wk						50 hr/year		
NS	30 min./day						Unavailable		
NB	100 min./wk						150 min./wk		
PE	5% (75 min./wk)						4–6%		
NL	6%						6% (50 hrs/yr)		

Figure 7.1. Recommended time allocations for physical education instruction by province, 2014 (note: PE = physical education, HE = health education; adapted from Kilborn, Lorusso, and Francis, 2016, 28)

Quantity of Physical Education, researchers have shown that the 150-minute standard is "really a political and/or health-related (connected to daily physical activity goals) one, rather than a research-based one."[7] Most provinces have a daily physical activity time requirement varying from twenty to thirty minutes per day for grades one to nine, though many only manage two to three classes per week ranging in time from thirty to forty-five minutes per class. Most high schools in Canada operate a two-semester year where students opt for four courses per semester, making it possible for students to get HPE every day for only one semester, unless subject combinations are put into effect. Despite the efforts of many dedicated physical educators, this speaks to the continuing marginalization of physical education as a subject area within the school systems. Among the various reasons offered are lack of government and school board support; school administrators' devaluation of physical education; lack of accountability measures to monitor the extent of physical education taking place; more focus on academic subjects, especially in high schools; low staff interest and support; and limited parent and community support. "Educators must stop believing and acting," suggest advocates, "as if one dimension of humanness (the cognitive aspect) is superior to the others (the physical and affective aspects)."[8]

More recently, wellness (or well-being) has taken on an increasingly important role in discussions concerning curricular revisions of school-based health and physical education programs. Although there is no universally agreed-upon definition of wellness, the literature suggests it is a holistic concept and that "achieving healthy school communities should rely on a multifaceted, whole-school approach known as comprehensive school health (CSH)."[9] Furthermore, well-being and wellness can be defined even more broadly, often incorporating aspects of physical, emotional, sexual, and spiritual health, as well as food literacy, self-awareness, relationship skills, and injury prevention. Our interest here, however, relates to how the variable concept of wellness is driving the reconceptualization of health and physical education curricula within Canadian schools. We use the province of Alberta as an example.

Alberta's current K–12 Physical Education curriculum and the K–9 Health and Life Skills curricula were last revised in 2000 and 2001 respectively. In 2003, the Alberta Commission on Learning recommended combining these two curricula into a single kindergarten to grade twelve wellness program. Eventually, and through an extensive consultation process, the Alberta government in 2009 brought forth a *Framework for Kindergarten to Grade 12 Wellness Education*.[10] Included were the five dimensions of wellness (social, emotional, spiritual, physical, and intellectual) within three key elements: health and physical education programs of study, wellness across the K–12 subject areas, as well as wellness-related courses. Multiple stakeholders, including parents, students, teachers, administrators, community members, First Nations, Métis, Inuit, and francophone groups were invited to collaborate in the development of an agreed-upon definition of wellness as a "balanced state of emotional, intellectual, physical, social, and spiritual well-being that enables students to reach their full potential in the school community. Personal wellness occurs with commitment to lifestyle choices based on healthy actions and attitudes."[11] Since this was a major revamp of the curriculum, Alberta Education decided to focus first on the senior level (grades ten to twelve); however, the revisions were not completed before the Progressive Conservative government in Alberta was defeated in 2015. The subsequent New Democratic Party government, although fully supportive of wellness education, were not in power long enough – they were defeated in 2019 – to accomplish any substantial curriculum revisions.

In the spring/summer of 2021, the Alberta government of the United Conservative Party, released a revised, draft curriculum for kindergarten to grade six.[12] There was immediate and intense public debate about all aspects of this curriculum, but our focus here is on the Physical Education and Wellness section, defined as "developing the whole individual and nurturing students in pursuing a healthy and active life." There is a return to the original (2003) recommendation to combine the content from two separate curricula (physical education/health and life skills) into an integrated curriculum with an additional focus on social-emotional learning, consent, and financial literacy. The term "physical activities" is used throughout along with "physical fitness" or "active living" goals. Criticism of the draft K–6 Physical Education and Wellness curriculum has been intense, pointing to questions about how previously separate curricula were combined and how they now align; its inaccessibility due to a lack of a systematic and logical arrangement of content; a lack of the whole-child focus; and most critical of all, the absence of current educational research in the field of health and physical education.[13] In particular, the "wellness" aspect of the draft curriculum has been criticized for reinforcing an emphasis on body weight and shape, and for "promoting problematic, binary, and externally measured indicators of health, rather than realistic, nuanced, and embodied experiences across multiple dimensions of health."[14] This is not surprising, given that the discourses of neoliberalism, such as competition, human capital, and individual responsibility, drive these curriculum changes. Within this context, the main purpose of school health and physical education, and why they have been combined, is to make "healthy citizens" who are self-regulating, informed, and capable of constructing their own healthy lifestyle and minimizing risky behaviours.[15] As a result, the rationale for physical education's existence in the core curriculum of schools is increasingly shifting from a physical activity and sport focus to a health focus. Still, most critiques of the Alberta curriculum draft on Physical Education and Wellness suggest that there needs to be a greater focus on "physical literacy," which recognizes that engaging in physical activity helps students develop skills, competence, and motivation to be active throughout their lives.

Physically Educated versus Physically Literate

The term "physical literacy" has a relatively long history, which can be traced back to the late nineteenth century, although in modern times its usage has become more frequent. For instance, in chapter 3 we discussed the work of François Delsarte, especially his principles of movement (posture, position, and gestures) that govern the use of the human body as an instrument of expression. Delsartean theory and practice were also significant to modern dance in that pioneers like Ted Shawn (1891–1972) drew upon his work in their performances and teaching. In the early 1950s, Shawn wrote a book about Delsarte in which he said: "I hope the day comes when all children, from their first start in primary grades, learn to use human movement as a language equally and along with their learning to communicate by speech and by writing. We would then have in a few generations a physical 'literate' adult population; for today, in spite of 'physical education' (which mostly confines itself largely to teaching athletic sports) we have mostly physical illiteracy."[16] Canadian Doris Plewes (see chapter 5) used the term in the 1950s when she travelled about the country promoting physical fitness: "Canadians are becoming increasingly aware of the importance of *physical literacy*, muscular and organic power, avoidance of premature loss of vigour and skill and are beginning to demand the tangible evidence that in and through physical education positive gains in physical powers are made each year."[17] On occasion, and for emphasis, Plewes also used the term "illiteracy" in reference to the lack of fitness. Historically, and to this day, physical literacy has been viewed "instrumentally as a means to combat the ills of modernization and secure better health and broad participation in life."[18]

British physical educator Margaret Whitehead has become the modern champion of physical literacy, beginning with her academic work in the early 1990s. She developed the concept through the philosophical study of monism, existentialism, and phenomenology. In other words, the mind/body cannot be separated (monism); humans create their being existentially through their lived experience (existentialism); and experience can only be understood from the standpoint of the individual who lives it (phenomenology). Therefore, Whitehead sees physical literacy as synonymous (embodied) with existence – what it is to be human – and not just as a tool for achieving other ends. Through her work, and especially in two edited books, she has promoted and extended the dialogue about physical literacy.[19] Often, and with her lead, a number of studies and conferences have taken place, leading in 2013 to the establishment of the International Physical Literacy Association. According to the Aspen Institute's 2014 global environmental scan of physical literacy initiatives, Canada is among the leaders of physical literacy initiatives that are delivered through sport and educational systems. The report noted that in Canada, physical literacy is considered the foundation for both elite sport and a healthy nation with the goal that every child should be physically literate by age twelve.[20] Committed to this foundation and the value of physical activity for every child, Whitehead focused upon those movement experiences most likely to propel that interest throughout life and asked how they could be imparted through physical education. "In short," she explained, "physical literacy can be seen as a disposition that supports life-long participation in physical activity."[21]

Seeking Optimism in a Contested Field

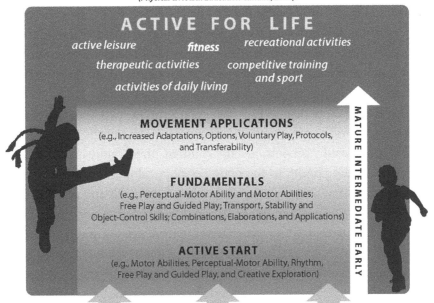

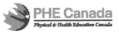

Figure 7.2. Physical literacy for life, a model for physical education promoted by PHE Canada (courtesy of PHE Canada)

Today, the definition of physical literacy used by the International Physical Literacy Association has broadened somewhat, but still retains its central tenets: "As appropriate to each individual, physical literacy can be described as the *motivation, confidence, physical competence, knowledge and understanding to value and take responsibility for engaging in physical activities for life.*"[22] The core principles that underlie this definition are that physical literacy is inclusive and accessible to all. Moreover, it represents an individual journey; it can be experienced in multiple contexts and environments; it needs to be cultivated through life; and finally, it contributes to the overall development of the whole person.[23]

Less institutionalized than its physical literacy counterpart, the notion of health literacy was adopted as part of PHE Canada's 2017–20 strategic plan with a focus upon achieving healthy schools, healthy children, and healthy communities. The view was that adding health to the notion of physical literacy would work to increase public awareness of the relationship between health and education and to foster workshops and wide-ranging curricula materials for teachers and teacher educators. It has also led, some contend, to the tendency for health educators and physical educators to operate like two ships passing in the night, with the claim that physical educators have been too focused on unlocking the movement competence door. In 2021, for example, American physical educators sought to further advance health and physical literacy in K–12 schools, higher education, and in dance and sport venues worldwide by establishing a National Academy of Health and Physical Literacy.

In some respects, the physical literacy movement has forced a rethinking of the type of activities implemented in many physical education programs, how they were being delivered, and the type of pedagogy used. The most recent (2019) Ontario Health and Physical Education Curriculum (Grades One to Eight) is an example of how both health and physical literacy are important and integral to the curriculum, and it is considered by many as an example of best practice since its 2019 refresh. PHE Canada uses a broadened definition of physical literacy: "Individuals who are physically literate move with competence in a wide variety of physical activities that benefit the development of the whole person." Moreover, physically literate individuals: (1) consistently develop the motivation and ability to understand, communicate, apply, and analyze different forms of movement; (2) demonstrate a variety of movements confidently, competently, creatively, and strategically across a wide range of health-related physical activities; and (3) make healthy, active choices throughout their lifespan that are both beneficial to, and respectful of their whole self, others, and the environment.[24] On the other hand, health literacy involves the skills needed to get, understand, and use information to make good decisions about health. The Ontario Health and Physical Education curriculum has four strands: Social-Emotional Learning Skills, Active Living, Movement Competence, and Healthy Living. The Movement Competence strand includes skills, concepts, and strategies, and it is here that physical literacy is most evident: "The development of fundamental movement skills in association with the application of movement concepts and principles provides the basic foundation for physical literacy."[25] Similarly, physical literacy (along with healthy and active living, social and community health, and mental well-being) is also an essential component of the K–10 physical and health education curriculum in British Columbia. Again, similar to the Ontario curriculum, the main component of physical literacy for each grade level is to "develop and demonstrate a variety of fundamental movement skills in a variety of physical activities and environments."[26] If this sounds familiar, we would remind readers of our earlier discussion about the origins of child-centred movement education by followers of modern dance exponent Rudolf Laban in the early 1950s; the debates that ensued; and the resistance that led to its eventual demise (see chapter 5). However, there is limited empirical evidence to substantiate the development of physical literacy in elementary schools.

Canada has become a leader in the physical literacy movement across multiple sectors, which obviously includes education, but also sport and recreation at all levels of government, as well as in the private sector. Experts argue that "collaboration between sport, recreation and education is necessary to empower Canadians to embark upon and benefit from their physical literacy journey."[27] There is consensus among some stakeholders for the use of the International Physical Literacy Association definition of physical literacy as stated above. The organizations collaborating on the definition include, for example, ParticipACTION, Sport for Life Society, PHE Canada, Canadian Parks and Recreation Association, Active for Life, and others. However, the notion of physical literacy has been taken up and interpreted differently depending on the main objectives of the organization. PHE Canada, for example, serves mainly physical education teachers, and their approach to physical literacy focuses on the holistic development of students. The Sport for Life Society, on the other hand, attempts to bridge gaps between sectors, create new collaborations with Canadian institutions, and mobilize their knowledge to communities across the country with the aim of creating a future in which absolutely everyone has access to quality sport and physical literacy experiences.[28] Its Long Term Athlete Development Plan recognizes physical literacy as the foundation for developing the skills, knowledge, and attitudes needed for Canadians to lead healthy, active lives. What is also interesting is that Sport for Life, in collaboration with the Coaching Association of Canada and HIGH FIVE® (which provides recreation professionals with training), offers a short course to qualify as a Physical Literacy Instructor.[29]

As mentioned earlier, several provincial jurisdictions in Canada have implemented physical literacy in their physical education curricula, which means that physical educators are now "challenged to deliver quality physical education programs rich in experiences that develop student physical literacy."[30] Some experts have suggested a pedagogical "models-based practice" as a means to overcome the serious limitations of the traditional sport-based, multi-activity form of physical education, which for many students deters rather than encourages a lifelong engagement with physical activity.[31] One well-known model is Sport Education, developed in the United States by physical educator Daryl Siedentop, which encourages students to become competent, literate, and enthusiastic sportspeople.[32] Other models include Teaching Games for Understanding, Cooperative Learning, or Teaching Personal and Social Responsibility.[33] It has been suggested that physical literacy become a pedagogical model as well, while others call for a "physical literacy praxis" to show how educators teaching physical education can effectively operationalize and implement physical literacy into school physical education programs with the goal of "moving, thinking, feeling, and doing (behavioral) individuals."[34]

Regardless of the model, trained physical education specialists are in the best position to implement it. However, physical education specialist positions continue to be removed from schools. At last count only 62 per cent of schools in Canada had a policy regarding the hiring of trained physical educators, and less than half of these schools had implemented this policy.[35] In some provinces, elementary-level physical education is one of the few disciplines in which no subject-specific teacher training is necessary. Classroom generalists repeatedly state that they do not feel comfortable teaching physical education. What then is the current state of physical education teacher training in Canada?

Training Physical Education Teachers

There are currently two structurally different systems of Physical Education Teacher Education (PETE) programs in Canada. Students can complete their programs "sequentially" with a PE/kinesiology/sport science four-year degree followed by pedagogy courses in a faculty of education (commonly referred to as an after-degree program). Alternatively, they can pursue an "integrated" degree (usually a Bachelor of Education in a faculty of education) with simultaneous coursework in both areas. The Canadian Council of University Physical Education and Kinesiology Administrators (CCUPEKA) accreditation standards are achieved differently in each type of program, although CCUPEKA does not accredit teacher certification degree status, given that administrators representing faculties or departments of education are not members of the organization. There are also concerns that CCUPEKA accreditation standards for PETE programs are still based primarily on performance-oriented discourses already established as characteristic of kinesiology-type programs. In other words, they are academic, scientific, technocratic, specific, and mechanic, rather than holistic, professional, societal, and contextual.

It should come as no surprise that in a survey designed to collect the profiles and opinions of PETE educators across Canada, almost all believed their most important role was to prepare future professionals to teach children and youth in schools, whereas many thought their institution was far more interested in (and rewarded) research related to physical education pedagogy.[36] There was also concern that an emphasis on performance-oriented courses in kinesiology departments outweighs the potential influence and impact of pedagogy courses, leading to the claim that some PETE programs are failing to adequately prepare teachers to meet the challenges of teaching students at either the elementary- or secondary-school level.

At the provincial level, and among physical education teachers themselves, more positive attitudes towards their training can be found. According to a study among Canadian physical education teachers in the Atlantic provinces on the future of physical education, they were largely satisfied with the state of quality daily physical education in their own provinces, and were especially appreciative of their initial practical training in schools.[37] They were most confident teaching sports, but spent little or no time on dance, gymnastics, or outdoor education, which suggested that PETE programs were failing in that regard. They did agree, however, that they were given inadequate instructional time and limited resources for teaching their subject, and also faced an ongoing lack of administrative support and general respect for their subject.

Among the many issues facing PETE are also basic questions about its name. Physical Education Sport Pedagogy (PESP) has been advanced as a new strategy to avoid further isolation from kinesiology departments by focusing upon a broader view of pedagogy that goes beyond school settings to other field-based settings such as the fitness industry, coaching, rehabilitation settings, and physical activity educational settings across the lifespan.[38] In some arenas, PESP is favoured over PETE, leading critics to observe that a disagreement over so fundamental an issue as its name might lead to the endangerment of both programs. Questions related to declining student enrolment in these programs, curriculum content, location of training, and the uneasy alignment with kinesiology continue to concern leaders in the field. The main challenges to the future of PETE/PESP include a lack of enlightened leadership to promote the subject, inadequate grounding of beginning teachers in the subject-matter knowledge needed to teach in schools, Canada's overemphasis on sport at the expense of daily exercise in schools, and the need for greater flexibility and proactivity in developing effective programs for the future. As one longtime expert put it: "we have academicised the field, we have actually shoved out to the margins, in some cases shoved out completely, the subject matter knowledge that teachers need to teach in schools."[39]

Physical Education versus Kinesiology in Higher Education

As Canadian universities became increasingly invested in research, their interest in supporting "less productive" professional faculties and departments has diminished across the country, especially where the training of physical educators is concerned. For example, in 2017 the School of Kinesiology and Health Studies at Queen's University in Ontario announced the closure of its Bachelor of Physical and Health Education undergraduate program. The rationale for this decision was as follows: the opportunities for physical education teachers within the school system had fallen dramatically; there were increasing demands for degrees in kinesiology and health studies; physical education programs were being replaced by kinesiology programs with very minor changes to the curriculum; the Queen's BPHE program failed to achieve the Canadian Council of University Physical Education and Kinesiology Administrators (CCUPEKA) accreditation; and none of the current PhD-level personnel held doctoral degrees in physical education and pedagogy or conducted research in this area.[40] Among the benefits to closure, noted the announcement, were the arrival of new faculty in biomechanics, motor control, and global health.

The slippage of physical education into and out of kinesiology in the curriculum offerings of colleges and universities, and the acknowledgment of declining interest in, or even the need for, physical education programs across Canada, underscored what had begun some decades earlier in relation to the fortunes of physical education in Canadian higher education. As we saw in chapter 6, the first two universities to introduce kinesiology into higher education in the late 1960s were Simon Fraser University in British Columbia and the University of Waterloo in Ontario. Fitness training specialist Norm Ashton, who developed the program at Waterloo, aptly called it the "non-professional study of human physical movement."[41] These were relatively new universities unhindered by a long history of academic traditions, and they were able to compete with other universities by offering a variety of innovative programs. At Simon Fraser University, kinesiology found its first roots in a Physical

Development Centre as part of the Faculty of Education, which led in 1972 to a Bachelor of Science (kinesiology) degree within the Faculty of Interdisciplinary Studies. Waterloo expanded its existing one-year program for physical education teachers following a three-year university degree in arts or science, to a four-year multidisciplinary approach to the study of human movement. Labelled kinesiology, it attracted a number of scientists (in biochemistry, biomechanics, motor learning, sport psychology, and sociology) to the department, which encouraged it some years later to offer an MSc and PhD.

Other kinesiology programs in higher education followed, often as a result of the declining demand for physical education teachers and the attraction of a wide variety of jobs in fields such as rehabilitation, ergonomics, and health promotion. While some older universities such as the University of Toronto and the University of Alberta maintained their faculties of physical education for some time, in the first decade of the twenty-first century kinesiology and human kinetics programs outnumbered physical education programs in Canada by more than two to one. By this time, the objectives of many kinesiology programs had come full circle, moving back to a multi-faceted professional focus, and replacing physical activity courses with research methods, laboratory, and clinical work experiences.

CCUPEKA, founded in 1971 to evaluate and set minimum standards for the curriculum, increasingly refocused its gaze from participation to performance as kinesiology moved towards the goal of training scientists and accredited health care professionals. The deans, directors, and "chairmen" of Canadian physical education university programs initially came together to socialize and discuss the challenges facing their field, one of which was to face down what they believed was the perceived reputation of physical educators among granting agencies as "ball bouncers in the gym."[42] Adding the "K" for kinesiology in 1995 was a move to formally accredit the specific content of both kinesiology and physical education programs. Today, CCUPEKA represents forty institutions across Canada of which only ten receive accreditation for physical education.[43]

The desire to promote kinesiology as a regulated health care profession has developed quickly and extensively across Canada. The Ontario Kinesiology Association was incorporated as a non-profit organization in 1981, and within a decade most other provinces had formed their own kinesiology associations.[44] Initiated in 1995, the Canadian Kinesiology Alliance/Alliance Canadienne de Kinésiologie (CKA/ACK) was federally incorporated in 2001 to promote kinesiology as a profession and to provide a national voice for kinesiologists working in the community. In Ontario, for example, the scope of practice in kinesiology is defined as "the assessment of movement, performance, and function; and the rehabilitation, prevention, and management of disorders to maintain, rehabilitate, and enhance movement, performance, and function in the areas of sport, recreation, work, exercise, and activities of daily living."[45] It is now a regulated health profession, and in order to apply to be certified as a kinesiologist in Ontario, the applicant must have a four-year university degree from a program approved by CCUPEKA. So far, Ontario is the only Canadian province or territory where legislation has been passed to regulate kinesiology as a profession though some other provinces are not far behind.[46] Indeed, this channelling of new kinesiologists into a health care profession may well have an impact upon the organization of kinesiology programs in higher education in the future.

Equity, Diversity, Inclusion, and Social Justice

A research study published in 2013 showed a profound lack of racial diversity as well as a prevalence of whiteness in Canadian faculties of kinesiology and physical education, and a similar study conducted several years later indicated that the situation had not significantly improved.[47] In the first study, it was found that 94 per cent of the faculty and staff were white. Racialized minority and Indigenous females were the most poorly represented with men outnumbering women by a ratio of nearly two to one. As for the students, the majority of undergraduates were white, but depending on the university there were small increments of racialized minorities and Indigenous students, but only one or two students with a disability. As axes of difference that warrant attention and analysis, gender and disability were privileged in course offerings within the curriculum at both the graduate and undergraduate levels of study, while race and sexuality remained on the margins As the authors of the 2013 study surmised: "It is our contention that both the predominance of whites and cultures of whiteness have had a significant influence on the character of pedagogical practice and knowledge production, as well as the recruitment and retention of Aboriginal and racialized minority students within the field of physical education."[48]

Seven years later, little had changed, and whiteness remained centred, dominant, and overlooked in physical education and kinesiology university faculties. The 2020 study examined eight kinesiology programs in Canada's top five "ethnically diverse" (South Asian, Chinese, and Black) cities: two universities in Ontario, three in Montreal, and one each in Vancouver, Calgary, and Ottawa. Data collected from the eight program websites showed that only 17 per cent of faculty appeared racialized or Indigenous, which is much lower than one might expect given the ethnic make-up of these cities. As with the previous study, issues of race, colonialism, and

BOX 7.1. EARLE F. ZEIGLER (1919–2018)

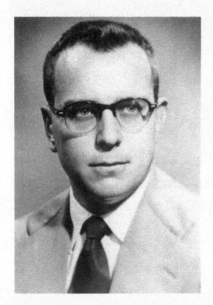

Figure 7.3. Earle F. Zeigler, early portrait (Bentley Historical Library, University of Michigan)

If there is anyone who best represents the changes that occurred in Canadian physical education in the twentieth and twenty-first centuries, it is Earle F. Zeigler – one of the most prolific, respected, and influential scholars of our time. Up until his death, he was still writing essays and books (in all 445 journal articles and sixty books).

Born in New York City, Zeigler obtained his early degrees in German followed by a PhD in the history and philosophy of education at Yale University, where he was a top-notch athlete in several sports. He also taught physical education, and coached football and wrestling while at Yale. A dual citizen of both Canada and the United States, he came to Ontario in 1949 as head of the physical education department at Western University until 1955. From there he went to the University of Michigan (1956–63) and then to the University of Illinois at Urbana-Champaign (1963–71). He returned to Western (as the first dean of the newly formed Faculty of Physical Education from 1971 to 1977), where he remained until his retirement in 1989. Along the way, he received many awards and recognition for his outstanding dedication and service to several professional and scholarly associations including the R. Tait McKenzie Honour Award in 1975, several awards from AAHPERD and other organizations, as well as three honorary doctorates.

After leaving Western he moved to Richmond, British Columbia, where he continued to write extensively, offering his opinion on a variety of topics. His output was astonishing in both volume and range. His family has kindly made available (until 2026) his later books and articles, many of which can be downloaded from http://earlezeigler.com.

One of the critically important pioneers in the sociocultural dimensions of sport and physical activity, Earle was influential in the establishment of the first professional societies dedicated to the history, sociology, philosophy, and comparative studies of sport. He supervised or examined over one hundred graduate students, many of whom became outstanding scholars and professional leaders in physical education.

> Earle was a passionate and devoted leader, and he served as the conscience of the profession and discipline of physical education for more than seventy-five years. In one of his final professional contributions, at age ninety-eight, he wrote: "Let's pledge ourselves to make still greater efforts to become vibrant and impactful through absolute dedication and commitment to our professional endeavours. Ours is a higher calling as we seek to improve the quality of life for all through the finest type of developmental physical activity in sport, exercise, and related expressive movement."*
>
>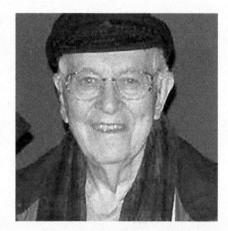
>
> Figure 7.4. Earle F. Zeigler, later portrait
>
> * Zeigler, "What Should the Field of Physical Activity Education Promote in the 21st Century?"

whiteness were often ignored in the curricula. In summary, the researchers found that "kinesiology programs in Canada's five most diverse cities changed minimally, and student narratives indicate a need for supporting anti-racist teaching and research that challenges the normalizing, centering, and overlooking of whiteness."[49]

More attention is now being paid to this issue. In June 2021, CCUPEKA issued a statement on Anti-Racism in Physical Education and Kinesiology indicating that it is "committed to equity, diversity, inclusion, and social justice through education as core values for all Canadian university Physical Education and Kinesiology programs." It also stated that CCUPEKA "stands in solidarity with all those who are fighting against racism, oppression, inequality, inequity, and injustice. CCUPEKA calls upon those in positions of power and privilege to reflect on their own experiences, biases, and privileges; to acknowledge that privilege often comes at the expense of Indigenous peoples, Black people, and other marginalized peoples; and to act to dismantle systemic racism and oppression."[50] Moreover, CCUPEKA's accreditation standards now require university programs to meaningfully and intentionally address challenges and barriers to participation and engagement in the work with underrepresented groups.

Although this position statement is a start, it is a far cry from the specific demands of the Physical and Health Education Canada Research Council, which in response to the Truth and Reconciliation Commission (TRC) called upon CCUPEKA to establish clear targets for the recruitment and retention of Indigenous and racialized minority scholars and students, with plans to ensure their success in the academy; include required courses addressing colonization, race, whiteness, and diversity; and provide professional development workshops related to anti-racism, cultures of whiteness, and Indigeneity for faculty, staff, and students.[51] In fact, it took CCUPEKA six years following the release of the TRC final report and calls to action to issue a position statement on truth and reconciliation in physical education and kinesiology: "CCUPEKA is committed to responding to the calls to action and honouring truth and reconciliation. In consultation and cooperation with Indigenous peoples, we commit to taking impactful steps using mechanisms of accreditation, education, and systemic change to support the learning and unlearning that promotes reconciliation, decolonization and Indigenization of Physical Education and Kinesiology programs."[52]

It should be noted, however, that "physical education" is not mentioned anywhere in the TRC calls to action. The recommendations focus entirely upon the policies of the Physical Activity and Sport Act – namely to promote physical activity as a fundamental element of health and well-being, reduce barriers to sports participation, increase the pursuit of excellence in sports, and build capacity in the Canadian sport system.[53] The TRC insisted that the act be amended to explicitly include Aboriginal peoples.[54] Nonetheless, within the Education section of the calls to action are two that are relevant to school physical education: first, end the discrepancy in federal education funding for First Nations children being educated on reserves compared with those being educated off reserves, and second, develop culturally appropriate curricula. It is estimated that First Nations schools funded by the federal government continue to receive approximately 30 to 40 per cent less funding than do provincially funded public schools, which means less opportunity for Indigenous children and youth to access quality, culturally relevant physical and health education programs in their communities. The impact of these disparities in funding and inequitable resources influence the delivery of quality physical education to Indigenous students in two significant ways: access to facilities and equipment, and quality of instruction.[55] As we have just discussed, there is a significant disparity in the number of Indigenous students training to be physical education teachers in kinesiology programs across the country. There is also a high turnover of non-Indigenous physical education teachers on reserves due to financial constraints (e.g., lower salary, inadequate space and facilities, inability to implement the curriculum) as well as the sometimes isolated locations.

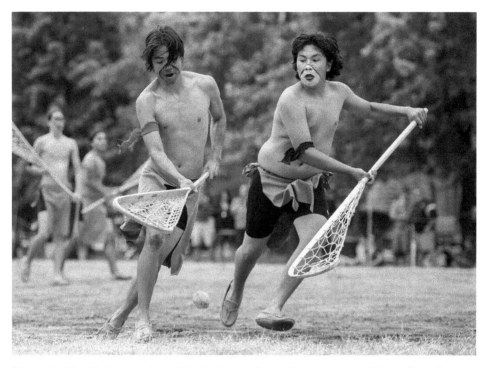

Figure 7.5. First Nations youth participating in a traditional lacrosse game in Montreal, Quebec, 2017 (The Canadian Press/Graham Hughes)

Although education for Indigenous students on reserve is governed by local First Nations, Métis, and Inuit authorities, the various provincial physical and health education curricula do not necessarily correspond to the needs and interests of students living in these contexts. The pathologizing of Indigenous peoples' health and physicality tends to result in the normalization of settler health, fixing perceived difficulties for them while excluding health conceptions held by Indigenous peoples. "Fit for what?" is an important question when considering the complex landscape of health and physical education in Canada. As we have discussed in previous chapters, settler forms of sport and physical education, especially in residential schools, were used as tools of assimilation, character development, and disease prevention that stood in stark contrast to the ways Indigenous people engaged in movement and healthy living. Physical cultural practices that were holistic, community oriented, land based, and purposeful were eliminated and replaced (if at all) by calisthenics, gymnastics, military drill, and competitive sports commonly found in the physical education curriculum of public schools.

Clearly, a rethink is needed concerning better ways to support the health, skills, and pleasure to be gained from meaningful, culturally appropriate, and relevant health and physical education curricula and pedagogies for Canada's Indigenous youth and their schools and communities. However, what exactly is meant by "culturally relevant" is not easy to define. According to experts, culturally relevant physical education can be described as four interrelated constructs: (1) the teacher as an ally, (2) who understands the students and their day-to-day cultural landscapes, (3) in order to provide a supportive learning environment, (4) that includes a meaningful and relevant curriculum.[56] Each of these aspects is interconnected and relational, and as a model it is designed to be applied interculturally across all student populations, not necessarily just Indigenous students. For the latter, it would need to be directed by and embedded with Indigenous perspectives and cultural values, although there is certainly value in non-Indigenous students learning about Indigenous culture.[57] As discussed earlier, physical literacy is now a key focus of most provincial physical education curricula, yet we know little about Indigenous peoples' meanings and experiences of physical literacy. Understanding these would go a long way to engaging Indigenous youth in culturally relevant physical education.[58] At the same time, introducing Indigenous perspectives on physical activity and health to physical education curricula everywhere would contribute significantly to reconciliation, while enriching students' understanding of the moving human body.

There is also a need for considerably more research not only on Indigenous children and youth, but also on Indigenous traditions, cultures, and perspectives in school-based health and physical education. A study designed to chart the English-language, peer-reviewed empirical literature related to these aspects in the Ontario school system between 2000 and 2020 identified alarmingly few articles.[59] Even then, the focus was mostly on elementary-aged Indigenous children in primarily remote northern communities but with little attention paid to Indigenous traditions, cultures, and perspectives. Obviously, there is a need to research diverse Indigenous communities, not just in Ontario but throughout Canada, to gain a better picture of the experience of Indigenous children and youth in all school-based health and physical education.

Of course, there are other interconnected diversities such as race, socioeconomic status, immigration/refugee background, gender identity, sexual orientation, religion, dis/ability (see next section), and body shape/size that also need be considered. This brings us to a discussion of what is called critical pedagogy in physical education, and the extent to which it can "identify, understand, and disrupt existing power relations so as the ensure equity, freedom, and justice for all."[60] Critical pedagogies, then, must also be pedagogies of social justice. In *Social Justice in Physical Education: Critical Reflections and Pedagogies for Change*, for example, the editors (Daniel Robinson and Lynn Randall) state their primary goal as "the

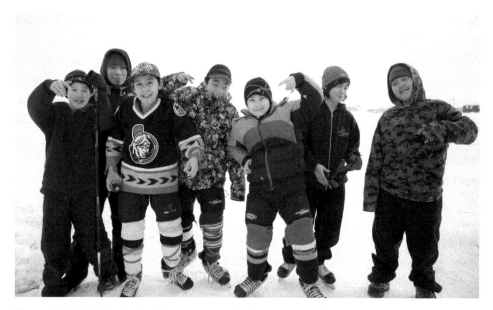

Figure 7.6. Ice Hockey in Gjoa Haven, an Inuit hamlet in Nunavut (ton koene/Alamy Stock Photo)

empowerment of physical education teachers, their students, and most importantly, those who have traditionally been on the margins."[61] They argue that the world and its students have changed a great deal, yet many physical education programs have not, which means that traditional practices and pedagogies need to be questioned and redesigned to be more inclusive and socially just. How exactly this can be done is the central question. One suggestion is that PETE should be designed to "shift prospective PE teachers from wherever they sit on a continuum, towards a position where social issues become a greater focus in their decision-making including teaching content, pedological choices, group structure, and assessment."[62] In this way, some teachers may position social justice to mean addressing individual concerns through humanistic teaching, whereas others may tackle structural inequities. Regardless, more has been written defending and advocating critical pedagogy than about how it might be operationalized, which is why *Social Justice in Physical Education* is valuable, certainly in the Canadian context. The editors' purpose is to "foster a critical reflection of the different realities, subjectivities, and possibilities that remain hidden or unknown to many," which eventually results in meaningful action.[63] They also hope readers will appreciate and come to a better understanding of intersectionality, or how social categorizations create overlapping and interdependent systems of discrimination or disadvantage. The book includes chapters about race, gender, sexuality, disability, mental health, Indigenous bodies, social class, religious minorities, immigrant students, transexual-intersex-cisgender issues, and finally the obesity discourse. Still, physical education teachers are quick to admit that they sometimes feel poorly informed and trained on diversity and inclusion issues.

The task of supporting equity and inclusion among students and faculty in Canadian universities and colleges has become multi-layered and complex for kinesiology and physical education in light of the increased internationalization of students, the nature of the subject matter (i.e., Eurocentric ideologies of meritocracy, individualism, and scientific objectivity that reflect the values of the dominant group), and the over-representation of whiteness in the faculty. Critics point to the status and everyday lived experiences of racialized scholars and students, calling attention to the normativity of whiteness that seems to remain entrenched across campuses at many levels, and more broadly across Canadian society. Transformation of programs and attitudes in relation to race and culture comes in ebbs and flows, and it takes hard work and keen awareness to move forward, but Canadian universities have responded in numerous ways to develop initiatives in equity, diversity, and inclusion.[64] In particular, hiring practices are being reorganized to target Black and Indigenous academics for leadership positions with funds being made available for curriculum revisions, more sensitive teaching strategies, and greater levels of support for students and faculty from diverse backgrounds (see Afterword).

Disability Inclusion through Adaptive Physical Activity

Adaptive physical activity, or what some prefer to call *adapted* physical activity, in which physical education plays a major role, is an interdisciplinary field drawing upon the research traditions of the social sciences, humanities, arts, and natural sciences.[65] We have said little in the foregoing chapters about the history of adaptive physical education, deciding it was better to consolidate the information in this section because the most important aspect for our purposes is the inclusion of children and youth experiencing disability in school-based physical education. Over the years there has been considerable rethinking concerning the language used in this field. Following some researchers, we prefer the term adapt*ive* as opposed to adapt*ed*. The term *adapted* implies that adaptation has occurred; whereas, *adaptive* indicates that practitioners are able to do or are doing something to foster thriving in others. In other words, it is the professional practitioner who should be adaptive, and not the person experiencing disability.[66]

Today, the term *person experiencing disability* is preferable to *person with a disability* or *disabled person* because it is "designed to acknowledge the wide variety of embodied sensations, social structures, cultural understandings, and identities that may relate to someone's disability experience."[67] We briefly outline some of the history of this multi-faceted field in Canada before discussing disability inclusion more thoroughly.

Although we have mentioned the famous Canadian physician, physical educator, and sculptor R. Tait McKenzie in previous chapters, he was perhaps most influential through his medical discourse on disability and physical activity. From the late 1880s until the years of the First World War, McKenzie focused his medical practice on the treatment of patients with physical disabilities, and at the same time, he wrote about his work in journal articles and books. For example, in his book *Exercise in Education and Medicine*, he included chapters concerning physical education for the blind and deaf, as well as for "mental and moral defectives," which may be the first instance of adaptive physical education explicated in any major text.[68] McKenzie provided useful suggestions as to how to adapt games, sports, and play to meet the needs of these children. However, in line with the prevailing view of the times, he accepted without question their institutionalization. During the war, especially in his treatment of injured and maimed military men, McKenzie used a range of physical therapies, but he also advocated physical activity through the use of exercise machines and gymnastics. His work, supported by female physical educators and massage therapists drawn to the war effort, was part of the physical rehabilitation and eventual vocational retraining of disabled soldiers. Despite the progressiveness of McKenzie's approach to disability, it was still very much in tune with the times: "that disabilities should be fixed in search of the 'normal' or ideal body; that rehabilitation was important to avoid economic decline; that education for those with a disability should be largely segregated and organised by experts with virtually no input from the person."[69]

It took another world war to bring about progressive change in how to consider the physical education needs of persons experiencing a disability. In the United States, for example, physical educators changed the name of the field from "correctives" to "adapted physical education," which in 1952 was accepted by the American Association for Health, Physical Education, and Recreation. Soon afterwards, the publication of the text *Adapted Physical Education* encouraged those working among individuals with a sensory and/or physical disability to provide more challenging activities for the participants.[70] In 1965, Patricia Austin, one of the first Canadian women physical educators to obtain a doctorate, completed her thesis by designing a physical education program for physically handicapped students (grades one to twelve) in a Flint, Michigan, school.[71] Returning to the University of Alberta, Austin was instrumental in promoting the role of physical education in children with learning disabilities, and was joined by colleagues Ted Wall and Jane Watkinson, especially in the development of a preschool play program for moderately mentally retarded children. For Austin, inclusion meant "there is a need to shift our position from one which approaches physical education as a content to be mastered to one which sees it as a personalized learning experience."[72]

Within Canadian educational systems, the 1960s brought the notion of "mainstreaming," which meant the integration of children with a disability into the regular classroom or gymnasium. Prior to this time, most of these students were in segregated settings such as special classes within regular schools, special schools, institutions, or even hospitals. Mainstreaming, however, was considered more suited to children with mild disabilities rather than the entire range, and then only after an assessment deemed it appropriate. As it continued into the 1970s and during the 1980s, the problems of mainstreaming became more evident because it was often implemented inappropriately with a lack of adequate staff, especially if students experiencing a severe disability with challenging and unique needs were also included.

For some, even mainstreaming did not go far enough, and other models were devised to make certain that *all* children experiencing a disability, no matter how severe, could be included in the regular school setting. In 1986, a national symposium was held in Jasper, Alberta, with the support of Fitness Canada, bringing together delegates from across the country to discuss physical activity and disability. One outcome was the formation in 1994 of the Active Living Alliance for Canadians with a Disability, which sponsored the "Moving to Inclusion" project to support the inclusion of children in physical education.[73] Over time, an understanding of inclusive physical education was maturing such that by the beginning of the twenty-first century the meaning of inclusive physical education was very clear. It meant "providing all students with disabilities the opportunity to participate in regular physical education with their peers, with supplementary aides and support services as needed to take full advantage of motor skill acquisition, fitness, knowledge of movement, and psycho-social well being, toward the outcome of preparing all students for an active lifestyle appropriate to their abilities and interests."[74]

Given this definition of inclusive physical education, what do we know about its implementation across Canadian provinces and territories at the various grade levels where physical education is actually taught in the curriculum? What do we know from the perspective of students experiencing disability who are engaged in inclusive physical education? As it turns out, neither question can be answered definitively or in much detail.[75] First, unlike the United States, there is no legislation in Canada forcing provincial governments or local school boards to protect the physical education

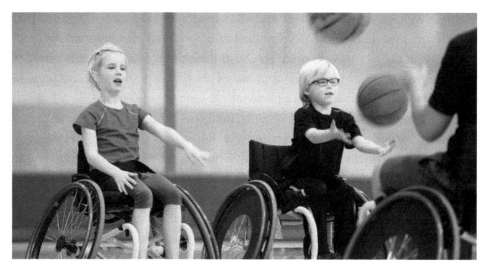

Figure 7.7. Children experiencing disability playing with basketballs (iStock)

needs of children experiencing disability. They must be trusted to do so, and there are no firm statistics to suggest that inclusive physical education is occurring widely in Canadian schools. Second, there is no formal certification to become an adaptive physical educator in Canada. Physical education students in Canadian universities sometimes have access to special courses in the field, especially where graduate programs are also available (for example at McGill University, the University of Alberta, and Lakehead University). Finally, and throughout most school systems, there is a lack of adequate supports – resource, moral, technical, and evaluation – so that physical educators attempting to be inclusive are usually on their own.[76]

As for what children experiencing disability think about their physical education and especially the notion of inclusion, again there are few studies. In one study, both positive and negative experiences in physical education classes were reported by elementary schoolchildren experiencing physical disabilities. "Good days," as they described them, included a sense of belonging, having opportunities for skilful participation, and sharing in the benefits of physical activity with their classmates; whereas "bad days" meant having their competence questioned by peers, being restricted in participation, and social isolation.[77] In another study that explored the perspectives of children experiencing disability participating in physical activity settings, their most important feelings about inclusion were gaining entry to play, feeling like a legitimate participant, and having friends.[78] Both studies confirm that, for children, it is the action of others that primarily contributes to whether or not they feel included in physical education and physical activity contexts.

Promoting Sport and Physical Activity for All

The first decades of the twenty-first century brought a reinvigoration of federal government funding targeted at promoting sport and physical activity well beyond the school environment. The successful Olympic bid to stage the 2010 Winter Olympic and Paralympic Games in Vancouver and Whistler encouraged the federal government to revive and strengthen various initiatives to promote competitive sport as well as physical activity. However, few of them made any effort to promote or link with school physical education.

The best known of the Vancouver/Whistler–inspired initiatives is Own the Podium (OTP). It was created to refocus Canadian institutions on competitive sport and provide research-focused funding for high-performance programs to help Canadian athletes win more medals in Vancouver and beyond. OTP was modelled on two previous Olympic-inspired programs, namely Game Plan developed for the 1976 Olympics and Best Ever for the 1988 Winter Olympics, both of which were phased out immediately after these games.[79] OTP funding was specifically directed at coaching and technical leadership, training and competition, sport science and medicine, and the organizational capacity to manage high-performance programs. With Canadian athletes winning a record fourteen gold medals in Vancouver-Whistler, the most of any country, OTP was continued. In addition to funding the specialized training of athletes preparing for major games, OTP has created Integrated Support Teams, including physiologists, sport psychologists, bio-mechanists, nutritionists, physical therapists, and physicians along with performance analysts. In recent years, OTP programs have continued to strengthen Canadian performances in international competitions. At the beleaguered Tokyo 2020 Olympic and Paralympic Games (postponed until 2021), Canadians finished eleventh overall, the best showing in thirty years. Women athletes, who were provided new opportunities to participate in a wider range of sports, were particularly successful. Yet OTP has come under fire for the way that it incentivizes winning at all costs. In the last few years, athletes in many of the Olympic sports have alleged sexual and other abuses in training and competition, so much so that the federal government has created a new Universal Code of Conduct to Prevent and Address Maltreatment in Sports, established the Office of the Sport Integrity Commissioner to provide an independent mechanism to investigate allegations, and promised a major overall of the way in which high-performance sports are funded, including OTP. It should also be noted that during the last few decades, while Canadian performances in international sports competition continued to improve, overall participation in sport and physical activity steadily fell.

ParticipACTION, well known to Canadians in the 1970s as discussed in chapter 6, was resurrected by the federal government in 2007, after more than a decade of neglect, with the provision of $5 million over two years to promote sport and physical activity among Canadians of all ages and abilities. Citing alarm over rising obesity levels and declining physical activity rates, the government announced support for the revival of ParticipACTION as a special measure designed to help Canadians develop healthier lifestyles. The primary focus was on social marketing, communications, and partnership synergy rather than physical activity program delivery. Three strategic priorities were identified: communications, capacity building, and knowledge exchange.[80] The new campaigns focused on promoting physical activity in daily life and making physical activity part of Canadian culture.

In many respects, it was the same old ParticipACTION – driving social marketing rather than providing actual programs or activities, albeit with the benefit of better monitoring and research. ParticipACTION's Report Cards on Physical Activity, for Children and Youth, for example, organized by one of its advisory groups, Action Healthy Kids Canada, were widely distributed and popular. By 2020, there were fourteen editions of these reports, which underscored the ongoing and dismal physical activity record of Canadian children and youth. They included the Canadian 24-Hour Movement Behaviour Guidelines for Children and Youth that encouraged the careful integration of physical activity, sedentary behaviour, and sleep each day and night.[81] Parents, teachers, exercise professionals, and pediatricians were called upon to disseminate and implement the guidelines and realize the ambitious vision of *Active Canada 20/20, A Physical Activity Strategy and Change Agenda for Canada*.[82] Its purpose was to engage decision makers and rally the collaborative, coordinated, and consistent efforts of all stakeholders at every level to reverse the decline in physical activity levels and the rise of sedentary behaviours. However, for physical educators it was basically yet another call to put Quality Daily Physical Education (see chapter 6) into action and to provide evidence to demonstrate the effectiveness of their school-based physical activity interventions.

In a critique of the adult version of the ParticipACTION report card for 2019, scholars point out that it "offers simplistic visions of complex health problems by excluding much with regard to class, gender, and ethnicity." It also fails to address the complexities that marginalized groups experience as stigma or obstacles to accessing education and/or health systems. In other words, these report cards neglect to tell the "stories of racialized pupils in Canadian schools, which teach how a body ought to be and act in the context of racism, assimilation, and humiliation." It also "silences the traumatic legacies invoked by the genocidal history of the Canadian government as enacted through Indigenous residential schools and sanitoriums."[83] In sum, the "deep divisions of intersecting and multiple oppressions and inter-embodiment of health are not acknowledged.[84] There was some improvement in the 2021 report card, which assigned letter grades to eighteen different indicators grouped into four categories: Daily Behaviours; Individual Characteristics; Spaces, Places and Cultural Norms; and Strategies and Investments. It also indicated throughout the report that national data are needed to better understand the physical activity levels of distinct population groups (e.g., ages, genders, people living with disabilities, Indigenous peoples, newcomers to Canada, individuals who are pregnant), which at least recognizes the problem.[85]

A variety of other interest groups developed around the promotion of sport and physical activity in the twenty-first century that also affected levels of support for physical education. For example, True Sport, Sport for Life, and the Sport Matters Group were examples of newly created organizations heavily supported and promulgated by Sport Canada. The proliferation of these resource-dependent organizations led to a series of unintended consequences, including a crowded policy space where many actors lobbied government with the consequent boundary-spanning quarrels. However, they allowed the federal government to retain some control within these pluralistic networks, and to affect the nature of the Canadian sport and physical education landscape. At the same time, it acknowledged traditional, jurisdictional structures and provincial/territorial organizations while strategically advocating for changes at the grassroots level. As a senior Sport Canada official commented: "Education is a provincial mandate jurisdiction and we're not in that game and yet we may want to be advocating for a change in the educational system."[86] Sport Canada's goal of "more steering, less rowing" depended, of course, on the ongoing will of the rowers (the national sports organizers) to steer their efforts away from high-performance sport and row in a more inclusive direction in support of broadly based sports and physical education programs.[87]

For several decades now, there has been an ongoing and lively debate about the effects of neoliberalism on publicly funded education in Canada.[88] To adequately sum up these critiques is impossible except to say that public education is under attack: it is being more frequently marketed, privatized, and commercialized. On a practical level, and to varying degrees across the country, neoliberal policies have decentralized provincial responsibilities for education to municipalities, reduced the power of school boards, destabilized organized labour among educators, privatized programming within the schools, and mandated a standardized curriculum and province-wide testing of students. Neoliberal reforms, say many educators, "often result in less time teaching, lower quality of teaching instruction, less diversity of subject matter, less pedagogical variance and less creativity in the classroom" (or the gymnasium).[89] But how, specifically, has school-based physical education changed under neoliberal policies? As far as we can tell, there are no specific Canadian studies as yet, although there is information from countries such as the United States, Australia, and the United Kingdom with similar educational systems. Examples from these countries point to the outsourcing, or the delegation of educational programming to organizations outside the education system (for example, so-called healthy eating outsourced to fast food franchises); gym equipment funded through partnerships with corporations in exchange for merchandising contracts. More seriously, where math, science, literacy, and technology are valued and supported, physical and outdoor education (also art, drama, music) are downplayed or disappear altogether. However, as the authors of one study observe: "empirical accounts of how various neoliberal policies may be influencing how expertise is understood and practiced are difficult to come upon."[90] This is an area that obviously requires more study especially within the Canadian context. We continue this line of thought in the last chapter as we outline our views of Canadian physical education in the future.

Afterword: Physical Education for the Future

> Historically, pandemics have forced humans to break with the past and imagine their world anew. This one is no different. It is a portal, a gateway between one world and the next. We can choose to walk through it, dragging the carcasses of our prejudice ... and dead ideas ... behind us. Or we can walk through lightly, with little luggage, ready to imagine another world. And ready to fight for it.
>
> Arundhati Roy, 2020

More than four years ago, when we began writing this book, we could never have imagined the world in which we now live. The global pandemic has fundamentally altered all levels of education and schooling from kindergarten to grade twelve and beyond. It has also had an unfortunate effect on physical education, physical activity, and sport participation, resulting in the dramatic loss of the fitness and resilience they provide. While it stimulated some encouraging innovations, such as the use of the internet for teaching activities and the closure of urban streets for walking, cycling, and rollerblading, it forced the closure of school and college gymnasiums, dance studios, coaching facilities, and sports fields, and relegated much of the teaching of the moving body to outside spaces or the internet. During the first year of the pandemic, Ontario principals, for example, reported a 90 per cent drop in after-school sports in elementary schools.[1] In one national survey, 69 per cent of parents reported that their children were showing the signs of being less physically fit, and 64 per cent of children reported that they were finding it difficult to reduce stress and anxiety.[2] A survey conducted by Canadian Women and Sport reported that 94 per cent of girls, aged thirteen to eighteen, were playing less with one-quarter of them saying that it was unlikely that they would take up sport again.[3] Although much of the cancelled activity has returned, physical activity levels remain extremely low, while the barriers of inequality, sexism, racism, and disability remain high. In its most recent report card, ParticipACTION reported that only 28 per cent of children and youth met the physical activity recommendations of the Canadian 24-Hour Movement Guidelines.[4] It will take creative ideas, significant new resources, and enormous determination to restore and enlarge opportunities, while making them more accessible, inclusive, equitable, and of higher quality.

What are the challenges now facing physical education teachers? In this Afterword, we look to the future of physical education in Canada. While the pandemic brought about a variety of concerns for the role and future of school-based physical and health education, it also forced change as teachers, school boards, provincial education authorities, colleges and universities, and indeed the entire population dealt with the realities of on-again, off-again closures, health and safety protocols, remote and asynchronous learning, and much else. Given these issues, the central theme of this chapter is to ask how physical educators might continue to navigate the post-pandemic future so as not to return completely to pre-pandemic versions of physical education. What has been learned during the pandemic, and as many are asking in other areas of life, how do we not only bring it back, but "bring it back better"?

As schools, colleges, and universities cautiously reopened, it became clear that sports and physical education needed to be championed and thoughtfully revised to address the fall-out among many children and youth from prolonged seclusion and decreased socializing among peers, families, and teachers. Greater efforts will be needed to ensure equitable opportunities in sport and physical education for learners from typically excluded populations, including girls, LGBTQ2S youth, those experiencing disabilities, as well as Indigenous, Black, and immigrant students. The hope is that sport, physical education, and education more broadly will be used to help build stronger bridges between and among communities, especially those in conflict, and to create windows of opportunity for dialogue and reconciliation. More than a few observers see challenges ahead for post-pandemic educational institutions given the many difficulties encountered by students and teachers in teaching and learning activities, and the deepening discussions prompted by the pandemic concerning inequities in education and their effects. At the same time, the opportunities to embrace the new flexible design principles that COVID-19 brought to the fore may provide a more robust and equitable environment in which to work and learn in the future. Storms like a pandemic present a rare chance to bring winds of change to physical education and challenge the long-held belief that the subject is impermeable to change. As the pandemic weakens there are promising innovations and efforts apparent on the physical education landscape. Among them is a reorientation towards the outdoors and its many benefits, a growing desire to enhance children's opportunities for play, the burgeoning use of new digital technologies to promote physical activity within and beyond schools, and a renewed enthusiasm among young physical education teachers to refashion approaches to curricula. There is also a new determination in higher education to develop physical education teacher education programs that include and learn from Indigenous knowledges and traditions.

Rediscovering the Benefits of the Outdoors

The prolonged lockdown period during the COVID-19 emergency affected young people's access to regular physical activity and recreational sporting activities, and in some arenas pressed a rethinking of ways to help children and youth continue living active and healthy lives with an urgent new focus upon fiscal constraints and mental health challenges. The 2020–1 school year, for example, provided PHE Canada with a unique opportunity to witness first-hand how physical educators across the country "stepped up, demonstrating time and time again their resiliency, innovation, and creativity to foster meaningful experiences for their students during a very difficult time."[5] Some observed that teachers were teaching outside whenever possible, and that there was an interweaving of outdoor education and land-based learning into physical education in particular. The hope is that teachers will continue to be supported in using outdoor learning environments like forests, streets, and parks to teach physical education.

Indeed, the COVID-19 pandemic has led to a rediscovery of the outdoors not only for physical and mental health, but also for enjoyment, fun, and relaxation, and a way to feel a renewed sense of normalcy. Launched in 2019, Outdoor Play Canada (OPC) is a network of advocates, practitioners, researchers, and organizations working together to "promote and preserve access to play in nature and the outdoors for all people living in Canada."[6] Through consultation, OPC has developed several priorities for the outdoor play sector, and among those most relevant to physical and health education are: promote the health, well-being, and developmental benefits of outdoor play; advocate for equity, diversity, and inclusion in outdoor play; and ensure that outdoor play initiatives are land-based and represent the diverse cultures, languages, and perspectives of Indigenous peoples. Another priority related to our discussion here is to "leverage engagement opportunities with the outdoors during and after COVID-19."[7]

To this end, OPC conducted an environmental scan of Canadian outdoor programs, projects, services, and activities during the COVID-19 pandemic, identifying almost eighty initiatives across the country.[8] They distributed a survey to these programs seeking input on their experiences adapting during the pandemic, the challenges faced, and best practices realized. Briefly, they found that most initiatives were largely recreation- and health-oriented, and aimed at supporting parents in getting children and youth outdoors. Although their greatest challenges were the new and ever-changing safety protocols, outdoor programming was naturally suited to minimizing health risk and adhering to the protocols. Most importantly, the greatest learning echoed by outdoor play providers was the reminder that children and youth thrive in the outdoors, which of course is an important message when supporting them in recovery from the pandemic.

Another child-centred, nature- and play-based, outdoor education program – the Forest/Nature School – also experienced increased interest and attendance during the pandemic. A recent survey of forest school practice in Canada showed that these programs vary in terms of size, age of children, type of outdoor setting, funding source, and schedule.[9] The exact number of these schools in Canada is unknown, yet they appear to have opened all across the country, predominately catering to urban families. The first outdoor nature program to utilize the Forest School label opened in Ottawa in 2007, while Forest School Canada was established in 2012.[10] The observed benefits to the children who attend these schools include better health, development of their social and physical skills as well as self-confidence, increased appreciation of nature, environmental awareness, and enhanced creativity. It is clear, however, that these schools and programs are not available to all children, given that the majority who attend are white and from families who can afford the tuition fees. Also, studies show that children with emotional, behavioural, and attentional challenges thrive in these forest schools, but there is a lack of funding to fully support children with significant needs. More effort is required among these schools in building positive relationships with First Nations, Métis, and Inuit to learn from their experiences and cultures.

More generally, outdoor education has been used as a broad term referring to organized learning that takes place outdoors. Canada has an extensive history of outdoor education, including programs in summer camps, kindergarten to grade twelve schools, and post-secondary institutions. Indeed, we have discussed some of this history, especially the rich heritage of Canadian summer camps for children and youth, in chapters 2, 3, and 4. The COVID-19 pandemic forced the reduction or cancellation of summer camp programs, especially in Ontario, where most are located. The Canadian Camping Association, a not-for-profit, national association of provincial camping associations representing nearly 800 camps across Canada, did everything in its power to seek government financial assistance in order to help its member camps survive.[11] Only time will tell how many of these camps will continue to exist in the future.

What we have not discussed is the kind of outdoor education taking place in schools, colleges, and universities. One difficulty is the limited research about these programs given the vastness of Canada, and the variety of existing programs. When they have been studied, there is often a focus on Ontario because of its extensive network of summer camps.[12] Furthermore, outdoor education programs, especially those within the educational setting, range widely from the urban experiences described earlier to self-propelled wilderness travel, often considered the pinnacle of Canadian outdoor education. Clearly, we need more systematic information about these programs, especially whether they too will survive the restrictions imposed by the pandemic, although it is to be hoped that the lure of the outdoors and its healthful benefits will remain or become a part of every Canadian's experience.

Physical and Health Education Using Digital Technologies

The need for and incorporation of online learning activities, which increased dramatically during the pandemic, affected all aspects of physical and health education. Teachers and health promoters were quick to recognize that social distancing measures, including school closures and stay-at-home recommendations, opened – indeed required – opportunities for looking to different ways of being active through various uses of technology. Yet in the transition needed from the well-established face-to-face instruction and environments to virtual ones, physical education encountered particular difficulties. Physical education teaching and learning are deeply rooted in physical movement and movement exploration, and there are significant inequalities in students' access to home computers and spaces where they could move and practise. For physical education teacher educators, the pandemic brought unprecedented challenges in the uses of technology, but it also opened up new opportunities to focus on the advantages of blended teaching, also known as hybrid learning, and the use of videos, visual aids, and culturally relevant online materials. According to some PHE Canada commentators, however, putting the "E" in online PE carried the real danger of reducing physical education to a narrow band of activities that could be learned through a YouTube playlist or repetitive fitness routine. They felt it lacked the wide variety of intangible skills that make up healthy, active, engaged, and well-rounded citizens in a rapidly changing world. At no point, they insisted, can physical education be replaced by simple fitness videos and programs, no matter how flashy and easy they may be. An online learning environment might serve in an emergency, but it is not generally effective for physical education.[13] We forget at our peril the benefits that accrue from physical learning in spacious, well-lit and serviced facilities, and high-quality specialized equipment. It is no secret that the best athletes depend on outstanding facilities.

Yet digital literacy has become a requirement for ever-younger students who are increasingly challenged to use digital techniques in their physical education classes, indeed all their classes, while at the same time not abusing the tools already at their disposal (e.g., social networking through TikTok, Instagram, and Twitter, and watching videos on YouTube). Instagram, for example, can be used to engage teenage girls in learning about their bodies, health, and well-being while resisting harmful dominant discourses about "perfect" slender and shapely bodies. Wearable technology (estimated to be a $95 billion industry) was number one for the fifth year running in the American College of Sports Medicine's worldwide survey of fitness trends for 2020. It included fitness trackers, smart watches, HR monitors, and GPS devices variously tracking heart rate, calories, and sitting and standing time. A year later, illustrating the effects of COVID-19, online training replaced wearable technology as the new number one in the survey with outdoor activities moving up into fourth place.[14] Here, too, widening income disparities severely reduce the ability of many children to benefit from these technologies.

Some researchers suggest that pedagogical questions will wane in importance as physical and health education digitizes itself, showing how critical technology and automation have become to the subject, though not necessarily to the PHE teacher who may not even be needed in computerized teacher-free delivery and new modes of data collection and accountability.[15] In light of the continued medicalization of everyday life, the possibility increases that digital technology could largely cut schools and teachers out of the health and physical education loop, allowing health authorities and related groups to more easily bypass teachers by posing health and physical activity as technological problems rather than pedagogical ones. Fitness trackers, for example, treat bodies as objects in need of constant attention and improvement, thus fostering an instrumental orientation towards movement that reinforces the mind as separate from and superior to the body. The effect could be to turn health and physical education into an instrument of social control in the future, a possibility that should continue to be resisted.

Uses are invented for and not created by state-of-the-art technologies, making new approaches to health and physical education attractive to students, such as "exergaming" or interactive fitness tools, which combine exercise and video games to create an interactive experience. Numerous self-tracking apps have been designed specifically for health and physical education teachers to use successfully with their students. However, there is a danger that the type of information about students' bodies generated by digital technologies will place too much emphasis on parental surveillance, and on students' obligation for ongoing self-improvement in relation to their size, body shape, and/or eating and exercise habits. As a result, schools and teachers using these technologies will need to pay closer attention to their broader implications, including issues of privacy and the ways in which the personal data of students could be used and/or exploited. As one expert warns, research into how and why digital technologies are being selected and used in physical and health education, and how the digital data they generate are appropriated for other purposes requires far more investigation.[16] As well, more information is needed regarding how particular digital technologies in physical education might assist students experiencing physical disabilities, many of whom faced additional challenges in the context of the pandemic. Indeed, it has become abundantly clear that all teaching needs to prepare students for a growing knowledge economy, the digital environment, and the social and cultural shifts that continually occur.

Ongoing Struggle over Health and Physical Education Curriculum Development

Educational curricula are the expression of complex historical and contemporary factors as well as timely interventions. These may include the purpose and effectiveness of former policies, the ambition and ideology of governments in power, the current and accepted state of knowledge, and also public opinion. As we have shown in previous chapters, health and physical education curricula, and their associated resource allocation, along with the effectiveness of their implementation, have the capacity to engage students and promote healthy, joyful physical activity, or to disengage or unduly regiment them by pushing the subjects to the fringes of school priorities. These continue to be important matters of both public and professional debate.

Historically, physical fitness testing has been, and continues to be, a source of controversy among physical educators. From the onset, agreement was lacking as to its definition. In the eyes of early test developers, physical fitness was best exemplified by athletic prowess. With the encouragement of the medical profession, this was followed by a strong focus on health-related fitness deemed necessary for a robust life (see chapter 5). Many accounts from past generations, however, provide less than fond memories of fitness testing as a result of inappropriate assessment practices, which caused personal anxiety and a loss of interest in physical activity.

We have seen in chapter 6 how the Canadian initiative ParticipACTION famously shamed its citizens by comparing them to aging Scandinavians, who were thought to know better how to sustain health-related physical fitness across their lifetimes. Despite continuing evidence that the social determinants of health are more important to health than lifestyle choices, the public and media have continued to focus on personal lifestyle choices as the key determinants of health. Within this context, health – increasingly defined by a variety of medical and lifestyle models – has been accommodated in physical education curricula in the last three decades or more. Indeed, we have seen how the promotion of these various models has played an important and continuing role in attempting to steer the agenda of physical and health education training as well as the nature and content of school and community programs.

In a 2014 study designed to ask what philosophies and values underlie individual provincial/territorial physical education curriculum policies in Canada, researchers created a policy analysis framework.[17] It identified three categories or models of curriculum policy: (1) *Traditional* reflected an emphasis on competitive sports and fitness, and individual behavioural change; (2) *Interactive/constructionist physical literacy* reflected a social/development approach to physical activity; (3) *Critical physical literacy* addressed empowerment, critical analysis, identifying power imbalances, questioning assumptions, advocacy, and action for social change. Their analysis found that all three categories were present to varying degrees in physical education policies across the country, although not surprisingly elements of critical physical literacy were the scarcest. Overall, the legacy of sports and medically defined fitness was the basis for physical education curriculum policies across the country. The choice of activities used to develop movement skills continued to be drawn more frequently from competitive team sports taught in school facilities designed for that purpose. Teachers still tend to be accused of sustaining the repetitive learning of skills and techniques associated with a core curriculum of sports dominated by traditional games, which may not reflect pupils' needs or the wider movement culture outside of the school. Indeed, some go so far as to argue that physical education in today's schools may not be "fit for purpose" in the twenty-first century.[18] The forms of physical culture that gave physical education-as-sport-techniques its cultural legitimacy in the mid-twentieth century such as amateurism have largely disappeared, and future demands for innovation and greater pupil autonomy may be difficult for physical educators to meet.

In an age of rising precarity (lacking in predictability, job security, material or psychological welfare), and its effects upon young people's ability to navigate various pathways to physical and health literacy, physical educators have turned increasingly to a focus on issues of health and well-being within their curricula to combat issues such as cyber-bullying, body shaming, poverty, racism, and gender discrimination.[19] It has pressed them to equate health promotion much more explicitly with physical education than was the case three or four decades ago. It also helps to explain why entrepreneurs and government officials from outside their field have managed so diligently to promote their influence within and outside of the school curricula, and into the detailed affairs and institutions of their communities. We have seen how, when ParticipACTION pressed for a 2020 physical activity plan claiming that less than half of Canadian children and youth were achieving their standard twenty-four-hour movement guidelines, Sport for Life Canada, the Indigenous Sport, Physical Activity and Recreation Council, the Childhood Obesity Foundation, PHE Canada, and various provincial physical education associations all jostled to deliver their versions of physical and health literacy that should be central to quality physical education programs.[20] When ParticipACTION celebrated its fiftieth birthday in 2021, the focus was necessarily turned upon the effects of the pandemic, the resulting mental health issues, and new ways to encourage and support Canadians to get up and move for the sake of their health. It was a prescient reminder of the staying power of long-standing, divisive debates among leading North American physical educators regarding education *of the physical* (emphasizing health, muscle, and physical fitness) or *education for the physical* (with attention to mind–body holism, and the social and cultural domains). In today's world, upended with the pressures brought by COVID-19, as well as a growing insistence on educational equity and justice, there are important arguments for physical educators to place considerable value on their pupils' health and fitness but always emphasizing the joyous satisfactions and modes of connectivity to be gained from play, games, sport, and dance.

Studies show that secondary school health and physical education curricula still silence and deny certain experiences, histories, and identities of Indigenous, Black, and new immigrant populations in their approaches to race and culture, while at the same time enabling other, primarily white perspectives to dominate. Indeed, whiteness clearly benefits those who already engage with Eurocentric practices of health and share similar values about healthy living and sporting practices. Even the most up-to-date curricula tend to focus on biomedical approaches to health intervention and ways of learning how to become a healthy, active, and engaged citizen with little consideration of the ways in which race and culture have shaped the content and messages conveyed. Furthermore, the teachers who develop and deliver health and physical education curricula, as well as the teacher educators within higher education institutions, are themselves largely embedded within systems still mostly dominated by white privilege, such that unconscious or conscious racial positioning remains unnoticed. As a result, the selection of health and physical activity knowledge, and teaching strategies appropriate for students in today's (and tomorrow's) world can become difficult and controversial. Where First Nations, Métis, and Inuit communities are concerned, stereotypical images of cultural health and healing practices through a Western biomedical framework carry a host of potential problems. These include obscuring the historical and ongoing role colonialism has played in the destruction of Indigenous societies, and the consequences for Indigenous health and well-being. Ontario's most recent health and physical education curriculum, for example, wrestles with these issues by providing an entry to learn more about students' culture and environment in relation to health, but a much greater effort is needed in the future to create a better and safe space for everyone.[21]

Higher Education Training in Physical and Health Education

While university faculties of education find their resources strained to offer substantive physical education teacher education (PETE) programs, kinesiology programs, which claim more scientific underpinnings, have seen increasing enrolments of students. They are attracted to the study of human movement as it relates to the enhancement of human performance, promotion of health, and the prevention and management of sports injuries and chronic disease. Indeed, more and more students are viewing their kinesiology degree as a stepping stone to further qualifications in the health science professions. They form the corpus of future physiotherapists, and strength and conditioning trainers. Many also aspire to postgraduate training to access credentials for health care professions such as dentistry, medicine, nursing, pharmacy, and occupational therapy. Now that Ontario has officially established kinesiology as a regulated health care profession, other provinces are working assiduously towards that goal. A related step has been for some kinesiology departments to align themselves with schools or faculties of Public Health, which from a curricular perspective leaves little room for sports-related or physical activity courses. This marks a return to much earlier notions of kinesiology dedicated to the anatomical and mechanical fundamentals of human movement, and it could well lead to a loss of identity or possibly the demise of the field. At the University of Alberta, for example, the Faculty of Kinesiology, Sport, and Recreation is now part of the all-encompassing College of Health Sciences (including Medicine and Dentistry, Nursing, Pharmacy and Pharmaceutical Sciences, Public Health, and Rehabilitation Medicine) with 770-plus faculty, and 7,200 undergraduate and graduate students. It is hoped that this arrangement might bring a "new level of interdisciplinary health science research and teaching that advances the full spectrum of human health and wellness."[22]

In 2021, according to the Canadian Council of University Physical Education and Kinesiology Administrators (CCUPEKA), there were twenty accredited university kinesiology programs across Canada with nine of these also accredited as physical education teacher education programs.[23] These realignments within departments and faculties in Canadian colleges and universities have had multiple effects including the selection and provision of knowledge deemed important for teacher educators to absorb, such that the discourses of performance (e.g., exercise physiology, anatomy, and sport medicine) have been privileged over pedagogical knowledge and skills. The developments are "a reflection of the extent to which, over the past half century, physical and health education professionals have gradually, and at time fervently, disavowed their roots in physical activity and sport, while at the same time marginalizing those who continue to pursue applied rather than basic research programs."[24]

The defining principle of curriculum reform and implementation requires trusting teachers as the experts in their craft. Key to their success is a system of teacher preparation that carefully selects future teachers with diverse backgrounds and includes organized practice teaching and systematic mentoring as a valuable part of their training. Unfortunately, this has not been reinforced by the ongoing distrust between schools and universities, or by the deployment of teacher training programs to faculties of education with decreasing support from kinesiology departments that favour research labs over courses concerned with the management of physical activity. Nor have these programs been assisted to any great degree by liaisons with university centres of dance and the creative arts, research centres of disability, or early childhood education, which all claim to value the importance of nurturing and training the moving body but may have little interest in connecting with physical educators. As an eminent historian of physical education pointed out when envisioning whether physical education could become the Renaissance field of the twenty-first century: "on many campuses, departments of physical education are often among the few remaining units concerned with whole, integral human beings – biologically, psychologically, socially, culturally, historically. We should capitalize on this!"[25]

Looking ahead, the manner in which the field of higher education is organized and supported is obviously critical for the preparation of future physical educators who need to be well trained to address the growing complexities of a post-pandemic, neoliberal world through a socially critical pedagogy. In some respects, more has been written about the need for critical pedagogy than how it can best be operationalized through teacher education programs, and teaching strategies and approaches. Critical pedagogy might best be seen as a way of thinking, or an opportunity to create a community of inquiry on what to value and how to act in relation to teachers and learners in physical education in a rapidly changing world. But the dialogue and reflection called for in critical pedagogy require assistance and ongoing practice for all physical educators in schools, communities, colleges, and universities. Thus, there is room to focus on the future selection, training, and support of socially critical teacher educators in Canadian higher education who are able to practise student-centred pedagogies in diverse communities, and to take a lead in designing and developing an education for a world of rapid change. Whatever form these take, they must be as tightly aligned as possible with the various dimensions of physical culture that all Canadians value and wish to transmit and renew in the future.

Meaningful Physical Education: A New Approach?

As we have seen previously, the current emphasis in many contexts is on what some view as a narrow set of utilitarian, health-based outcomes for young people, where disease prevention through personal fitness is privileged over the joy of movement. The aim of some physical educators, however, is for children "to walk through the doors of a gym or dance studio or enter onto a field, hiking trail, bike path, or body of water and be filled with a sense of excitement, joy, and adventure rather than dread, boredom, or fear."[26] They argue that physical education is better positioned as an opportunity for students to engage in active participation in ways that make experiences more meaningful and enrich their lives. Therefore, the primary theme of *meaningful physical education* is "to support students in coming to value physical education through experiencing meaningfulness," which means "interpreting an experience as having personal significance and recognizing ways participation enhances the quality of their lives."[27] Of course, this child- and student-centred approach is not something new, and we would remind readers of our analysis of movement education, including creative dance, that came to Canada after the Second World War and prevailed, especially at the elementary level, into the 1980s (see chapter 5). But it does ask school administrators to think creatively about how their school and its teachers can become assisted, as well as more invested, in broadening physical activity opportunities that can be fruitful for all pupils during their time at school.

Meaningful physical education stems in part from the ideas posed by American sports philosopher Scott Kretchmar in his articles published in the early 2000s.[28]

He differentiated between joy-oriented physical education, grounded in meaning, and health-oriented physical education, grounded in biological and physiological facts related to heart rate, caloric expenditure, range of motion, and the like (in other words, the mandates of efficiency). Although it is possible, sometimes necessary, to have both, in Kretchmar's view joy-grounded physical education should have priority over any health-focused program.

Canadian and Irish physical educators have broadened meaningful experiences in physical education to include social interaction, challenge, fun, motor competence, personally relevant learning, and delight. They have also created LAMPE, the online presence of the Learning About Meaningful Physical Education research project, which contains sources, documents, research papers, blogs, and podcasts.[29] The first phase of this longitudinal research and teaching project focused on ways to prepare future physical education teachers and coaches to foster meaningful engagement in physical activity through physical education and youth sport. The second and current phase involves developing an approach to meaningful physical education that will be implemented and refined by a sample of teachers working mainly in primary/elementary schools.[30]

Indigeneity and EDI Initiatives: Still a Long Way to Go

Public discussions about Indigenous sport and physical education are typically inserted into equity, diversity, and inclusion (EDI) categories. Certainly, there are overlapping issues of concern, such as increasing the number of Indigenous students and staff in university faculties of kinesiology, sport, and/or physical education (see chapter 7) as well as addressing racism. However, framing Indigenous physical education and sport as an EDI issue poses fundamental challenges for Indigenous people.[31] Not only does it reinforce colonial beliefs, practices, and structures about sport and physical education, it often marginalizes the critical ways in which Indigenous people are using sport and physical activity for Indigenous nation-building and cultural revitalization. Therefore, Indigenous sport and physical education should be understood and examined apart from EDI frameworks and pitfalls. Sometimes (see below) it makes sense to include both in an exploratory study or task force, although it is important to keep them separate.

More than two decades into the twenty-first century, what are Canadian university departments, schools, and faculties of kinesiology, sport, recreation, and physical education doing (or intending to do) with regard to creating and enhancing pathways to Indigenous achievement? Although a systematic survey was not possible, it is clear there is a good deal of variation in commitment within these programs, ranging from doing nothing, to just getting started, and, most importantly, to implementing serious and thoughtful Indigenous engagement. What we can provide are a few examples particularly of the latter. It should also be noted that university units often address these issues in their strategic plans, although many do not, and it is sometimes difficult to know exactly what has or has not been implemented.

Nonetheless, the first step is often a comprehensive study or task force, and the University of Toronto's Faculty of Kinesiology and Physical Education is an excellent example. Prompted in part by the Calls to Action of the Truth and Reconciliation Commission of Canada, their Task Force on Race and Indigeneity operated from May 2016 to November 2018 with the final report released in early December 2018. The decision to study race and Indigeneity together was deliberate because of the need to "acknowledge the trauma of colonialism and racism within Canadian culture generally, and within the field of Kinesiology and Physical Education specifically." The Task Force also recognized "the potential and opportunity for a more productive, equitable, just and fair Faculty of KPE if policies and practices are developed and implemented using the insights of anti-racist, de-colonizing and Indigenizing philosophies and praxis."[32] Finally, although the focus, discussion, and recommendations from the Task Force concerned race and Indigeneity first and foremost, it also examined ways in which race and Indigeneity were necessarily connected to – or intersect with – other aspects of society and identity, such as gender, sexuality, social class, and ability/disability.

The University of Toronto task force also clearly defined equity, diversity, and inclusion, which is helpful to this discussion. *Equity* is the "fair and respectful treatment of all people and involves the creation of opportunities and reduction of disparities in opportunities and outcomes for diverse communities ... these disparities are rooted in historical and contemporary injustices and disadvantages." *Diversity* is the "demographic mix of the university community and involves recognizing and respecting everyone's unique qualities and attributes, but focuses particularly on groups that remain underrepresented." Finally, *inclusion* means creating an environment where everyone feels welcome and respected, especially those from underrepresented groups. It is also important to note that "while an inclusive group is by definition diverse, a diverse group is not always inclusive" and an inclusive university "strives for equity and respects, accepts, and values difference."[33]

The recommendations of the University of Toronto task force were comprehensive, yet at the same time specific, and grouped thematically into seven categories: Academics, Curriculum and Programming, Communications, Data Collection, Recruitment, Relationships, Space, and Training.[34] We encourage readers to examine them carefully as well as the follow-up 2019–20 *Equity Report*, which was a measure of progress in recruitment, curricular and co-curricular programs, research and scholarship, and infrastructure from the perspective of Indigeneity, as well as equity, diversity, and inclusion.[35]

Establishing a task force and conducting an internal study can often elicit support and welcome change concerning EDI and social justice. The Faculty of Education at the University of British Columbia, for example, through their 2021 *Task Force on Race, Indigeneity and Social Justice*, provided "recommendations and actions to systemically improve the experiences and outcomes of Indigenous and racialized students, employees, and community members" within their faculty.[36] Responding to concerns in the task force recommendations, the School of Kinesiology pointed to its Indigenous Studies in Kinesiology program designed to introduce students, faculty, and staff to Indigenous understandings of health and well-being, and "provide comprehensive insight into the complex social, cultural, historical, and economic factors that shape healthy living within Indigenous communities."[37] Furthermore, a full-time Indigenous Student Adviser was hired along with a new Indigenous faculty member to support and enhance Indigenous-focused curricula offerings that will be required for all incoming kinesiology students.

The Faculty of Kinesiology and Recreation Management (FKRM) at the University of Manitoba is further along in an Indigenization process primarily because, in 2015, this university approved a planning framework of five major priorities to guide the university's decision making through to 2020, one of which was "Creating Pathways to Indigenous Achievement." FKRM's strategic plan for 2015–20 (extended to 2022) contains over ninety references to Indigenous or Indigeneity.[38] Out of twenty-seven faculty in the FKRM, four are Indigenous, including one who also serves as the Director for Indigenous Engagement. Inspired by the Truth and Reconciliation Commission's calls to action, FKRM is committed to working with Indigenous community elders, leaders, key stakeholders, and the university's Office of Indigenous Achievement to reclaim the transformative potential of physical activity, human movement, sport, recreation, and leisure as understood through the distinct cultural lens of Manitoba's Indigenous peoples.

Other Canadian university programs in kinesiology and physical education are just getting started with regard to considering Indigeneity initiatives and EDI. The University of Alberta's Faculty of Kinesiology, Sport, and Recreation, for example, has for some time maintained a certificate program in Aboriginal Sport and Recreation administered jointly by that Faculty and the Faculty of Native Studies. It is open to students enrolled in degree programs in either of the two units.[39] In 2022, the Faculty of Kinesiology, Sport, and Recreation established an Indigenous Initiatives and Equity, Diversity, and Inclusion Action Committee (II & EDI).

One positive way forward to contribute to and learn from Indigenous perspectives on the development of physically educated youth calls for a Two-Eyed seeing approach, whereby from one eye you can view the strengths of Indigenous ways of knowing and from the other estimate the utility of Western perspectives. The approach requires one to draw on the strengths of both perspectives to help create a shared understanding of salient issues related to being active, staying healthy, and developing life skills and sporting interests in today's society.[40] As a framework, Two-Eyed seeing can provide opportunities to bring together both Indigenous and Western knowledge systems once it is understood that Indigenous and non-Indigenous children and youth are more likely to succeed when the knowledge they possess and the competencies they have can be incorporated into the fabric of both schools and communities. In the spirit of fully respecting the treaty partnerships we form with the Indigenous peoples, we must find new ways of imparting Indigenous knowledge of the land and the body, and their forms of physical education, games, and dances to Canadian students. At the same time, we must better understand and critique the ways in which the dominant narratives of Western medicine and science have shaped the understandings and everyday practices in health and physical activity.

Overall, there appears to be a growing interest among Indigenous students in studying health and physical education, kinesiology and exercise science, recreation and leisure studies at the post-secondary level. For example, Indspire (a national Indigenous registered charity that invests in the education of First Nations, Inuit, and Métis people) receives on average about 170 applications each year for student funding in these fields of study. Despite calls for increased federal sources to advance these and other reconciliation issues, however, they can only support less than 30 per cent of their financial needs.[41] It is imperative, therefore, that departments, schools, and faculties of kinesiology, physical education, and recreation across Canada continue to find ways to entice these potential Indigenous students into their programs, and once there, support them in every way possible.

To look optimistically towards a future for physical education, we can imagine a society where Canadian children and youth have quality instruction appropriate to their needs, gender, culture, and abilities without undue cost or hardship. It should be educational in the truest sense by enabling them to acquire the knowledge, skills, and confidence to direct their own lifelong health practices, competently pursue whatever forms of physical activity they desire, and live with confidence and respect in a diverse society. Such instruction should be provided by a specialist sensitive to and trained to address individual and group differences and excite child-centred learning. Such a society must recognize and fund physical education as an essential right of citizenship, and a basic component of population health. It is imperative that we ensure that physical education across all levels pays full attention to diversity in its multiple forms, seeks innovative research and healthy development initiatives, and focuses on a full range of social justice and human rights concerns. How else can we provide all Canadian youth the joys and pleasures of a physical education that is student-centred, community-oriented, collaborative, flexible, evidence-based, and led by caring and well-educated teachers?

We began this history with Egerton Ryerson's vision for universal physical education in a free and accessible public school system as a requirement for Canadian citizenship. While the realization of Ryerson's vision was severely undermined by ideology and resources, subsequent generations pursued it ambitiously, providing opportunity for many. During the interwar period, through the Strathcona Trust, the federal and provincial governments cooperated to make a version of physical education the most widely taught elementary school subject in Canada. At the same time, outside the schools, other groups, institutions, and entrepreneurs provided a great variety of other opportunities, some of which, such as physical activity in the natural environment, significantly influenced the school system. The last sixty years have witnessed further experimentation, innovation, and expansion of opportunities, despite rapid, sometimes bewildering, social, economic, and technological change. That being said, survey research indicates that only a minority of Canadian children and youth enjoy quality physical education that meets their needs, and those who do are disproportionately from the white, urban middle and upper classes.

The vision of universal physical education in a free and accessible public school system is as valid as ever, although we would frame this as an inalienable right of citizenship rather than a requirement. The Canadian government, on behalf of all governments in Canada – federal, provincial, territorial, and municipal – has formally recognized physical education as a "fundamental right" in the eloquent *International Charter of Physical Education, Physical Activity and Sport*. Among its twelve articles, it promises opportunities free of discrimination, planned with democratic participation, delivered by qualified personnel, with adequate and safe facilities and equipment, protections against maltreatment and abuse, and high ethical standards.[42] Canadians must continue to push their governments to provide such opportunities, while contributing their own ideas, experiences, and energies to the outcome.

Appendix: R. Tait McKenzie Honour Award Winners

This award is PHE Canada's most prestigious honour and is named after the distinguished Canadian physician, sculptor, and physical educator, Dr. R. Tait McKenzie. The award epitomizes McKenzie's professional ideals, his service to humanity, and his dedication to the advancement of knowledge and understanding of physical and health education, recreation, and dance. As of 2023, the award was renamed the R. Tait McKenzie Lifetime Achievement Award.

1948 – Montreal

C.R. Blackstock, Newmarket, Ontario*
Ethel Mary Cartwright, Saskatoon, Saskatchewan
J. Howard Crocker, London, Ontario
Arthur S. Lamb, Montreal, Quebec
Doris W. Plewes, Ottawa, Ontario

1950 – Vancouver

Silas Armstrong, Toronto, Ontario
"Morrie" M. Bruker, Montreal, Quebec
E.W. Griffiths, Saskatoon, Saskatchewan
Robert Jarman, Winnipeg, Manitoba
Jack G. Lang, Montreal, Quebec*

Joseph H. Ross, Calgary, Alberta
Florence A. Somers, Toronto, Ontario

1952 – Toronto

Jules Gilbert, Montreal, Quebec*
Oscar Pearson, Toronto, Ontario
Wray Youmans, Winnipeg, Manitoba

1955 – Winnipeg

Mary R. Barker, Toronto, Ontario*
A.J. "Alph" Dulude, Ottawa, Ontario*
Iveagh Munro, Montreal, Quebec*

1957 – Halifax

Captain William Bowie, Montreal
Cecile Grenier, Neil, Quebec*
Alberta Hastie, Edmonton, Alberta

1959 – Edmonton

Rev. Father M. Montpetit, Quebec*
N. Rae Speirs, Toronto, Ontario*

1961 – Hamilton

Lorne Brown, Vancouver, British Columbia
Helen L. Bryans, Toronto, Ontario
J.B. Kirkpatrick, Montreal, Quebec*
Stanley T. Spicer, Fredericton, New Brunswick*
F.S. Urquhart, Montreal, Quebec

1963 – Saskatoon

William A. Hutton, Edmonton, Alberta (Posthumously awarded)
Elsie M. Macfarland, Edmonton, Alberta*

Hugh A. Noble, Halifax, Nova Scotia*
Ella B. Sexton, Toronto, Ontario*
Maurice L. Van Vliet, Edmonton, Alberta*
Gordon A. Wright, Toronto, Ontario*

1965 – Fredericton

M. Gladys Bean, Montreal, Quebec*
Arthur W.E. Eriksson, Edmonton, Alberta*
J. Wesley McVicar, Toronto, Ontario*
John H. Passmore, Toronto, Ontario*
Lucien Plante, Montreal, Quebec (Posthumously awarded)
W. Donald Smith, Edmonton, Alberta

1967 – Montreal

A. May Brown, Vancouver, British Columbia*
Helen Gurney, Toronto, Ontario*
Maxwell L. Howell, Edmonton, Alberta
William J. L'Heureux, London, Ontario*
John W. Meagher, Fredericton, New Brunswick*

1969 – Victoria

Alan F. Affleck, Edmonton, Alberta
Fred L. Bartlett, Kingston, Ontario (Posthumously awarded)
N.A. "Pete" Beach, Toronto, Ontario*
Elsie Gauer, Winnipeg, Manitoba
William A.R. Orban, Ottawa, Ontario
Robert F. Osborne, Vancouver, British Columbia*

1971 – Waterloo

Patricia L. Austin, Edmonton, Alberta
D.B. "Bing" Caswell, North York, Ontario
Nora Chatwin, Toronto, Ontario*
John R. Life, Toronto, Ontario
Marian H. Penney, Vancouver, British Columbia*

Robert H. Routledge, Edmonton, Alberta (Posthumously awarded)
E.W. "Wally" Stinson, Saskatoon, Saskatchewan

1973 – Calgary

Hart M. Devenney, Toronto, Ontario
Luther Goodwin, Calgary, Alberta
Rose Hill, Hamilton, Ontario*
W.F.R. "Frank" Kennedy, Winnipeg (Posthumously awarded)
John F. Mayell, Calgary, Alberta
Marion Ross, Kingston, Ontario*
Dorothy G. Walker, Truro, Nova Scotia*
Michael S. Yuhasz, London, Ontario

1974 – Ottawa

Stuart A. Bird, Edmonton, Alberta*
Stewart A. Davidson, Ottawa, Ontario
Patricia A. Lawson, Saskatoon, Saskatchewan
Howard R. Nixon, Saskatoon, Saskatchewan
Albert W. Thiessen, Toronto, Ontario
Joseph Willard, Ottawa, Ontario

1975 – Saskatoon

Jean M. Stirling, Toronto, Ontario
Earle F. Zeigler, London, Ontario

1976 – Quebec

David M. Boswell, Charlottetown, Prince Edward Island
John J. Keay, Toronto, Ontario
Russ Kisby, Toronto, Ontario
Fernand Landry, Quebec
Bryce M. Taylor, Toronto, Ontario

1977 – Wolfville

Donald A. Bailey, Saskatoon, Saskatchewan
Pasquale J. "Pat" Galasso, Windsor, Ontario
George Grant, Victoria, British Columbia*

1978 – Edmonton

Fred L. Martens, Victoria, British Columbia
M. Vance Toner, Moncton, New Brunswick

1979 – Winnipeg

Dorothy J. Harris, Edmonton, Alberta

1980 – St. John's

Evelyn M. Cudmore, Charlottetown, Prince Edward Island*
Donald MacIntosh, Kingston, Ontario
Donald M. Newton, Calgary, Alberta
Emmanuel "Em" Orlick, Newark, NJ, USA

1981 – Victoria

Ruby Anderson, Edmonton, Alberta
Audrey Bayles Hester, Ottawa, Ontario
Donald MacGregor, Toronto, Ontario
Archie McKinnon, Victoria, British Columbia
Murray F.R. Smith, Edmonton, Alberta

1982 – Montreal

James F. Leys, Almonte, Ontario*
F.M. Van Wagner, Montreal, Quebec*
George A. Wearring, London, Ontario

1983 – Toronto

No Awards Presented – Fiftieth Anniversary

1984 – Ottawa

R. Gerald Glassford, Edmonton, Alberta
Robert P. Hillier, Mount Pearl, Newfoundland & Labrador
Arthur Sheedy, Montreal, Quebec
Donald H. Williams, Calgary, Alberta

1985 – London

Joyce L. Boorman, Edmonton, Alberta
Mary E. Keyes, Hamilton, Ontario
Herbert McLachlin, Edmonton, Alberta
Richard J. Moriarty, Windsor, Ontario
Norman W. West, London, Ontario

1986 – Charlottetown

Wendy J. Dahlgren, Winnipeg, Manitoba
Juri V. Daniel, Toronto, Ontario

1987 – Vancouver

Carl J. Troester, USA
Thomas Bedecki, Ottawa, Ontario
Gordon Brandreth, Vancouver, British Columbia
Iris Bliss Hamilton, Toronto, Ontario
John James Jackson, Victoria, British Columbia

1988 – Edmonton

George Edward Longstaff, Coquitlam, British Columbia
Norman Jack MacKenzie, Regina, Saskatchewan

1989 – Halifax

Norma Adams, Dartmouth, Nova Scotia
K. Wayne Somerville, Kitchener, Ontario
Harold David Turkington, Victoria, British Columbia
Verna Jean Wilson, St. Catharines, Ontario

1991 – Kingston

Daniel G. Soucie, Ottawa, Ontario
Jennifer A.T. Wall, Montreal, Quebec
Eric F. Broom, Vancouver, British Columbia
Sheila Hedges-Anderson, St. John's, Newfoundland & Labrador
Warren Campbell, Scarborough, Ontario

1992 – Winnipeg

Richard (Dick) Lapage, Winnipeg, Manitoba

1993 – Moncton

Thomas F. Hanley, Fredericton, New Brunswick
Janette M. Vallance, Edmonton, Alberta

1994 – Victoria

Colin Higgs, St. John's, Newfoundland & Labrador
Shirley Hoad, Mississauga, Ontario
Stuart Robbins, Georgetown, Ontario
Kirk Albert Walter Wipper, Toronto, Ontario

1995 – Saskatoon

Dan Cooney, Calgary, Alberta

1996 – St. John's

Saul Ross, Ottawa, Ontario

1997 – Red Deer

Colin Lumby, Calgary, Alberta
Andrea Borys, Edmonton, Alberta

1998 – Saskatoon

Farida Gabbani, Truro, Nova Scotia
Garald Bowie, Alberta
Morag (Mo) Mackendrick, Surrey, British Columbia
Kenneth Ian Taylor, New Brunswick

1999 – Wolfville

Dr. C. Inge Andreen, British Columbia
Gerald Redmond, Alberta
Ken Loehndorf, Saskatchewan

2000 – Orillia

Moira Luke, British Columbia
Harold George Sawchuk, Ontario
Heather Morse, Nova Scotia

2002 – Banff

Rick Bell, Victoria, British Columbia
Nancy Francis (Murray), Welland, Ontario
Val Olesky, Edmonton, Alberta
Linda Thompson, St. Albert, Alberta

2003 – Winnipeg

Ian Craigon, Black Creek, British Columbia
David Fitzpatrick, Winnipeg, Manitoba
Garth Wade, Fredericton, New Brunswick

2005 – Regina

Andy Anderson, Toronto, Ontario

2007 – Moncton

Nicholas Forsberg, Regina, Saskatchewan
Andrew Pipe, Ottawa, Ontario
Norman Russell, Fredericton, New Brunswick

2010 – Toronto

Nancy Melnychuk, Alberta
Garth Turtle, Prince Edward Island
Myra Stephen, Ontario

2012 – Halifax

Sandra Gibbons, British Columbia
Ellen Singleton, Ontario

2013 – Manitoba

Grant McManes, Manitoba

2015 – Banff

James Mandigo, Ontario

2017 – St. John's

Ted Temertzoglou, Ontario

2018 – Whistler

Joy Butler, British Columbia

2019 – Montreal

Douglas Gleddie, Alberta

2020

M. Louise Humbert, Saskatchewan

2022

Leisha Strachan, Manitoba

2023 – Charlottetown

Janice Forsyth, British Columbia
Sylvain Turcotte, Quebec

---

* Indicates that there is a taped, oral history interview of this individual in the Stewart A. Davidson fonds available through Library and Archives Canada (Reference No. R5644-0-7-E).

Notes

Introduction

1. For an excellent historical summary, see Vertinsky, "A Question of the Head and the Heart."
2. Truth and Reconciliation Commission, *Final Report*.
3. For example, see Dashuk, *Clearing the Plains*; Graham, *The Mush Hole*; Greer, *Property and Dispossession*; Harris, *A Bounded Land*; Kelm, *Colonizing Bodies*; Miller, *Shingwauk's Vision*; Milloy, *A National Crime*; and Smith, *Seen but Not Seen*.
4. Canadian Historical Association, "A Syllabus for History after the TRC," https://cha-shc.ca/_uploads/6165982cda40d.pdf (accessed 3 January 2022).
5. Truth and Reconciliation Commission, *Canada's Residential Schools: Reconciliation*, 16.
6. Truth and Reconciliation Commission, *Honouring the Truth*, 331.
7. Ibid., 336.
8. Greer, "Settler Colonialism and Beyond."
9. Truth and Reconciliation Commission, *Canada's Residential Schools: Reconciliation*, 17.
10. Cited by Eisen, "Games and Sporting Diversions," 59.
11. Beers, *Lacrosse: The National Game of Canada*, 8–9.
12. For a history of lacrosse from an Indigenous perspective, see Downey, *The Creator's Game*.
13. Greer, *Property and Dispossession*.
14. For a history of this journal, now called *Sport History Review*, see Hall, "Fifty Years of Sport."
15. Library and Archives Canada reference number R5644-0-7-E.
16. Davidson, "New Projects/Nouveaux projets," 46.
17. The last interviewee did not pass away until 2021. She was Dorothy Walker Robbins from Nova Scotia, who was just a month short of her 101st birthday when she died.
18. Kirk, "Schooling Bodies through Physical Education," 477.

1. Ryerson and His Vision

1. *Canadian Sport Policy 2012*, 7.
2. While Ryerson continually referred to the area over which he held responsibility for education as Upper Canada, strictly speaking the colony of Upper Canada was joined with Lower Canada in 1841 to form the Province of Canada, and the portion previously known as Upper Canada became Canada West.
3. Ryerson, *"The Story of My Life,"* 537–8.
4. Gidney, R.D., "RYERSON, EGERTON."
5. Greer, *Property and Dispossession*; Russell, *Canada's Odyssey*.
6. de la Cour, Morgan, and Valverde, "Gender Regulation and State Formation."
7. Ryerson, *Report on a System of Public Elementary Instruction*, 20.
8. Gidney and Millar, "From Voluntarism to State Schooling."
9. Curtis, *Building the Educational State*, 56; R.D. Gidney, "Centralization and Education"; Prentice, *The School Promoters*.
10. Ryerson, *Report on a System of Public Elementary Instruction*, viii. Emphasis in the original.
11. Ibid., 58–9.
12. Ryerson, "Physical Training in Schools," 65.
13. Morrow, "Selected Topics in the History of Physical Education in Ontario," 36.
14. Cited in Prentice, *The School Promoters*, 29.
15. Cited in ibid., 35.
16. "Physical Education – Vocal Music," *Journal of Education for Upper Canada* 12, no. 5 (1859): 66.
17. "Harriet Martineau on Female Education – Calisthenics," *Journal of Education for Upper Canada* 13, no. 1 (1860): 11.
18. *Report to the Chief Superintendent of Schools*, Queen's Printer, Fredericton, New Brunswick, 1873, 11 and cited by Pearl-Cartu, "Social and Political Changes," 19.
19. Ryerson, "Military Drill in Public Schools," 113.
20. Ryerson, *"The Story of My Life,"* 64.
21. Smith, *Mississauga Portraits*, 19.
22. For a clear explanation of Egerton Ryerson's relationship with the Mississauga, and a plea for further scholarship, see Smith, "Egerton Ryerson and the Mississauga."
23. Cited in Milloy, *A National Crime*, 11.
24. Leslie, "The Bagot Commission," 39–40.
25. Ryerson, "Report by Dr. Ryerson on Industrial Schools."
26. Cited in Prochner, "Placing a School at the Tail of a Plough," 54. Prochner provides a detailed historical account of Hofwyl, based on the observations of many visitors to the school especially during the 1820s and 1830s.
27. Ryerson, *Report on a System of Public Elementary Instruction*, 20–1.
28. Graham, *The Mush Hole*, provides a detailed history of both the Mohawk Institute and the Mount Elgin Indian Residential Schools.
29. Prochner, "Placing the School at the Tail of the Plough," 60.
30. Indian Affairs, Province of Canada, *Report for the Half-Year Ended 30th June, 1864* (Quebec: Hunter, Rose, 1865), 26.
31. Creighton, *The Road to Confederation*; Waite, *The Confederation Debates*.
32. Miller, *Compact, Contract, Covenant*; Dashuk, *Clearing the Plains*.
33. McKenzie, "Frederick S. Barnjum and His Work"; "Physical Education," *Journal of Education, Province of Quebec* 12, no. 1 (1868): 9.

34 Barnjum, "Physical Education," 384, 386–7.
35 Originally from the *Montreal Evening Telegraph*, 12 January 1867, and cited in Slack, "The Development of Physical Education," 2–3.
36 Hébert, "BEAUDRY, CYRILLE."
37 Moody, "SAWYER, ARTEMAS WYMAN"; Moody, "GRAVES, MARY ELIZABETH."
38 Grenier, "BURGESS, THOMAS JOSEPH WORKMAN"; Rogers, "MACKIESON, JOHN"; and Kiefer, "DYMOND, ALFRED HUTCHINSON."
39 Downey, *The Creator's Game*, 74–7.
40 Kidd, "Muscular Christianity."
41 Metcalfe, *Canada Learns to Play*; see also Bouchier, *For the Love of the Game*.
42 Hall, *The Girl and the Game*.
43 Janson, *Emparons-nous du sport*; Kidd, *The Struggle for Canadian Sport*, 146–83.
44 Cited in Hunt, "A History of Physical Education," 18–19.
45 Ross, *The Y.M.C.A. in Canada*, 93.
46 A good example is the Boys' Brigade. Founded in Great Britain in 1883, it soon spread across the British Empire – in Canada by 1896, there were some 5,000 boys involved in over 100 companies affiliated with a church, mission, or other Christian group. Patriotism to the British Empire and faith in Christianity went together as boys were taught to honour Queen Victoria and to fear God. Military training and drill combined with athletics (cricket, football, gymnastics, and swimming) were the main physical activities. See Hopkins, "Youthful Canada, and the Boys' Brigade."
47 Ryerson, "Papers on Military School Drill," 149.
48 Burke, "Good for the Boy and the Nation," 75–89.
49 Cited in "Military Drill at Schools," *Journal of Education, Province of Quebec* 18, no. 9 (1874): 143.
50 Morrow, "Selected Topics in the History of Physical Education in Ontario," 47–51.
51 Burke, "Good for the Boy and the Nation," 22–3.
52 Morrow, "Selected Topics in the History of Physical Education in Ontario," 52.
53 Houghton, *Physical Culture*, 11.
54 Feminist historians have termed the vitalists "moral physiologists," because they substituted their own social vision for empirical science. They also point out that the vitalists conveniently ignored the extent of women's work during their childbearing years in households, agriculture, and industry. See Vertinsky, *The Eternally Wounded Woman*, and Lenskyj, "Femininity First."
55 Titley, "Indian Residential Schools in Western Canada," 135.
56 Miller, *Shingwauk's Vision*, 102.
57 Davin, *Report on Industrial Schools*, 1.
58 *Statistics Respecting Indian Schools*, 63–6.
59 Information summarized from report submitted by the Sisters of St. Joseph, Shingwauk Home, Sault Ste. Marie, Ontario, in Dominion of Canada, *Annual Report Department of Indian Affairs for the Year Ended 30th June, 1895* (Ottawa, 1896), 20–1.
60 Department of Indian Affairs, *Sessional Papers (No. 12)*, Standard Courses of Study, 1890, 171.
61 Department of Indian Affairs, *Sessional Papers (No. 14)*, Programme of Studies for Indian Schools, 1895, 246–7.
62 Dominion of Canada, *Annual Report Department of Indian Affairs for the Year Ended 30th June, 1896* (Ottawa, 1897), 125.
63 Dominion of Canada, *Annual Report Department of Indian Affairs for the Year Ended 30th June, 1897* (Ottawa, 1898), 244–5.

64 See Graham, *The Mush Hole*, especially pages 9, 23, 90–4. See also Habkirk, "From Indian Boys to Canadian Men," 227.
65 Dominion of Canada, *Annual Report Department of Indian Affairs for the Year Ended 31st December, 1888* (Ottawa, 1889), 146–7.
66 Dominion of Canada, *Annual Report Department of Indian Affairs for the Year Ended 31st December, 1889* (Ottawa, 1890), 296.
67 Dominion of Canada, *Annual Report Department of Indian Affairs for the Year Ended 31st December, 1895* (Ottawa, 1896), 114.

2. Towards a Pan-Canadian Curriculum

1 Axelrod, *The Promise of Schooling*, vii.
2 Harrigan, "The Schooling of Boys and Girls in Canada."
3 Johnson, "The Ryersonian Influence"; see also McNutt, "Shifting Objectives."
4 *Leader* (Toronto), 14 August 1861, cited by Gidney and Millar, "From Voluntarism to State Schooling," 468.
5 Cited in Titley, "Indian Residential Schools in Western Canada," 147.
6 Hunt, "A History of Physical Education," 3.
7 McNutt, "Shifting Objectives," 36.
8 Cited in Mott, "Confronting 'Modern' Problems Through Play," 57.
9 Axelrod, *The Promise of Schooling*, 116.
10 Social Darwinism is the theory that human groups and races are subject to the same laws of natural selection as Charles Darwin perceived in plants and animals in nature. It was used to justify political conservatism, imperialism, and racism and to discourage intervention and reform.
11 James L. Hughes's address to the young women of the normal school and the Faculty of Education, University of Toronto, 1909, cited in Berger, *The Sense of Power*, 257. See also Ellis, "HUGHES, JAMES LAUGHLIN."
12 Cited in ibid., 255.
13 There is a film about Lord Strathcona and the Strathcona Trust made in 1951 by Crawley Films Limited called *His Name Was Smith*. It is available through Library and Archives Canada (ISN 435457).
14 Cartwright, "Physical Education and the Strathcona Trust," 306.
15 Morrow, "Selected Topics in the History of Physical Education, 100–4.
16 *Syllabus of Physical Exercises for Schools*, v.
17 Morrow, "Selected Topics in the History of Physical Education," 224.
18 *Syllabus of Physical Training for Schools 1919*, 4.
19 Morrow, "Selected Topics in the History of Physical Education," 191.
20 Ibid., 220.
21 Personal communication from George Tomkins, professor of education, University of British Columbia to Bruce Kidd, 21 October 1982, in Bruce Kidd Fonds, University of Toronto Archives, University of Toronto, https://discoverarchives.library.utoronto.ca/index.php/bruce-kidd-fonds.
22 Bryce, *Report of the Indian Schools*, 18.
23 Ibid., 19.
24 Smith, *Seen but Not Seen*, 119. In 1913, Scott was appointed superintendent in charge of Indian Affairs, a position he held until 1932, when he finally retired.

25 Dominion of Canada, *Annual Report of the Department of Indian Affairs for the Year Ended March 31, 1910* (Ottawa, 1911), 274.
26 Dominion of Canada, *Annual Report of the Department of Indian Affairs for the Year Ended March 31, 1930* (Ottawa, 1931), 13. However, according to Miller, *Shingwauk's Vision* (462–3n67), since some students below the age of six and beyond fifteen were in residential schools, this calculation exaggerates the proportion of students in the institutions.
27 *Calisthenics and Games Prescribed for Use in All Indian Schools*, 3.
28 Ibid., 5.
29 Ibid., 17.
30 "Memorandum for the Guidance of Teachers in Indian Schools," Dominion of Canada, *Annual Report of the Department of Indian Affairs for the Year Ended March 31, 1911* (Ottawa, 1911), 439.
31 "Memorandum for the Guidance," 439.
32 Dominion of Canada, *Annual Report of the Department of Indian Affairs for the Year Ended March 31, 1912* (Ottawa, 1913), 330.
33 Dominion of Canada, *Annual Report of the Department of Indian Affairs for the Year Ended March 31, 1924* (Ottawa, 1924), 15.
34 Morrow, "Selected Topics in the History of Physical Education," 196.
35 Janson, "SCOTT, HENRI-THOMAS."
36 Morrow, "Selected Topics in the History of Physical Education," 205.
37 Gidney, *Tending the Student Body*, 18.
38 Minutes of the Executive of the Board of Governors, University of Alberta, 14 October 1913 and 6 June 1914.
39 Reid, *From Bloomers to Body Mass Index*, 88.
40 Habkirk, "From Indian Boys to Canadian Men."
41 Dominion of Canada, *Annual Report of the Department of Indian Affairs for the Year Ended June 30, 1896* (Ottawa, 1897), 321. See also chapter 1 of this volume, n45.
42 Dominion of Canada, *Annual Report of the Department of Indian Affairs for the Year Ended June 30th, 1904* (Ottawa, 1905), 325.
43 Graham, *The Mushhole*, 105–6.
44 Putnam and Weir, *Survey of the School System*, 395.
45 McNeill, *Keeping Together in Time*, 2.
46 Ibid., 152.
47 Putnam and Weir, *Survey of the School System*, 395–6.
48 Ibid., 226.
49 Ibid., *Survey of the School System*, 47.
50 Eaton, "The Life and Professional Contributions of Arthur Stanley Lamb," 32.
51 Lamb, "Physical Education," 159.
52 Ibid., 161
53 Cartwright, "Physical Education as a Profession." Several early MSPE graduates went on to stellar careers in physical education. For example, Zerada Slack completed a BA degree at McGill (1919–21) and a diploma from MSPE (1924–5). She taught at McGill (1928–39), Mount Allison (1939–42), and the University of Toronto (1945–65). Iveagh Munro attended MSPE (1922–3), and after several years of teaching obtained a master's degree from Columbia University. She returned to McGill for the remainder of her career (1939–66). Marion Ross attended MSPE (1925–6), followed by "Y" work in various cities, and then a long career at Queen's University (1934–71). There are extensive interviews available for these women. For Slack, see

https://discoverarchives.library.utoronto.ca/index.php/slack-zerada-oral-history (accessed 11 April 2022). For Munro and Ross, see the Stewart Davidson fonds, Library and Archives Canada, Items 435189 and 435320 respectively.
54 Walton, "The Life and Professional Contributions of Ethel Mary Cartwright," 54.
55 See, for example, Cartwright, "Athletics and Physical Education for Girls;" Cartwright, "Physical Education and Its Place in the School;" Cartwright, "The Place of Physical Education"; and Cartwright, "Physical Education and the Strathcona Trust."
56 Cartwright, "Physical Education and Its Place in the School," 112.
57 Ibid., 114.
58 Walton, "The Life and Professional Contributions of Ethel Mary Cartwright," 59. See also Reid, *From Bloomers to Body Mass Index*, 49–70.
59 Walton, "The Life and Contributions of Ethel Mary Cartwright," 92–114. See also Reid, *From Bloomers to Body Mass Index*, 71–92.
60 Kidd, *The Struggle for Canadian Sport*, 127–8; and interview with Joyce Plumptre Tyrrell, 10 June 1989. Tyrrell was a student and colleague of Lamb's at McGill.
61 Neil, "A History of Physical Education," 204–5; Webb. *The Challenge of Change in Physical Education*, 72; "Report of the Physical Education Committee of the Senate," in *Principal's Report*, Queen's University, Kingston, Canada, 1920–1, 43–4.
62 Clark, "Physical Education," 239.
63 Gidney, *Tending the Student Body*, 57.
64 *Third Congress of the Universities of the British Empire*, 1926, 168–73.
65 It should also be noted that all students were required to show "evidence of successful vaccination within the past seven years," and if not, they were required to be vaccinated.
66 For a useful analysis of Hall's *Adolescence* from a modern, psychological perspective, see Arnett, "G. Stanley Hall's Adolescence."
67 On the influence of G. Stanley Hall on early physical education and the playground movement in the United States, see Gagen, "Making America Flesh."
68 MacDonald, *Sons of the Empire*, 12.
69 Ross, *The Y.M.C.A. in Canada*, 191.
70 Our discussion about the YWCA in Canada has benefited greatly from the historical work of Diana Pedersen beginning with her master's thesis (1981) and her PhD dissertation (1987), both completed at Carleton University. She also published numerous articles and book chapters about the YWCA, and among them are: "Keeping Our Good Girls Good"; "The Photographic Record of the Canadian YWCA"; "Building Today for the Womanhood of Tomorrow"; "The Power of True Christian Women."
71 For the exact statistics, see Byl, "Directing Physical Education in the Canadian YWCAs," 141.
72 "Ernest Thompson Seton's Boys," *Ladies Home Journal*, May 1902, 15; June 1902, 15; July 1902, 17; August 1902, 16; September 1902, 15; October 1902, 14; November 1902, 15.
73 Anderson, "Ernest Thompson Seton and the Woodcraft Indians," 43. There has been a tremendous amount written about Seton's movement and his life. One of the most comprehensive and well-written sources is Anderson, *The Chief*.
74 Anderson, *The Chief*, 131.
75 Edwards, *Taylor Statten*, 88–90.
76 Baden-Powell, *Scouting for* Boys, xiv and xx.
77 Over the years, there have been suggestions that to some extent Baden-Powell was guilty of plagiarism, and specifically from Seton's *The Birch-Bark Roll of the Woodcraft Indians* (1903).
78 Dirks, "Canada's Boys – An Imperial or National Asset," 115.
79 Statten, "Canadian Standard Efficiency Training for Boys."

80 Macleod, "A Live Vaccine," 21. See also Ross, *The Y.M.C.A. in Canada*, 201–7.
81 Baden-Powell, "The Girl Guide Movement," 173.
82 Lamb, "Physical Education," 162.
83 For histories of the CGIT in Canada, see Prang, "The Girl God Would Have Me Be"; Blais, "The Complete Feminine Personality"; Marr, "Church Teen Clubs, Feminized Organizations." For a comparison of the Girl Guides and the CGIT, see Dirks, "Shaping Canada's Women."
84 Dirks, "Shaping Canada's Women," 157.
85 Blais, "The Complete Feminine Personality," 35.
86 Prang, "The Girl God Would Have Me Be," 161.
87 Gurney, *The CAHPER Story 1933–1983*, 13.
88 Neil, "A History of Physical Education," 48–9.

3. The Margaret Eaton School: Forty Years of Women's Physical Education

1 Meagher, "Professional Preparation," 67.
2 A settlement house was a kind of community centre set up to help people living in crowded immigrant neighbourhoods. Early graduates of the Margaret Eaton School of Literature and Expression taught music, gymnastics, and elocution, as well as performing in, or directing settlement plays and other entertainments. For a useful history, see James, "Reforming Reform."
3 There is a considerable amount of available historical information about the Margaret Eaton School. See a dissertation by Lathrop, "Elegance and Expression, Sweat and Strength," in addition to her published papers: "Elegance and Expression, Sweat and Strength: A Portrait of the Margaret Eaton Schools"; "Strap an Axe to Your Belt"; and Hallman and Lathrop, "Sustaining the Fire." See also the work of John Byl, especially his dissertation, "The Margaret Eaton School, 1901–1942," as well as his published papers: "Why Physical Educators Should Know about the Margaret Eaton School," and "Directing Physical Education in the Canadian YWCAs." He is also responsible for collecting and making available a remarkable digital archive about the Margaret Eaton School: https://libguides.redeemer.ca/MES (accessed 15 December 2021). See also Byl, "SCOTT, EMMA PRISCILLA (Raff; Nasmith)," Jackson, *A Brief History*, and also a chapter by Murray, "Making the Modern."
4 Nicholas, *The Modern Girl*, 4.
5 Ibid., 117.
6 Fletcher, *Women First*.
7 Posse, *The Special Kinesiology*. Posse's manual contained some 400 pages of tables and commands to assist the teacher of Swedish gymnastics in every phase of a lesson.
8 "Physical Education," *Montreal Weekly Witness*, 10 October 1899, 18.
9 Cited in Slack, "Development of Physical Education," 10–11.
10 Cited in Burdett, "The High School for Girls," 35.
11 Vendla H. Holmstrom, "Children and Breathing," *Boston Daily Globe*, 6 February 1916, SM13.
12 Schwarz, "Torque: The New Kinesthetic," 73.
13 Murray, "Making the Modern," 40.
14 A wonderful example of this is the famous movie *Metropolis* (1927), which illustrated the deadly mechanical dance of workers forced to operate the machines like robots. In 2001, the film was inscribed on UNESCO's Memory of the World Register, the first film to be so recognized.
15 Vertinsky, "Transatlantic Traffic."
16 Ruyter, "American Delsartism," 2015. See also Ruyter, *The Cultivation of Body*.
17 Cited in Ruyter, "American Delsartism," 2018. See also Walsh, *Eugenics and Physical Culture*, especially chapter 2.

18 Ruyter, "American Delsartism," 2022.
19 Veder, "Expressive Efficiencies."
20 *Proceedings of the American Association*, 84. See also Veder, "Expressive Efficiencies," 826–7.
21 McKenzie, *Exercise in Education*, 136.
22 For a thorough explanation concerning the principles of Dalcroze eurythmics, see Pennington, *The Importance of Being Rhythmic*.
23 Elie Marcuse, "La Grace et la Force," *L'Illustration*, 22 March 1913, 39–41.
24 *Congrès Internationale de l'Éducation*. See especially papers by Dr. Danjou and Dr. Nicole Girard-Mangin.
25 Emma Scott's birthdate has been erroneously reported in various sources as 1880. Although no birth certificate was found, her death certificate shows that she was born on 3 August 1869.
26 Her husband, William Bryant Raff, whom she married in Owen Sound, Ontario, on 6 June 1894, was in his early thirties when he died on 5 July 1897 of tuberculosis. Their daughter, Dorothy Victoria Scott Raff, was born on 23 October 1896 in Aspen, Colorado.
27 For more on this issue, see Lathrop's dissertation, "Elegance and Expression, Sweat and Strength," 55–64.
28 Ibid., 44–5.
29 Ibid., 65–6.
30 Chris Bateman, "A Brief History of the Margaret Eaton School in Toronto." http://www.blogto.com/city/2012/01/a_brief_history_of_the_margaret_eaton_school_in_toronto/ (accessed 13 December 2021).
31 Cited in Gerber, *Innovators and Institutions*, 291. See also Walsh, *Eugenics and Physical Culture*, especially chapter 3.
32 For information about George Gallie Nasmith, see https://cabbagetowner.com/tbt-april-22-1915-nasmith/ (accessed 13 December 2021). Their marriage took place in Toronto on 21 January 1916. On the marriage certificate, Nasmith is noted as thirty-eight and Scott Raff as forty, when actually she was forty-six.
33 Jackson, *A Brief History of Three Schools*, 10.
34 Lathrop, "Elegance and Expression, Sweat and Strength," 91.
35 Regarding the complicated financial arrangements between the Eaton family and the MES over its lifetime, see Byl, "The Margaret Eaton School, 1901–1942," 368–411.
36 Hallman and Lathrop, "Sustaining the Fire."
37 Hamilton, *The Call of the Algonquin*, 6. The Chautauqua Summer School in the United States was second only to the Harvard Summer School in its influence on teacher training, and a variety of gymnastic systems were taught there.
38 Hamilton, *The Call of the Algonquin*, 6.
39 Lathrop, "Strap an Axe to Your Belt."
40 Hamilton, *The Call of the Algonquin*, 174.
41 For an extended discussion of "playing Indian" at summer camp, see Wall, *The Nature of Nurture*, 216–50.
42 Hamilton, *The Call of the Algonquin*, 21.
43 Ibid., 177.
44 Ibid., 149.
45 Ibid., 90. See also Lathrop, "Elegance and Expression, Sweat and Strength," 178–9.
46 Verbrugge, *Active Bodies*, 25–6. Little has been written about this concern within early Canadian women's physical education.
47 Byl, "The Margaret Eaton School, 1901–1942," 342.
48 Cited in ibid., 389.

49 Somers, "Ideals for Girls' Athletics," 10.
50 In particular, see Hall, *The Girl and the Game*, 119–25, and Kidd, *The Struggle for Canadian Sport*, 119–25.
51 Verbrugge, *Active Bodies*, 47.
52 Lenskyj, *Out of Bounds*, 18.
53 Marian Henderson Penney is a good example. She attended OCE in 1931, where she was strongly influenced by Helen Bryans and her philosophy. Penney taught physical education in secondary schools in both London and Toronto, but after the war moved west to take up a position at the University of British Columbia, where she remained for the rest of her career. See Hall, *The Girl and the Game*, 122–3, and the Marian Penney interview (Stewart Davidson fonds, Library and Archives Canada, Item number 435326).
54 Bryans, "Secondary School Curriculum for Girls."
55 Lathrop, "Elegance and Expression, Sweat and Strength," 247.
56 Byl, "The Margaret Eaton School, 1901–1942," 378–80.
57 Cited in ibid., 384.
58 Cited in Lathrop, "Elegance and Expression, Sweat and Strength," 261.
59 Ibid., 271.
60 Ibid., 202.
61 See note 3.

4. Fit for Living

1 Mosby, "Administering Colonial Science."
2 Blackstock, "The Canadian Association for Health, Physical Education, and Recreation," 277.
3 Plewes, "Affiliated Organizations," 273.
4 For more on this issue, see Gurney. *The CAHPER Story 1933–1983*, 15.
5 Plewes, "Affiliated Organizations," 273.
6 Lamb, "Physical Education in Canada."
7 Lamb, "Looking Ahead in Physical Education," 9.
8 At this time, there were nine Canadian provinces. Newfoundland and Labrador did not enter Confederation until 1949. The study that follows did not involve the Northwest Territories or the Yukon.
9 Murray, "The Status of Physical Education."
10 "Danish Gymnasts Accorded Warm Welcome in the City," *Calgary Daily Herald*, 30 October 1931, 12. See Bonde, "Globalization *before* Globalization." Also, in *Gymnastics and Politics*, Bonde has written extensively about Bukh's gymnastic work and its liberating male aesthetic, but he also reminds us of Bukh's collaboration with the Nazis and his admiration of fascism, which inevitably affected the nature of his gymnastic work and its mobilizing power.
11 Murray, "The Status of Physical Education," 65.
12 See Neil, "History of Physical Education," 110–24. See also the interview with Lang conducted by Stuart Davidson in 1978 (Stewart Davidson fonds, Library and Archives Canada, Item number 435184).
13 There is also an interview (in French) with René Bélisle in the Stewart Davidson fonds, Library and Archives Canada, Item number 435191.
14 Morrow, "Selected Topics in the History of Physical Education," 238.
15 For more information about this course, see ibid., 240–50.
16 Wipper, *Retrospect and Prospect*. See also Lathrop, "Elegance and Expression, Sweat and Strength," 248–54.

17 Dominion of Canada, *Annual Report of the Department of Indian Affairs for the Year Ended March 31, 1932* (Ottawa, 1932), 11.
18 Department of Mines and Resources, Canada, *Report of Indian Affairs Branch for the Fiscal Year Ended March 31, 1938.*
19 Te Hiwi, "Physical Culture as Citizenship Education." See also Te Hiwi, "Unlike Their Playmates of Civilization."
20 Te Hiwi, "Physical Culture as Citizenship Education," 56.
21 From a pamphlet about the Sioux Lookout School designed to attract prospective students and staff described in Te Hiwi, "Unlike their Playmates of Civilization," 109.
22 Te Hiwi, "Physical Culture as Citizenship Education," 65.
23 Milloy's report was published as a book, which we quote from here: Milloy, *A National Crime*, xxxviii.
24 Miller, *Shingwauk's Vision*, 7–8. Located in Sault Ste Marie, Ontario, Shingwauk Indian Residential School ceased to operate in 1971 and is now the site of Algoma University.
25 Kelm, *Colonizing Bodies*, 57.
26 These were the conclusions from a national survey of day and residential schools conducted in 1956, so that conditions were likely even worse prior to the Second World War. See Truth and Reconciliation Commission, *Canada's Residential Schools: The History, Part 2 1939 to 2000*, 468.
27 British Columbia's Pro-Rec program has been studied extensively. The most thorough source is a dissertation by Schrodt, which also includes reference to the studies that preceded it. See Schrodt, "A History of Pro-Rec." There is also useful information on the internet; see, for example, https://scoutmagazine.ca/2019/11/18/the-origins-of-vancouvers-fitness-fetish/ (accessed 5 November 2021).
28 Eisenhardt, "Department of Recreational and Physical Education."
29 Macdonald, *Strong, Beautiful and Modern*, 136.
30 "Miss P. Stack Opens League," *Globe*, 26 September 1935, 10.
31 For an excellent analysis, see Vertinsky, "Building the Body Beautiful."
32 For more information about the League, see Matthews, "They Had Such a Lot of Fun." See also Stack, *Zest for Life*, and Vertinsky, "Building the Body Beautiful."
33 Eisenhardt, "Dominion-Provincial Youth Training Programme."
34 Schrodt, "Federal Programmes of Physical Recreation and Fitness."
35 For more on the early history of the OAC camp, see Kidd, "Making the Pros Pay," and McMurray, "The Organizational Growth and Development."
36 Kidd, *The Struggle for Canadian Sport*, 253.
37 West, "Physical Fitness, Sport and the Federal Government," 34.
38 "Health Training in Schools," 178.
39 West, "Physical Fitness, Sport and the Federal Government," 35.
40 Canadian Youth Commission, *Youth & Recreation*, 74–5.
41 Lamb, "National Physical Fitness," 29. He also provided a breakdown of the distribution of the grant to the provinces, provided only after a province established an organization for the purpose of promoting physical fitness and entered into an agreement with the federal government.
42 Eisenhardt, "Canada's National Fitness Act," 230.
43 Ibid., 187.
44 Axelrod, "Spying on the Young in Depression and War," 53.
45 Comacchio, *The Dominion of Youth*, 197.
46 By 1933 there were 1,015 Guide Companies, with 24,537 girls enrolled, and 95 Ranger companies (older Guides, over sixteen) with 1,699 girls. The 1937 annual report showed 50,784 members. Cited in Comacchio, *The Dominion of Youth*, 274n49.

47 Ibid., 203–4.
48 Department of Mines and Resources, Canada, *Report of Indian Affairs Branch for the Fiscal Year Ended March 31, 1942* (Ottawa: King's Printer, 1943), 135, 154–5.
49 Ross, *The Y.M.C.A. in Canada*, 393–5.
50 Ambrose, "Collecting Youth Opinion," 65.
51 Canadian Youth Commission, *Youth & Health*; and *Youth & Recreation*.
52 Canadian Youth Commission, *Youth & Recreation*, 49.
53 Ibid., 76. The CYC committee on recreation was chaired by Murray G. Ross of the National Council of YMCAs, who in all likelihood authored much of this report.
54 Canadian Youth Commission, *Youth & Health*, Appendix D, 64–9.
55 Ibid., Appendix F, 91–2.
56 Ibid., 20–1.
57 Comacchio, *The Dominion of Youth*, 203. For a detailed, historical examination of the commission, see Ambrose, "The Canadian Youth Commission."
58 The Member of Parliament was Conservative Tommy Church of Toronto's Broadview riding. Cited in Macdonald, *Strong, Beautiful and Modern*, 139.

5. Setting a Heroic Agenda – Realizing the Possibilities

1 Trained as a physical educator in England, Jarman came to Winnipeg in 1928 to assist in the reorganization of physical training in the city's schools. He was persuaded to remain in Canada, and from 1929 until 1951 was Director of Physical Education for the Winnipeg School Division (see Fitzpatrick, "The Socialization Goal").
2 The full text of Jarman's speech can be found in Plewes, "Canadian News," *Journal of Health and Physical Education* 16, no. 7 (1945): 397.
3 Eisenhardt, "Canada's National Fitness Act," 230.
4 West, "Physical Fitness, Sport and the Federal Government."
5 Plewes, "Canadian News." *Journal of Health and Physical Education* 16, no. 6 (1945), 336.
6 "Department Appoints Well Known B.C. Physical Director," *Bulletin of CAHPER* 17, no.1 (1949): 6.
7 Cited in West, "Physical Fitness, Sport and the Federal Government," 41.
8 Schrodt, "A History of Pro-Rec," 313–22.
9 Bruce Kidd notes that Plewes was "bright, funny, and inspirational" and that she was feared within the civil service especially by men. One deputy minister even hid under his desk when she came to see him (Kidd, *A Runner's Journey*, 106). As important as Plewes's position and influence were, we know little about her. Born in 1898 in Wallaceburg, Ontario, she received her early schooling in Chatham, after which she trained as a teacher. Beginning in the mid-1920s, she taught in elementary and secondary schools in London, Ontario. She completed post-graduate studies at Columbia University, attaining a master's degree, followed by a doctorate in 1943. Her EdD dissertation was "A Course of Study in Health, Physical Education, and Recreation, London, Ontario (Kindergarten to Grade XIII)." In 1946 she took a full-time position with the federal government, where she remained with the civil service until her retirement in the late 1960s. Her last position (in 1964) was establishing what became the Sport Information Resource Centre (SIRC). Plewes was also an amateur painter, and she is referenced in the *Biographical Index of Artists in Canada* (2003). She died in 1994 at the age of ninety-six.
10 "Present Standards Make for Physical 'Illiteracy.'" *Lethbridge Herald*, 28 July 1954, 19. Unfortunately, there does not appear to be published proceedings for this conference.

11 With regard to the Kraus-Weber test and the controversy about it, see Orban, "The Fitness Movement."
12 Interview with W.J. L'Heureux conducted by Stewart Davidson in 1979 (Stewart Davidson fonds, Library and Archives Canada, Item number 435315). These films are available in Library and Archives Canada. For example, for "No. 1 Skating" in the "How to Play Hockey" series, see http://central.bac-lac.gc.ca/.redirect?app=filvidandsou&id=123114&lang=eng (accessed 10 June 2022).
13 See "Scrub to Keep Fit," *Globe and Mail*, 2 December 1957, 14.
14 Plewes, "Physical Fitness – Its Problems and Implications."
15 Mossman, *Lloyd Percival*, 21.
16 Ibid., 25.
17 Percival, "Our Flabby Muscles."
18 Mossman, *Lloyd Percival*, 135–9. Listen also to the CBC Ideas radio program about Percival: https://www.cbc.ca/radio/ideas/lloyd-percival-canada-s-sports-prophet-1.6318337 (accessed 2 March 2022).
19 The correspondence between Zeigler and Percival was published as "Sports College Director Explains Product Research," *Journal of CAHPER* 19, no. 1 (1953): 9–14.
20 Some sources indicate that Prince Philip was installed as the "honorary" president of the Canadian Medical Association. He was indeed the president for the 1959–60 year, although he designated his deputy, Dr. E. Kirk Lyon of Leamington, Ontario, to act on his behalf.
21 "The Duke of Edinburgh's Presidential Address to the Canadian Medical Association," obtained from the Canadian Medical Association Archives Material. See also "Installation of the President," *Canadian Medical Association Journal* 81, no. 2 (1959): 116–18.
22 "The Duke of Edinburgh's Presidential Address."
23 "A Nation of Weaklings," *Globe and Mail*, 13 September 1960, 6.
24 The most complete analysis of the origins of Bill C-131 and its early impact can be found in Macintosh, Bedecki, and Franks, *Sport and Politics in Canada*, chapters 2 and 3.
25 *CAHPER Fitness-Performance Test Manual*.
26 *Physical Work Capacity of Canadian Children*.
27 See Macintosh, Bedecki, and Franks, *Sport and Politics in Canada*, 62–76.
28 "Edmonton Branch Examines Alberta's School Physical Education," *CAHPER Bulletin* 15, no. 6 (1948): 3, 5–6.
29 Province of Manitoba, *Education and Recreation*. See also Fitzpatrick, "The Socialization Goal," 96–110.
30 Potts, "The Development of Physical Education in Nova Scotia," 26–7.
31 For more information, see taped interviews with Hugh Noble and Dorothy Walker conducted by Stuart Davidson in 1978 (Stuart Davidson fonds, Library and Archives Canada, Items number 435199 and 435198). See also the delightful documentary film, *When All the People Play*, made in 1948 by the National Film Board. It focuses on the people of Annapolis Royal, Nova Scotia, and their efforts to create a recreation centre (https://www.nfb.ca/film/when_all_people_play/).
32 Plewes, "Canadian News." *Journal of Health and Physical Education* 16, no. 4 (1945): 204. Plewes's columns began in 1945 with volume16, no. 3 and continued until volume 17, no. 10 (1946), at which time she moved to Ottawa to take up a full-time position in Health and Welfare. The column was continued, but more sporadically, by Hart Devenney, director of physical fitness in Manitoba, until volume 19, no. 5 in 1948. Together they provide an interesting and informative account of physical education and recreation throughout Canada in the immediate postwar period.

33 Plewes, "Physical Fitness – Its Problems and Implications," 56.
34 Ibid.
35 Sexton, "Teacher Recruitment in Physical Education."
36 See Wright, "Youth Leadership through Camping." One author, Ann Hall, attended the OALC camp in 1958, and without a doubt it was instrumental in her decision to become a physical education teacher. This camp still exists today as the Ontario Educational Leadership Centre.
37 Plewes, "Physical Fitness – Its Problems and Implications," 58. See also Plewes, "Canadians: Rugged or Ragged?"
38 Hill, "The English Concept of Basic Movement."
39 Ministry of Education, *Moving and Growing*.
40 Ministry of Education, *Planning the Programme*. Most of the photographs in both volumes were taken by Austrian-born photographer Edith Tudor-Hart, who in 1934 fled Vienna and came to London, England. She also worked as a low-level Soviet operative in Austria and Great Britain (see Forbes, "'Tracking' Edith Tudor-Hart").
41 Plewes, "Physical Education in the Primary School."
42 For a concise, yet informative, history of movement education in Ontario between 1940 and 1970, see Lathrop, "Contested Terrain." For more detail, see Lathrop's master's thesis under Anna H. Course, "Movement Education." For a broader discussion of the rise and fall of the "female tradition" in Ontario elementary school physical education, see Francis and Lathrop, "Children Who Drill."
43 Tyrrell, "Watch Britain," 15.
44 Duncan, "A Report from England," 21. See also Reid and Duncan, "Anglo-American Course."
45 The key individuals were Nora Chatwin, Sheila Stanley, Mary Liddell, and Rose Hill.
46 Chatwin remembers these days in a wonderful interview conducted by Stuart Davidson in 1978 (Stewart Davidson fonds, Library and Archives Canada, Item number 435298).
47 Chatwin, "The Pioneers of 1968."
48 Ontario Department of Education, *Physical Education Primary Division Grades*, and *Physical Education Junior Division Grades*.
49 Stanley, *Physical Education*. Stanley taught in elementary schools and secondary schools in British Columbia before moving to Ontario in 1952, where she met Nora Chatwin. In 1954, Stanley visited schools in England observing classes in dance and gymnastics, and she also attended a summer course that included Laban as an instructor.
50 Kirchner also published *Physical Education for Elementary School Children* in 1966, which by 1998 was in its tenth edition.
51 Lathrop and Drake, "The Canadian Climber."
52 Valerie Proyer was a graduate of I.M. Marsh College in Liverpool. She arrived in Nova Scotia in 1951 and eventually completed a graduate degree at McGill. In 1969 she went to Lakehead University as an Associate Professor. See Proyer, "Formal and Educational Gymnastics – Why the Dichotomy?"
53 Potts, "The Development of Physical Education in Nova Scotia," 76–81.
54 Interview with Anne Tilley in Vancouver in April 2015 as part of a study of British teachers who came to Canada to teach movement education.
55 See Vertinsky, "Transatlantic Traffic in Expressive Movement." It should also be noted that Dorothy Harris, dance pioneer at the University of Alberta, studied with Margaret H'Doubler at the University of Wisconsin in the late 1940s.
56 Hussey and Murray, "Anglo-American Workshop." See also Reid and Duncan, "Anglo-American Course."

57 Hill, "Programme Improvement in Modern Dance," 8. Hill counted fourteen universities, but by the end of 1965, there were nineteen universities in Canada offering undergraduate degree programs in physical education. How many of these offered modern dance in their curriculum is not known.
58 Lathrop, "Contested Terrain," 178.
59 Simons, "Educational Gymnastics," 26.
60 Clearly, "Progress – Real or Imagined?" 10.
61 Anderson, "Movement Educators – Beware!" 43.
62 For an excellent account, see Kirk, *Defining Physical Education*.
63 Munrow, *Pure and Applied Gymnastics*.
64 For more detail, see Fletcher, *Women First*.
65 Neatby, *So Little for the Mind*, 16, 265, 267.
66 Barrett, "Movement Education in the 80s."
67 Lawther, *The Learning and Performance of Physical Skills*, 110.
68 Zeigler, *History of Physical Education and Sport*, 278.
69 Forsyth, *Reclaiming Tom Longboat*, 48.
70 For the actual job advertisement, see ibid., 49.
71 *Indian School Bulletin* 4, no. 4 (1950): 18–19. In this announcement, it mentions that Eisenhardt spent the last year as "Secretary to an International Commission on Educational Reconstruction." Eisenhardt's job with the United Nations was abolished in April 1948, and he was reassigned to the Commission for International Educational Reconstruction (which already had a secretary in Washington, DC). By March 1949, this organization had shut down and transferred its work to UNESCO.
72 *Indian School Bulletin* 2, no. (1948): 2. See also Forsyth and Heine, "The Only Good Thing That Happened at School."
73 Forsyth and Heine, "The Only Good Thing That Happened at School," 220.
74 Department of Citizenship and Immigration, Report of Indian Affairs Branch for the Fiscal Year Ended March 31, 1950, 86.
75 We are indebted to Janice Forsyth for sharing some of her detailed analyses of Eisenhardt's inspection of residential and day schools. Also shared was an interview she conducted with Eisenhardt in 2004, just months before he died at the age of ninety-seven. For further information, see also Forsyth and Heine, "A Higher Degree of Social Organization," 267–9; and Forsyth, *Reclaiming Tom Longboat*, 54–61.
76 Eisenhardt, "The Canadian Red Man of Today," 10.
77 Charlotte Whitton, "Lo! The Poor Indian!," *Evening Citizen* (Ottawa), 7 September 1950, 2.
78 Eisenhardt was immediately hired by Canadair Ltd. in Montreal to oversee its employee fitness program, but was soon fired as a "security risk" because he had been blacklisted by a secret RCMP investigation. In 1954, he took a job with Dominion Life, where he remained for the rest of his working life. He also remained fit his entire life through running and jogging, and eventually he received several honours for his fitness work. He died in 2004 at the age of ninety-eight.
79 Truth and Reconciliation Commission of Canada, *Canada's Residential Schools: The History, Part 2 1939 to 2000*, 17.
80 Forsyth and Heine, "The Only Good Thing That Happened at School," 211.
81 Truth and Reconciliation Commission of Canada, *Canada's Residential Schools: The History, Part 2 1939 to 2000*, 465.
82 Ibid., 468. Note the specific examples of underfunding on pp. 468–70.
83 Barnes was principal between 1952 and 1955, abolishing the half-day system and ending the use of student labour on the farm. He appears not to have had any training or experience in physical

education. However, he completed a master's degree at Stanford University in 1955 with the title "A Comparative Study of the Mental Ability of Indian Children."
84 Barnes, "Physical Education Programme for Indian Schools."
85 Braden and Forsyth, "A Rink at This School."
86 For an informative analysis of residential school photography, see McCracken, "Archival Photographs in Perspective." See also McKee and Forsyth, "Witnessing Painful Pasts."
87 McCracken, "Archival Photographs in Perspective," 170.
88 Giancarlo et al., "Methodology and Indigenous Memory."
89 Harrigan, Patrick J., *Finding Their Place*, 6.

6. Changing Times and New Initiatives

1 *Living and Learning.*
2 *Report of the Royal Commission on Aboriginal Peoples: Gathering Strength*, 531–2.
3 "The Constitution Act, 1982, Part II, Rights of the Aboriginal Peoples of Canada, Section 35 (1)" in *The Constitution Acts 1867 to 1982*. Ottawa: Government of Canada, 2021, 56. See also: https://laws-lois.justice.gc.ca/eng/const/page-13.html#h-53.
4 *Report of the Royal Commission on Aboriginal Peoples: Perspectives and Realities*, 160–6. See also Winther, "A Comprehensive Overview."
5 *Report of the Royal Commission on the Status of Women*, 187.
6 Macintosh, "The Challenges Facing Physical Education," 3.
7 Kidd and Associates, *Physical Recreation in Canada*. Available in the Bruce Kidd fonds, University of Toronto Archives, https://discoverarchives.library.utoronto.ca/index.php/bruce-kidd-fonds.
8 Macintosh, "The Challenges Facing Physical Education," 4.
9 Davidson, "Current Status of Health, Physical Education and Recreation."
10 See, for example, Macintosh, "The Challenges Facing Physical Education," 6; Pennington et al., "Education through Challenge and Adventure," 77–82.
11 Bailey, "Exercise, Fitness and Physical Education," 427–8; Hall, "Physical Education for the Future."
12 Laffage-Cosnier and Vivier, "The French Snow Class."
13 These points are attributed to a 1969 interview with Dr. H. Perie, Chief of the Medical Services of the Ministry of Youth and Sports in Paris, cited by Bailey, "Exercise, Fitness and Physical Education," 427–8.
14 Laffage-Cosnier, Hugedet, and Vivier, "Nature and Sport in Education."
15 Ibid., 187.
16 Martens, Fred L., "Daily Physical Education."
17 Ibid., 56.
18 Ibid., 57. Emphasis in original.
19 Shephard and Trudeau, "Quality Daily Physical Education."
20 Davidson, "Current Status of Health, Physical Education and Recreation," 27.
21 Donnelly and Starkes, "Review of the Hamilton Board of Education."
22 Daly, Kidd, and Orchard, *New Directions in Physical Education*.
23 Bailey, "Exercise, Fitness and Physical Education," 425. Emphasis in original.
24 Ibid., 429.
25 Shephard, *Endurance Fitness*, 274.
26 Drover, "ParticipACTION: A Legacy in Motion," 60–1. See also Drover, "ParticipACTION, Healthism, and the Crafting of a Social Memory." She provides an excellent, detailed account

of the early history of ParticipACTION. See also the ParticipACTION Archive Project at http://digital.scaa.sk.ca/gallery/participaction/english/home.html (accessed 11 November 2021).
27 Drover, "ParticipACTION: A Legacy in Motion (1971–1999)," 1–2.
28 *National Report on New Perspectives*, 5.
29 Ibid., 4.
30 The kit, for grades K–12, was called "Planning a Quality School Physical Education Program." It included a guide, charts, and worksheets, and was distributed through CAHPER in 1988.
31 Docherty and Yore, "Health Activity Program (HAP)."
32 Even when provinces stipulate curricula, the amount and quality of actual teaching can be uncertain. See, for example, Petherick, "Curriculum, Pedagogy and Embodied Experience," which provides a fascinating account of the problems in the formulation of curricula by a provincial ministry of education and the actual instruction in a classroom.
33 Martens, "Daily Physical Education," 55.
34 Janzen, "The Status of Physical Education," 6.
35 McDermott, "Thrash Yourself Thursday," 412.
36 These are the same tests discussed in chapter 5. See *CAHPER Fitness-Performance Test Manual*.
37 Shephard and Trudeau, "Quality Daily Physical Education," 109.
38 Francis and Lathrop, "Here We Go round the Mulberry Bush," 28.
39 *Syllabus of Physical Exercises for Schools*, 152–5.
40 *Syllabus of Physical Training for Schools 1933*, 61–3.
41 Francis and Lathrop, "From Dancing Girls to Elder Statesmen." See also Francis, "Birthday Candles for the PHE Canada Dance."
42 See, for example, Kirchner, *Physical Education for Elementary School Children*; Kirchner, Cunningham and Warrell, *Introduction to Movement Education*; Stanley, *Physical Education*; and Wall and Murray, *Children and Movement*.
43 In 2008, after much debate, CAHPERD changed its name to PHE Canada.
44 Macintosh and King, *The Role of Interscholastic Sports*, 17–23, 27–33, 42–3.
45 Ibid., 37–8.
46 For an extended discussion of this dilemma and feminists' efforts to address it, see Hall, *The Girl and the Game*, chapter 7.
47 Vertinsky, "Reclaiming Space, Revisioning the Body," 378.
48 Macintosh and King, *The Role of Interscholastic Sports*, 62–4.
49 Macintosh and King, *The Role of Interscholastic Sports*, 188.
50 Hall, *The Girl and the Game*, 263–5.
51 Hall and Richardson, *Fair Ball*, 56–62. See also Norman, Donnelly, and Kidd, "Gender Inequality in Canadian Interuniversity Sport."
52 For a complete list, see Davidson, "Current Status of Health, Physical Education and Recreation," 50–7.
53 Henry, "Physical Education: An Academic Discipline."
54 Park, "A Long and Productive Career," 300.
55 Ziegler, "Jacks-of-All-Trades and Masters of None?"
56 For an interesting account of this period in Canadian universities, see "The Reconstruction of the Physical Education Profession" in Macintosh and Whitson, *The Game Planners*, 108–21. See also Whitson and Macintosh, "The Scientization of Physical Education."
57 Harrigan, *Finding Their Place*, 40–51. See also https://www.ccupeka.org/accreditation/ (accessed 21 October 2021).
58 Canadian Council of University Physical Education and Kinesiology Administrators, "Position Statement."

59 Ogrodnik, "Sport Participation in Canada, 1998."
60 See, for example, People for Education, "Fundraising and Fees in Ontario's Schools," 2018, https://peopleforeducation.ca/wp-content/uploads/2018/02/AR18_Fundraising_WEB.pdf (accessed on 21 October 2021).

7. Seeking Optimism in a Contested Field

1 Varpalotai and Singleton, "So Little for the Body," 1.
2 *The ParticipACTION Report Card on Physical Activity for Children and Youth*, 2018, https://www.participaction.com/en-ca/resources/report-card (accessed 12 January 2022).
3 For access to all provincial physical education and health curricula, see https://phecanada.ca/about/physical-and-health-education-curriculum-canada (accessed 21 November 2020). Curriculum development tends to be on an eight–ten-year cycle but it does vary by province and territory.
4 Kilborn, Lorusso, and Francis, "An Analysis of Canadian Physical Education," 24. See also table 1.1, Physical Education Curricula across Canada, in Robinson and Randall, *Teaching Physical Education Today*, 15–18.
5 Kilborn, Lorusso, and Francis, "An Analysis of Canadian Physical Education," 43–4.
6 See https://phecanada.ca/inspire/quality-daily-physical-education-award-program/qdpe-award-standards (accessed on 14 November 2021).
7 Robinson et al., "Canada's 150-Minute 'Standard' in Physical Education," 241. See also, the Physical Education and Daily Physical Activity Requirements for each province or territory at https://phecanada.ca/about/physical-and-health-education-curriculum-canada (accessed 21 November 2021).
8 Robinson et al., "Canada's 150-Minute 'Standard' in Physical Education," 241.
9 Alberta Teachers' Association, "School Wellness and Well-Being," iii.
10 *Framework for Kindergarten to Grade 12 Wellness Education*. See also Kilborn, "Kindergarten to Grade 12 Wellness Education."
11 *Framework for Kindergarten to Grade 12 Wellness Education*, 3.
12 See also "The Guiding Framework for the Design and Development of Kindergarten to Grade 12 Provincial Curriculum," Alberta Education, Government of Alberta, 2020. The Physical Education and Wellness section is on p. 11. The full draft curriculum is available at https://curriculum.learnalberta.ca/curriculum/en/c/pdek (accessed 2 November 2021).
13 For example, see review posted on the Healthy Schools LAB website: https://hslab.ca/2021/04/14/review-alberta-educations-draft-k-6-physical-education-and-wellness-curriculum/ (accessed 2 November 2021).
14 See "An Open Letter to All Alberta Parents of School-Aged Children – Kindergarten to Grade 6 Curriculum," from the Werklund School of Education, University of Calgary, https://werklund.ucalgary.ca/research/body-image-lab/open-letter-all-alberta-parents-school-aged-children (accessed 2 November 2021).
15 Philpot, "Critical Pedagogies in PETE," 316–17. Neoliberal initiatives are characterized by free-market policies, deregulation, encouragement of private enterprise and consumer choice, small(er) government, the outsourcing of government services to private providers, personal responsibility, and entrepreneurial initiative.
16 Shawn, *Every Little Movement*, 89–90.
17 Plewes, "Physical Fitness – Its Problems and Implications for Physical Education," 57.
18 Cairney, Kiez, Roetert, and Kriellaars, "A 20th-Century Narrative," 82.
19 Whitehead, *Physical Literacy throughout the Lifecourse* and *Physical Literacy across the World*.

20 The Aspen Institute Project Play, Physical Literacy: A Global Environmental Scan, 2014, http://plreport.projectplay.us/introduction-1/.
21 Whitehead, "Under the Critical Eye," 63.
22 Whitehead, *Physical Literacy across the World*, 8 (emphasis in the original). This is also the definition used by the International Physical Literacy Association.
23 Sheehan, Robinson, and Randall, "Physical Literacy in Canada," 127.
24 PHE Canada brochure, "What Is the Relationship between Physical Education and Physical Literacy?," https://phecanada.ca/activate/physical-literacy (accessed 2 November 2021).
25 *Health and Physical Education*, The Ontario Curriculum, Grades 1–8. Queen's Printer of Ontario, 2019, 31.
26 Province of British Columbia, "Physical and Health Education K–10 – Curricular Competencies," July 2019, https://curriculum.gov.bc.ca/sites/curriculum.gov.bc.ca/files/curriculum/continuous-views/en_phe_k-10_curricular_competencies.pdf (accessed 15 November 2021).
27 Sheehan, Robinson, and Randall, "Physical Literacy in Canada," 131.
28 Sport for Life, https://sportforlife.ca/about-us/ (accessed 3 November 2021).
29 "Physical Literacy Instructor Program," https://physicallit.wpengine.com/physical-literacy-instructor-program/ (accessed 15 November 2021).
30 Gleddie and Morgan, "Physical Literacy Praxis," 32.
31 Kirk, "Educational Value and Models-Based Practice."
32 Siedentop, *Sport Education*.
33 There is an extensive literature about models-based physical education, but much of it refers to models developed in the United States. See, for example, Landi, Fitzpatrick, and McGlashan, "Models Based Practices in Physical Education."
34 Gleddie and Morgan, "Physical Literacy Praxis," 45.
35 Sheehan, Robinson, and Randall, "Physical Literacy in Canada," 130.
36 Melnychuk et al., "Physical Education Teacher Education (PETE) in Canada."
37 Robinson and Randall, "Smooth Sailing or Stormy Seas?" It should be pointed out, however, that the sample represented only one-fifth of the population of PE teachers in Atlantic Canada even though all were invited to participate.
38 Solmon, "Physical Education and Sport Pedagogy." For a comprehensive text about physical education pedagogies, see Ennis, *Routledge Handbook*.
39 Lorusso and Richards, "Expert Perspectives on the Future," 124.
40 "Proposal for the Closure of the Bachelor of Physical and Health Education Programs."
41 Elliot, "Forty Years of Kinesiology," 155. Elliot provides an interesting and informative history of Kinesiology from a Canadian perspective.
42 https://www.ccupeka.org/history/ (accessed 20 November 2021). At the first official meeting in 1971, there were eight representatives from Ontario, four from the West, four from the Maritimes, and four from Quebec in attendance. See also Harrigan, *Finding Their Place*.
43 For a list of CCUPEKA-accredited Kinesiology and Physical Education institutions, as well how accreditation is achieved, see https://www.ccupeka.org/accreditation/ (accessed 20 November 2021).
44 *Kinesiology across Canada* 1, no. 1 (2000): 1–12.
45 Cited in Elliot, "Forty Years of Kinesiology," 160.
46 For the CCUPEKA position statement on the role of kinesiologists, see https://www.ccupeka.org/wp-content/uploads/2019/04/ACA_Position_Statement_F2.pdf (accessed 6 December 2021).
47 Douglas and Halas, "The Wages of Whiteness;" Nachman, Joseph, and Fusco, "What If What the Professor Knows Is Not Diverse Enough for Us?"

48 Douglas and Halas, "The Wages of Whiteness," 456.
49 Nachman, Joseph, and Fusco, "What If What the Professor Knows Is Not Diverse Enough for Us?," 10.
50 See https://www.ccupeka.org/statements/ (accessed 23 November 2021).
51 Fletcher, Lorusso, and Halas, "Redesigning Physical Education in Canada," 138. For efforts at the University of Manitoba to address these issues, see Halas, "Decolonizing Physical and Health Education Teacher Education," and "R. Tait McKenzie Scholar's Address."
52 See https://www.ccupeka.org/statements/ (accessed 23 November 2021).
53 For a description of the Physical Activity and Sport Act, see https://laws-lois.justice.gc.ca/eng/acts/p-13.4/page-1.html#h-392649 (accessed 20 June 2022).
54 See calls 87–91 under "Sports and Reconciliation" in *Truth and Reconciliation Commission of Canada: Calls to Action*, 2015.
55 Halas, McRae, and Carpenter, "The Quality and Cultural Relevance of Physical Education."
56 Ibid., 197. See also Robinson, Borden, and Robinson. "Charting a Course for Culturally Responsive Physical Education."
57 See, for example, Kalyn, "Indigenous Knowledge and Physical Education"; and Lorusso et al., "Learning to Infuse Indigenous Content in Physical Education."
58 Nesdoly, Gleddie, and McHugh, "An Exploration of Indigenous Peoples' Perspectives." See also Dubnewick, Hopper, Spence, and McHugh, "There's a Cultural Pride through Our Games."
59 Lorusso, Markham, and Forsyth, "Indigenous Youth in Ontario."
60 Robinson and Randall, *Social Justice in Physical Education*, 4.
61 Ibid., 6.
62 Philpot, Gerdin, and Smith, "Socially Critical PE," 142.
63 Robinson and Randall, *Social Justice in Physical Education*, 7.
64 Tamtik and Guenter, "Policy Analysis of Equity, Diversity and Inclusion."
65 Goodwin and Causgrove Dunn, "Revisiting Our Research Assumptions." See also Reid and Stanish, "Professional and Disciplinary Status," 224.
66 Goodwin and Howe, "Framing Cross-Cultural Ethical Practice."
67 Peers, Spencer-Cavaliere, and Eales, "Say What You Mean," 275.
68 Mason, "R. Tait McKenzie's Medical Work," 54.
69 Reid and Jobling, "R. Tait McKenzie," 240–1.
70 Daniels, *Adapted Physical Education*. See also Wall, "The History of Adapted Physical Activity in Canada."
71 Austin, "A Conceptual Structure of Physical Education."
72 Austin, "The Forgotten Child."
73 Reid, "Moving toward Inclusion." See also the "Moving to Inclusion Online Learning Tool" currently available through the Active Living Alliance for Canadians with a Disability website: https://ala.ca/moving-inclusion (accessed 14 February 2022).
74 Goodwin, Watkinson, and Fitzpatrick, "Inclusive Physical Education," 192.
75 Harvey, "Adapted and Inclusive Physical Education," provides the most detailed and up-to-date overview of adapted and inclusive physical education in Canada.
76 Harvey, "Adapted and Inclusive Physical Education," also provides advice on concrete steps towards inclusion. See also Goodwin, Gustafson, and Hamilton, "The Experience of Disability in Physical Education."
77 Goodwin and Watkinson, "Inclusive Physical Education."
78 Spencer-Cavaliere and Watkinson, "Inclusion Understood from the Perspectives."
79 In February 2004, Canada's thirteen Winter National Sport Organizations, the Canadian Olympic Committee, the Canadian Paralympic Committee, Sport Canada, Win Sport Canada,

and the Vancouver Olympic Committee organized to develop Own the Podium on a not-for-profit basis.
80 For a detailed examination of these strategic priorities see Faulkner et al., "Exploring the Impact of the 'New' ParticipACTION."
81 Faulkner et al., "Canadian 24-Hour Movement Guidelines."
82 The *Active Canada 20/20* document is available at https://sirc.ca/wp-content/uploads/2019/12/Active-Canada-2020-_-FinalE-May-2012.pdf (accessed 1 February 2022).
83 MacNeill and Kriger, "Bartering with Fate," 104.
84 Ibid., 109.
85 ParticipACTION, *The Future Is Physical*.
86 Cited in Dowling and Washington, "The Governing of Governance," 467.
87 Ibid., 463–5.
88 See note 15 for a definition of neoliberalism.
89 Carpenter, Weber, and Schugurensky, "Views from the Blackboard," 160.
90 Enright, Kirk, and Macdonald, "Expertise, Neoliberal Governmentality," 209.

Afterword: Physical Education for the Future

1 People for Education, *Challenges and Innovations: 2020–21 Annual Report on Ontario Schools*, 8. https://peopleforeducation.ca/wp-content/uploads/2021/10/2020-21-AOSS-Final-Report-Published-110721.pdf (accessed 16 February 2022).
2 *Jump Start State of Sport Report*, March 2021, 6. https://cdn.shopify.com/s/files/1/0122/8124/9892/files/Jumpstart_State_of_Sport_Report_March_2021.pdf?v=1616793836 (accessed 16 February 2022).
3 Canadian Women & Sport, *COVID Alert: Pandemic Impact upon Girls in Sport*, July 2021, 7, 23. https://womenandsport.ca/wp-content/uploads/2021/07/COVID-Alert-final-English-July-2021.pdf (accessed 16 February 2022).
4 ParticipACTION, *Lost & Found: Pandemic-Related Challenges and Opportunities for Physical Activity*, October 2022, 19. https://www.participaction.com/the-science/children-and-youth-report-card/ (accessed 25 April, 2023).
5 PHE Canada, "Imagined Possibilities for the Future: What Will You Hang on to Post-Pandemic?" https://phecanada.ca/connecting/blog/imagined-possibilities-future-what-will-you-hang-post-pandemic (accessed 26 January 2022).
6 Outdoor Play Canada. *Outdoor Play in Canada*.
7 Ibid., 25.
8 For a full list of the outdoor play programs, projects, and activities found in the environmental scan, see Appendix B in ibid.
9 Boileau and Dabaja, "Forest School Practice in Canada." See also Harwood et al., "Exploring the National Scope of Outdoor Nature-Based."
10 Forest School Canada is part of the Child and Nature Alliance of Canada. See https://childnature.ca/ (accessed 26 January 2022).
11 See, for example, https://ccamping.org/covid-19-resources/ (accessed 27 January 2022).
12 For a current survey of outdoor education programs across Canada, see Asfeldt et al., "Outdoor Education in Canada." See also Purc-Stephenson et al., "We Are Wilderness Explorers," as well as Priest and Asfeldt, "The History of Outdoor Learning."
13 PHE Canada, https://phecanada.ca/connecting/blog/putting-e-online-physical-education-thinking-beyond-push-ups-and-jumping-jacks (accessed 16 February 2022).

14 ISPO, Study of trends in the fitness market, https://www.ispo.com/en/taxonomy/term/8146/top-10-fitness-trends-american-college-sports-medicine-acsm-international-survey (accessed 16 February 2022).
15 Gard, "eHPE: A History of the Future."
16 Lupton, "Data Assemblages, Sentient Schools."
17 Thomson and Robertson, "Fit for What?"
18 Kirk, "Physical Education Futures."
19 Kirk, *Precarity, Critical Pedagogy and Physical Education*.
20 Spence, "Active Canada 20/20."
21 See Petherick, "Race and Culture in the Secondary."
22 https://www.ualberta.ca/health-sciences/index.html (accessed 8 February 2022).
23 https://www.ccupeka.org/accreditation/ (accessed 8 February 2022). Brock University is also an accredited physical education institution, but not for kinesiology.
24 Forbes and Livingston, "Roots, Rifts, and Reorientations, 55.
25 Park, "The Second 100 Years," 18.
26 Fletcher, Ní Chróinín, Gleddie, and Beni, *Meaningful Physical Education*, 5.
27 Ibid., 4–5.
28 In particular, see Kretchmar, "Ten Reasons for Quality Physical Education" and "What to Do with Meaning?"
29 See LAMPE at https://meaningfulpe.wordpress.com/ (accessed 21 February 2022).
30 Some of this research has been published in Fletcher, Ní Chróinín, Gleddie, and Beni, *Meaningful Physical Education*, a practical book oriented towards guiding the application of meaningful physical education by practitioners.
31 Forsyth, "Land, Rights, and Reciprocity."
32 University of Toronto, Faculty of Kinesiology and Physical Education, *Task Force on Race and Indigeneity*, 3.
33 Ibid., 11.
34 Ibid., 12–18.
35 University of Toronto, Faculty of Kinesiology and Physical Education, *Equity Report 2019–2020*. See also Joseph and Kriger, "Towards a Decolonizing Kinesiology."
36 University of British Columbia, Faculty of Education, *Task Force on Race, Indigeneity and Social Justice Final Report*, 2.
37 https://indigenous.kin.educ.ubc.ca/ (accessed 25 February 2022).
38 See University of Manitoba, Faculty of Kinesiology and Recreation Management, *Strategic Plan 2015–2020*, 12–15, for how the FKRM supports the University of Manitoba's commitment to Indigenous achievement.
39 https://www.ualberta.ca/kinesiology-sport-recreation/programs/undergraduate-programs/certificates/certificate-in-aboriginal-sport-and-recreation.html (accessed 25 February 2022).
40 Bruner et al., "Indigenous Youth Development through Sport."
41 Statistics supplied by Indspire show that in 2020–1, the number of funded applicants in Kinesiology, Sport, or Recreation was 165 with a financial need of $1,720,517. The amount awarded was $499,440, representing only 29 per cent of their financial needs.
42 UNESCO, *International Charter of Physical Education, Physical Activity and Sport*.

Bibliography

Alberta Teachers' Association. "School Wellness and Well-Being Initiatives across Canada: Environmental Scan and Literature Review." Edmonton: Alberta Teachers' Association, 2019.
Ambrose, Linda M. "The Canadian Youth Commission: Planning for Youth and Social Welfare in the Post-War Era." PhD diss. University of Waterloo, 1992.
– "Collecting Youth Opinion: The Research of the Canadian Youth Commission, 1943–1945." In *Dimensions of Childhood: Essays on the History of Children and Youth in Canada*, edited by Russell Smandych, Gordon Dodds, and Alvin Esau, 63–83. University of Manitoba: Legal Research Institute, 1991.
Anderson, C.S. "Movement Educators – Beware!" *CAHPER Journal* 45, no.1 (1978): 42–4.
Anderson, H. Allen. *The Chief: Ernest Thompson Seton and the Changing West*. College Station: Texas A & M University Press, 1986.
– "Ernest Thompson Seton and the Woodcraft Indians." *Journal of American Culture* 8, no. 1 (1985), 43–50.
Arnett, Jeffrey Jensen. "G. Stanley Hall's *Adolescence*: Brilliance and Nonsense." *History of Psychology* 9, no. 3 (2006): 186–97.
Asfeldt, Morten, Rebecca Purc-Stephenson, Mikaela Rawleigh, and Sydney Thackeray. "Outdoor Education in Canada: A Qualitative Investigation," *Journal of Adventure Education and Outdoor Learning* 21, no. 4 (2021): 297–310.
Austin, Patricia Louise. "A Conceptual Structure of Physical Education for the School Program." PhD diss., Michigan State University, 1965.
– "The Forgotten Child." In *The R. Tait McKenzie Memorial Addresses*, edited by Stewart A. Davidson and Peggy Blackstock, 35–41. CAHPER, 1980.
Axelrod, Paul. *The Promise of Schooling: Education in Canada, 1800–1914*. Toronto: University of Toronto Press, 1997.
– "Spying on the Young in Depression and War: Students Youth Groups and the RCMP, 1935–1942." *Labour/Le Travail* 35 (Spring 1995): 43–63.
Baden-Powell, Lady. "The Girl Guide Movement," *Proceedings of the Sixty-Second Annual Convention of the Ontario Educational Association*, Toronto, 2–5 April 1923, 169–73.

Baden-Powell, Robert. *Scouting for Boys: A Handbook for Instruction in Good Citizenship.* Edited with an Introduction and Notes by Elleke Boehmer. Oxford, UK: Oxford University Press, 2005.
Bailey, D.A. "Exercise, Fitness and Physical Education for the Growing Child – A Concern." *Canadian Journal of Public Health/Revue Canadienne de Santé Publique* 64, no. 5 (1973): 421–30.
Baker, Kellie. "Confessions of a Teacher with Two Left Feet: Using Self-Study to Examine the Challenges of Teaching Dance in PETE." *Asia-Pacific Journal of Health, Sport and Physical Education* 6, no.3 (2015): 221–32.
Barnes, Findlay. "Physical Education Programme for Indian Schools." *Indian School Bulletin* 11, no. 3 (1957): 8–9.
Barnjum, Frederick S. "Physical Education." *The Educational Record of the Province of Quebec* 1, no. 9 (1881): 384–7.
Barrett, Kate. "Movement Education in the 80s: Direction? Or Demise?" *Proceedings of the Contemporary Elementary and Middle School Physical Education Conference*, Georgia State University, 15–17 January 1981, 4–13.
Beers, W.G. *Lacrosse: The National Game of Canada.* Montreal: Dawson Brothers, 1869.
Berger, Carl. *The Sense of Power: Studies in the Ideas of Canadian Imperialism 1867–1914.* 2nd ed. Toronto: University of Toronto Press, 2013.
Blackstock, C.R. "The Canadian Association for Health, Physical Education, and Recreation." In *Physical Education in Canada*, edited by M. L. van Vliet, 276–91. Scarborough, ON: Prentice-Hall, 1965.
Blais, Gabrielle. "'The Complete Feminine Personality': Female Adolescence in the Canadian Girls in Training (CGIT) 1915–1955." MA thesis, University of Ottawa, 1986.
Boileau, Elizabeth Y.S., and Ziad F. Dabaja. "Forest School Practice in Canada: A Survey Study." *Journal of Outdoor and Environmental Education* 23, no. 3 (2020): 225–40.
Bonde, Hans. "Globalization *Before* Globalization: Niels Bukh and the American Connection." *International Journal of the History of Sport* 26, no. 13 (2009): 1999–2014.
– *Gymnastics and Politics. Niels Bukh and Male Aesthetics.* University of Copenhagen: Museum Tusculanum Press, 2006.
Bouchier, Nancy B. *For the Love of the Game: Amateur Sport in Small-Town Ontario, 1938–1895.* Montreal and Kingston: McGill-Queen's University Press, 2003.
Bruner, Mark W., Robert Lovelace, Sean Hillier, Colin Baillie, Brenda G. Bruner, Kathy Hare, Christine Head, Aaron Paibomsai, Keiran Peltier, and Lucie Lévesque. "Indigenous Youth Development through Sport and Physical Activity: Sharing Voices, Stories, and Experiences." *International Journal of Indigenous Health* 14, no. 2 (2019): 224–51.
Bryans, Helen. "Secondary School Curriculum for Girls." In *Physical Education in Canada*, edited by M.L. Van Vliet, 124–39. Scarborough, ON: Prentice-Hall, 1965.
Bryce, P.H. *Report of the Indian Schools of Manitoba and the Northwest Territories.* Ottawa: Government Printing Bureau, 1907.
Burdett, Gillian Mary. "The High School for Girls, Montreal 1875–1914." MA thesis. McGill University, 1963.
Burke, Garry J. "Good for the Boy and the Nation: Drill and the Cadet Movement in Ontario Public Schools 1865–1911." PhD diss., University of Toronto, 1996.
Byl, John. "Directing Physical Education in the Canadian YWCAs: Margaret Eaton School's Influence, 1901–1947." *Sport History Review* 27, no. 2 (1996): 139–54.
– "The Margaret Eaton School, 1901–1942: Women's Education in Elocution, Drama and Physical Education." PhD diss., State University of New York at Buffalo, 1992.

- "SCOTT, EMMA PRISCILLA (Raff; Nasmith)," in *Dictionary of Canadian Biography*, vol. 16, University of Toronto/Université Laval, 2003–. Accessed 18 February 2022. http://www.biographi.ca/en/bio/scott_emma_priscilla_16E.html.
- "Why Physical Educators Should Know about the Margaret Eaton School." *CAHPER Journal* 59, no. 1 (1993): 10–13.

CAHPER Fitness-Performance Test Manual. Canadian Association of Health, Physical Education and Recreation, 1966.

Cairney, John, Tia Kiez, E. Paul Roetert, and Dean Kriellaars. "A 20th-Century Narrative on the Origins of the Physical Literacy Construct," *Journal of Teaching in Physical Education* 38, no. 2 (2019): 79–83.

Calisthenics and Games Prescribed for Use in All Indian Schools. Ottawa: Government Printing Bureau, 1910.

Canadian Council of University Physical Education and Kinesiology Administrators. "Position Statement: The Role of Kinesiologists and the Promotion of Physical Activity and Exercise in the Canadian Health Care System." October 2014.

Canadian Sport Policy 2012. Endorsed by Federal, Provincial and Territorial Ministers responsible for sport, physical activity and recreation, 27 June 2012, Inuvik, Northwest Territories.

Canadian Youth Commission. *Youth & Health: A Positive Health Programme for Canada*. Toronto: Ryerson Press, 1944.
- *Youth & Recreation: New Plans for New Times*. Toronto: Ryerson Press, 1946.

Carpenter, Sara, Nadya Weber, and Daniel Schugurensky. "Views from the Blackboard: Neoliberal Education Reforms and the Practice of Teaching in Ontario, Canada." *Globalization, Societies and Education* 10, no. 2 (2014): 145–61.

Cartwright, Ethel Mary. "Athletics and Physical Education for Girls." In *Proceedings of the Sixty-Second Annual Convention of the Ontario Educational Association*, 274–81. Toronto: Clarkson W. James, 1923.
- "Physical Education and Its Place in the School; the Function of the Strathcona Trust; and the Training of Teachers." Dominion Educational Association, *Proceedings of the Eighth Convention of the Association*, Ottawa, ON, 20–3 August 1913, 109–23.
- "Physical Education and the Strathcona Trust." *The School: A Magazine Devoted to Elementary and Secondary Education* 4, no. 4 (1916): 306–10.
- "Physical Education as a Profession for College Graduates." *McGill News* 2, no. 4 (1921): 20.
- "The Place of Physical Education in the School and Home Curriculum." In *Proceedings of the Sixty-Second Annual Convention of the Ontario Educational Association*, 291–300. Toronto: Clarkson W. James, 1923.

Chatwin, Nora. "The Pioneers of 1968." *Journal of CAHPER* 35, no. 2 (1968–9): 13–14.

Clark, Ruth. "Physical Education." *Queen's Quarterly* 27 (1 July 1919): 234–9.

Clearly, Brian O. "Progress – Real or Imagined?" *Journal of CAHPER* 20, no.8 (1955): 9–11.

Comacchio, Cynthia. *The Dominion of Youth: Adolescence and the Making of Modern Canada 1920–1950*. Waterloo, ON: Wilfrid Laurier University Press, 2006.

Congrès Internationale de l'Éducation Physique Rapports. Paris 17–20 Mars 1913. Paris: J.-B. Baillière et Fils, 1913.

Cosentino, Frank, and Maxwell L. Howell. *A History of Physical Education in Canada*. Toronto: General Publishing, 1971.

Course, Anna H. "Movement Education: A Study of Cultural Diffusion." MA thesis, University of Western Ontario, 1989.

Creighton, Donald. *The Road to Confederation: The Emergence of Canada, 1863–1867*. Don Mills, ON: Oxford University Press, 2012.

Curtis, Bruce. *Building the Educational State: Canada West, 1836–1871.* London, ON: Althouse Press, 1988.
Daly, Jack, Bruce Kidd, and Jim Orchard. *New Directions in Physical Education for Manitoba Schools.* Winnipeg, MB: Queen's Printer, 1975.
Daniels, Arthur Simpson. *Adapted Physical Education.* New York: Harper, 1954.
Dashuk, James. *Clearing the Plains: Disease, Politics of Starvation, and the Loss of Indigenous Life.* New Edition. Regina: University of Regina Press, 2019.
Davidson, Stewart A. "Current Status of Health, Physical Education and Recreation 1977." Documentary statement prepared for the International Council on Health, Physical Education and Recreation, Mexico City, 18 July 1977. Ottawa: CAHPER, 1977.
– "New Projects/Nouveaux projets. Pioneers in Physical Education and Sport in Canada." *Oral History Forum/D'histoire orale* 4, no. 2 (1980): 46–7.
Davin, Nicholas Flood. *Report on Industrial Schools for Indians and Half-Breeds.* Report to the Minister of the Interior, Ottawa, 14 March 1879.
de la Cour, Lykke, Cecelia Morgan, and Marianne Valverde. "Gender Regulation and State Formation in Nineteen Century Canada." In *Colonial Leviathan: State Formation in Mid-Nineteenth-Century Canada*, edited by Allan Greer and Ian Radforth, 163–91. Toronto: University of Toronto Press, 1992.
Detellier, Élise. *Mises au jeu: Les sports féminins à Montréal 1919–1961.* Montreal: Les Éditions du remue-ménage, 2015.
Dirks, Patricia. "Canada's Boys – An Imperial or National Asset? Responses to Baden-Powell's Boy Scout Movement in Pre-War Canada." In *Canada and the British World: Culture, Migration, and Identity*, edited by Phillip Buckner and R. Douglas Francis, 111–28. Vancouver: University of British Columbia Press, 2006.
– "Shaping Canada's Women: Canadian Girls in Training versus Girl Guides." In *Framing Our Past: Canadian Women's History in the Twentieth Century*, edited by Sharon Anne Cook, Lorna R. McLean, and Kate O'Rourke, 155–9. Montreal and Kingston: McGill-Queen's University Press, 2001.
Docherty, David, and Larry Yore. "Health Activity Program (HAP) Bridging the Health Gap." *Promotion, Journal of the B.C. Physical Education Teachers' Association* 24, no. 6 (1980): 28–30.
Donnelly, Peter, and Janet Starkes. "Review of the Hamilton Board of Education Elementary Itinerant Physical Education Programme." Unpublished manuscript, McMaster University, School of Physical Education and Athletics, 1983.
Douglas, Delia D., and Joannie M. Halas. "The Wages of Whiteness: Confronting the Nature of Ivory Tower Racism and the Implications for Physical Education." *Sport, Education and Society* 18, no. 4 (2013): 453–74.
Dowling, Mathew, and Marvin Washington. "The Governing of Governance: Metagovernance and the Creation of New Organizational Forms within Canadian Sport," *Managing Sport and Leisure* 22, no.6 (2017), 458–71.
Downey, Allan. *The Creator's Game: Lacrosse, Identity, and Indigenous Nationhood.* Vancouver: UBC Press, 2018.
Drover, Victoria Lamb. "ParticipACTION: A Legacy in Motion (1971–1999)." PhD diss., University of Saskatchewan, 2016.
– "ParticipACTION, Healthism, and the Crafting of a Social Memory (1971–1999)." *Journal of the Canadian Historical Association/Revue de la Société historique du Canada* 25, no. 1 (2014): 277–306.
Dubnewick, Michael, Tristan Hopper, John C. Spence, and Tara-Leigh F. McHugh. "'There's a Cultural Pride through Our Games': Enhancing the Sport Experiences of Indigenous Youth in

Canada through Participation in Traditional Games." *Journal of Sport and Social Issues* 42, no. 4 (2018): 207–26.

Duncan, Ruth. "A Report from England," *Journal of CAHPER* 22, no. 5 (1956): 19–21.

Eaton, John D. "The Life and Professional Contributions of Arthur Stanley Lamb, MD, to Physical Education in Canada." PhD diss., Ohio State University, 1964.

Edwards, C.A.M. *Taylor Statten: A Biography*. Toronto: Ryerson, 1960.

Eisen, George. "Games and Sporting Diversions of the North American Indians as Reflected in American Historical Writings of the Sixteenth and Seventeenth Centuries." *Canadian Journal of History of Sport and Physical Education* 9, no. 1 (1978): 58–85.

Eisenhardt, Ian. "Canada's National Fitness Act." *Journal of Health and Physical Education* 16, no. 4 (1945): 186–7, 229–30.

– "The Canadian Red Man of Today." *Journal of the American Association for Health, Physical Education, and Recreation* 22, no. 6 (1951): 9–10.

– "Department of Recreational and Physical Education, Government of British Columbia." *Canadian Physical Education Association Bulletin* 4, no. 10 (1936): 2–4.

– "Dominion-Provincial Youth Training Programme." *Canadian Physical Education Association Bulletin* 8, no. 3 (1941): 1.

Elliot, Digby. "Forty Years of Kinesiology: A Canadian Perspective." *Quest* 59, no.1 (2007): 154–62.

Ellis, Jason. "HUGHES, JAMES LAUGHLIN." In *Dictionary of Canadian Biography*. Vol. 16. University of Toronto/Université Laval, 2003–. Accessed 18 April 2023. http://www.biographi.ca/en/bio/hughes_james_16E.html.

Ennis, Catherine D., ed. *Routledge Handbook of Physical Education Pedagogies*. London and New York: Routledge, 2017.

Enright, Eimear, David Kirk, and Doune Macdonald. "Expertise, Neoliberal Governmentality and the Outsourcing of Health and Physical Education." *Discourse: Studies in the Cultural Politics of Education* 4, no. 2 (2020): 206–22.

Faulkner, Guy, Lauren White, Negin Riazi, Amy E. Latimer-Cheung, and Mark S. Tremblay. "Canadian 24-Hour Movement Guidelines for Children and Youth: Exploring the Perceptions of Stakeholders Regarding Their Acceptability, Barriers to Uptake, and Dissemination." *Applied Physiology, Nutrition, and Metabolism* 41, no. 6 (2016): S303–S310.

Faulkner, Guy, Lira Yun, Mark S. Tremblay, and John C. Spence. "Exploring the Impact of the 'New' ParticipACTION: Overview and Introduction of the Special Issue." *Health Promotion and Chronic Disease Prevention in Canada* 38, no. 4 (April 2018): 153–61.

Fitzpatrick, David A. "The Socialization Goal of Manitoba Public School Physical Education." MEd thesis, University of Manitoba, 1989.

Fletcher, Sheila. *Women First: The Female Tradition in English Physical Education 1880–1980*. London: Athlone Press, 1984.

Fletcher, Tim, Jenna Lorusso, and Joannie Halas. "Redesigning Physical Education in Canada." In *Redesigning Physical Education: An Equity Approach in Which Every Child Matters*, edited by Hal A. Lawson, 134–44. London and New York: Routledge, 2018.

Fletcher, Tim, Déirdre Ní Chróinín, Douglas Gleddie, and Stephanie Beni. *Meaningful Physical Education: An Approach to Teaching and Learning*. London and New York: Routledge, 2021.

Forbes, Duncan. "'Tracking' Edith Tudor-Hart." *History Workshop Journal* 84 (Autumn 2017): 235–47.

Forbes, Susan L., and Lori A. Livingston. "Roots, Rifts, and Reorientations: Rediscovering the Common Community of Inquiry." In *Pedagogy in Motion: A Community of Inquiry for Human Movement Studies*, edited by Ellen Singleton and Aniko Varpalotai, 45–63. London, ON: Althouse Press, 2012.

Forsyth, Janice. "Land, Rights, and Reciprocity: Indigenous Sport Is Not an EDI Issue." Webinar lecture to School of Kinesiology, Faculty of Education, University of British Columbia, 25 November 2020.

– *Reclaiming Tom Longboat: Indigenous Self-Determination in Canadian Sport*. Regina, SK: University of Regina Press, 2020.

Forsyth, Janice, and Michael Heine. "'A Higher Degree of Social Organization': Jan Eisenhardt and Canadian Aboriginal Sport Policy in the 1950s." *Journal of Sport History* 35, no. 2 (2008): 261–77.

– "'The Only Good Thing That Happened at School': Colonising Narratives of Sport in the *Indian School Bulletin*." *British Journal of Canadian Studies* 30, no. 2 (2017): 205–25.

Framework for Kindergarten to Grade 12 Wellness Education. Alberta: Alberta Education Curriculum Branch, 2009.

Francis, Nancy R. "Birthday Candles for the PHE Canada Dance Education Advisory Committee! Celebrating the First Three Decades: 1965–1995." *Physical and Health Education Journal* 80, no. 1 (2014): 41–4.

Francis, Nancy R., and Anna H. Lathrop. "'Children Who Drill, Seldom Are Ill.' Drill, Movement and Sport: The Rise and Fall of a 'Female Tradition' in Ontario Elementary Physical Education – 1850s to 2000." *Historical Studies in Education/Revue d'histoire de l'éducation* 23, no 1 (2011): 61–80.

– "From Dancing Girls to Elder Statesmen." *Physical and Health Education Journal* 84, no. 2 (2018): 1–25.

– "'Here We Go 'round the Mulberry Bush': Problematizing 'Progress' in Ontario's Elementary School Dance Curriculum: 1900 to 2000." *Journal of Dance Education* 14, no. 1 (2014): 27–34.

Gagen, Elizabeth A. "Making America Flesh: Physicality and Nationhood in Early Twentieth-Century Reform." *Cultural Geographies* 11 (2004): 417–42.

Gard, Michael. "eHPE: A History of the Future." *Sport, Education and Society* 19, no. 6 (2014): 827–85.

Gerber, Ellen W. *Innovators and Institutions in Physical Education*. Philadelphia: Lea & Febiger, 1971.

Giancarlo, Alexandra, Janice Forsyth, Braden Te Hiwi, and Taylor McKee. "Methodology and Indigenous Memory: Using Photographs to Anchor Critical Reflections on Indian Residential School Experiences." *Visual Studies* 36, no. 4–5 (2021): 406–20.

Gidney, Catherine. *Tending the Student Body: Youth, Health, and the Modern University*. Toronto: University of Toronto Press, 2015.

Gidney, R.D. "Centralization and Education: The Origins of an Ontario Tradition." *Journal of Canadian Studies* 7, no. 4 (1972): 33–48.

– "RYERSON, EGERTON." In *Dictionary of Canadian Biography*, vol. 11. University of Toronto/Université Laval, 2003–. Accessed 24 May 2021, http://www.biographi.ca/en/bio/ryerson_egerton_11E.html.

Gidney, R.D., and W.P.J. Millar. "From Voluntarism to State Schooling: The Creation of the Public School System in Ontario." *Canadian Historical Review* 66, no. 4 (1985): 443–73.

Gleddie, Douglas L., and Andrew Morgan. "Physical Literacy Praxis: A Theoretical Framework for Transformative Physical Education." *Prospects* 50, no. 1/2 (2021): 31–53.

Goodwin, Donna L., and Janice Causgrove Dunn. "Revisiting Our Research Assumptions 20 Years On: The Role of Interdisciplinarity." *Adapted Physical Activity Quarterly* 35, no. 3 (2018): 249–53.

Goodwin, Donna L., Paul Gustafson, and Brianne N. Hamilton. "The Experience of Disability in Physical Education." In *Stones in the Sneaker: Active Theory for Secondary School Physical and Health Educators*, edited by Ellen Singleton and Aniko Varpalotai, 223–53. London, ON: Althouse Press, 2006.

Goodwin, Donna L., and P. David Howe. "Framing Cross-Cultural Ethical Practice in Adapt[ive] Physical Activity." *Quest* 68, no. 1 (2016): 43–54.
Goodwin Donna L., and E. Jane Watkinson. "Inclusive Physical Education from the Perspective of Students with Physical Disabilities." *Adapted Physical Activity Quarterly* 17, no. 2 (2000): 144–60.
Goodwin, Donna L., E. Jane Watkinson, and David A. Fitzpatrick. "Inclusive Physical Education: A Conceptual Framework." In *Adapted Physical Activity*, edited by Robert D. Steadward, Garry D. Wheeler, and Jane Watkinson, 189–212. Edmonton: University of Alberta Press, 2003.
Graham, Elizabeth. *The Mush Hole: Life at Two Indian Residential Schools.* Waterloo, ON: Heffle Publishing, 1997.
Greer, Allan. *Property and Dispossession: Natives, Empires and Land in Early Modern North America.* Cambridge, UK: Cambridge University Press, 2018.
– "Settler Colonialism and Beyond." *Journal of the Canadian Historical Association/Revue de la Société historique du Canada*, 30, no. 1 (2019): 61–86.
Grenier, Guy. "BURGESS, THOMAS JOSEPH WORKMAN." In *Dictionary of Canadian Biography*, vol. 15. University of Toronto/Université Laval, 2003–. Accessed 20 March 2021, http://www.biographi.ca/en/bio/burgess_thomas_joseph_workman_15E.html.
Gurney, Helen. *The CAHPER Story 1933–1983.* Ottawa: Canadian Association for Health, Physical Education and Recreation, 1983.
Habkirk, Evan J. "From Indian Boys to Canadian Men? The Use of Cadet Drill in the Canadian Indian Residential School System." *British Journal of Canadian Studies* 30, no. 2 (2017): 227–47.
Halas, Joannie. "Decolonizing Physical and Health Education Teacher Education." Paper presented at the Canadian Society for the Study Education Conference, University of British Columbia, 1–6 June 2019.
– "R. Tait McKenzie Scholar's Address: Physical and Health Education as a Transformative Pathway to Truth and Reconciliation with Aboriginal Peoples." *Physical and Health Education Journal* 79, no. 3 (2013): 41–9.
Halas, Joannie, Heather McRae, and Amy Carpenter. "The Quality and Cultural Relevance of Physical Education for Aboriginal Youth: Challenges and Opportunities." In *Aboriginal Peoples and Sport in Canada*, edited by Janice Forsyth and Audrey R. Giles, 182–205. Vancouver: UBC Press, 2013.
Hall, M. Ann. "Fifty Years of Sport History Review." In *Routledge Handbook of Sport History*, edited by Murray G. Philips, Douglas Booth, and Carly Adams, 332–8. London and New York: Routledge, 2022.
– *The Girl and the Game: A History of Women's Sport in Canada*, 2nd ed. Toronto: University of Toronto Press, 2016.
– "Physical Education for the Future." *CAHPER Journal* 37, no. 5 (1971): 4–7.
Hall, M. Ann, and Dorothy Richardson. *Fair Ball: Towards Sex Equality in Canadian Sport.* Ottawa: Canadian Advisory Council on the Status of Women, 1982.
Hallman, Dianne M., and Anna H. Lathrop. "Sustaining the Fire of 'Scholarly Passion.'" In *Women Teaching, Women Learning: Historical Perspectives*, edited by Elizabeth M. Smyth and Paula Bourne, 45–64. Toronto: Inanna Publications & Education, 2006.
Hamilton, Mary G. *The Call of the Algonquin: A Biography of a Summer Camp.* Toronto: Ryerson Press, 1958.
Harrigan, Patrick J. *Finding Their Place: The History of the Canadian Council of University Physical Education and Kinesiology Administrators (CCUPEKA).* The Canadian Council of University Physical Education and Kinesiology Administrators in conjunction with Patrick J. Harrigan (University of Waterloo) and the Faculty of Physical Education and Health, University of Toronto, 2004.

- "The Schooling of Boys and Girls in Canada." *Journal of Social History* 23, no. 4 (1990): 803–16.
Harris, Cole. *A Bounded Land: Reflections on Settler Colonialism in Canada*. Vancouver: UBC Press, 2020.
Harvey, William. "Adapted and Inclusive Physical Education." In *Teaching Physical Education Today: Canadian Perspectives*, edited by Daniel B. Robinson and Lynn Randall, 137–52. Toronto: Thompson Educational Publishing, 2014.
Harwood, Debra, Elizabeth Boileau, Ziad Dabaja, and Mark Julien. "Exploring the National Scope of Outdoor Nature-Based Early Learning Programs in Canada: Findings from a Large-Scale Survey Study." *International Journal of Holistic Early Learning and Development* 6 (2020): 1–24.
"Health Training in Schools." *Canadian Public Health Journal* 33, no. 4 (1942): 178–9.
Hébert, Léo-Paul. "BEAUDRY, CYRILLE." In *Dictionary of Canadian Biography*, vol. 13. University of Toronto/Université Laval, 2003–. Accessed 20 March 2021. http://www.biographi.ca/en/bio/beaudry_cyrille_13E.html.
Henry, Franklin M. "Physical Education: An Academic Discipline." *Journal of Health, Physical Education, Recreation* 35, no. 7 (1964): 32–3, 69.
Hill, Rose. "The English Concept of Basic Movement Training." *Journal of CAHPER* 26, no. 4 (1960): 18–20.
- "Programme Improvement in Modern Dance." *Journal of CAHPER* 32, no. 5 (1966): 8, 23–5.
Hopkins, J. Castell. "Youthful Canada, and the Boys' Brigade." *Canadian Magazine* 4, no. 6 (1895): 551–6.
Houghton, E.B. *Physical Culture: First Book of Exercises in Drill, Calisthenics, and Gymnastics*. Toronto: Warwick & Sons, 1886.
Hunt, Edmund Arthur. "A History of Physical Education in the Public Schools of British Columbia from 1918 to 1967." MA thesis, University of Washington, 1967.
Hussey, Delia, and Ruth Murray. "Anglo-American Workshop in Elementary Physical Education." *Journal of Health, Physical Education, Recreation* 27, no. 8 (1956): 22–3.
Jackson, Dorothy. *A Brief History of Three Schools*. Toronto: University of Toronto, 1953.
James, Cathy. "Reforming Reform: Toronto's Settlement House Movement, 1900–20." *Canadian Historical Review* 82, no. 1 (2001): 55–90.
Janson, Gilles. *Emparons-nous du sport: Les Canadiens français et le sport au XIXe siècle*. Montreal: Guérin, 1995.
- "SCOTT, HENRI-THOMAS (baptized Thomas-Henri)." In *Dictionary of Canadian Biography*, vol. 15. Accessed 29 April 2021. University of Toronto/Université Laval, 2003–. http://www.biographi.ca/en/bio/scott_henri_thomas_15E.html.
Janzen, Henry. "The Status of Physical Education in Canadian Public Schools." *CAHPERD Journal* 61, no. 3 (1995): 5–9.
Johnson, F. Henry. "The Ryersonian Influence on the Public School System of British Columbia." *BC Studies* 10 (Summer 1971): 26–34.
Joseph, Janelle, and Debra Kriger. "Towards a Decolonizing Kinesiology Ethics Model." *Quest* 73, no. 2 (2021): 192–208.
Kalyn, Brenda. "Indigenous Knowledge and Physical Education. In *Teaching Physical Education Today*, edited by Daniel B. Robinson and Lynn Randall, 153–76. Toronto: Thompson Educational Publishing, 2014.
Kay, Cheryl. "'Two-Eyed Seeing': Moving from Paralysis to Action in Understanding the Legacy of Indian Residential Schools in British Columbia, Canada." *Journal of Dance Education* 17 no. 3 (2017): 106–14.
Kelm, Mary-Ellen. *Colonizing Bodies: Aboriginal Health and Healing in British Columbia, 1900–1950*. Vancouver: University of British Columbia Press, 1998.

Keyes, Mary E. "John Howard Crocker, LL. D, 1870–1959." MA thesis, University of Western Ontario, 1964.
Kidd. Bruce. "'Making the Pros Pay' for Amateur Sports: The Ontario Athletic Commission, 1920–1947." *Sport in Society* 16, no. 4 (2013): 533–52.
- "Muscular Christianity and Value-Centred Sport: The Legacy of Tom Brown in Canada." *International Journal of the History of Sport* 23, no. 5 (2006): 701–13.
- *A Runner's Journey*. Toronto: Aevo UTP, 2021.
- *The Struggle for Canadian Sport*. Toronto: University of Toronto Press, 1996.
Kidd, Bruce, and Associates. *Physical Recreation in Canada*. A Report Prepared for the Committee on Youth, Office of the Secretary of State, July 1970.
Kiefer, Nancy. "DYMOND, ALFRED HUTCHINSON." In *Dictionary of Canadian Biography*, vol. 13. University of Toronto/Université Laval, 2003–. Accessed 20 March 2021. http://www.biographi.ca/en/bio/dymond_alfred_hutchinson_13E.html.
Kilborn, Michelle. "Kindergarten to Grade 12 Wellness Education in Alberta: Health and Physical Education Curriculum." *Physical & Health Education Journal* 78, no. 1 (2012): 15–21.
Kilborn, Michelle, Jenna Lorusso, and Nancy Francis. "An Analysis of Canadian Physical Education Curricula." *European Physical Education Review* 22, no. 1 (2016): 23–46.
Kirchner, Glenn. *Physical Education for Elementary School Children*. Dubuque, IA: W.C. Brown, 1966.
Kirchner, Glenn, Jean Cunningham, and Eileen Warrell. *Introduction to Movement Education: An Individualized Approach to Teaching Physical Education*. Dubuque, IA: W.C. Brown, 1970.
Kirk, David. *Defining Physical Education: The Social Construction of a School Subject in Postwar Britain*. London and New York: Routledge, 1992.
- "Educational Value and Models-Based Practice in Physical Education." *Educational Philosophy and Theory* 45, no. 9 (2013): 973–86.
- "A New Critical Pedagogy for Physical Education in 'Turbulent Times': What Are the Possibilities?" In *Critical Research in Sport, Health and Physical Education: How to Make a Difference*, edited by Richard Pringle, Håkan Larsson, and Göran Gerdin, 106–18. London and New York: Routledge, 2019.
- *Physical Education Futures*. London and New York: Routledge, 2010.
- "Physical Education Futures: Can We Reform Physical Education in the 21st Century?" *eJRIEPS* [Online] 27 (2012). Accessed 11 January 2022. https://journals.openedition.org/ejrieps/3222.
- *Precarity, Critical Pedagogy and Physical Education*. London and New York: Routledge, 2019.
- "Schooling Bodies through Physical Education: Insights from Social Epistemology and Curriculum History." *Studies in Philosophy and Education* 20, no. 6 (2001): 475–87.
Kretchmar, R. Scott. "Ten Reasons for Quality Physical Education." *Journal of Physical Education, Recreation and Dance* 77, no. 9 (2006): 6–9.
- "What to Do with Meaning? A Research Conundrum for the 21st Century." *Quest* 59, no. 4 (2007): 373–83.
Laban, Rudolf. *Modern Educational Dance*. 3rd ed. London: Macdonald and Evans, 1980.
Laffage-Cosnier, Sébastien, Willy Hugedet, and Christian Vivier. "Nature and Sport in Education: The Migration of a School Model from France to Canada (1953–1995)." *Paedagogica Historica* 56, nos. 1–2 (2020): 182–99.
Laffage-Cosnier, Sébastien, and Christian Vivier. "The French Snow Class: How the Focus of a School Innovation Changed from Physical Education to Academic Learning (1953–1981)." *Loisir et Société / Society and Leisure* 38, no. 3 (2015): 330–46.
Lamb, Arthur S. "Looking Ahead in Physical Education." *Bulletin of the Canadian Physical Education Association* 3, no. 7 (1935): 5–9.

- "National Physical Fitness: A Duty and Opportunity." *Canadian Welfare* 19, no. 8 (1944): 27–30.
- "Physical Education." In *Proceedings of the Sixty-Second Annual Convention of the Ontario Educational Association*, 159–68. Toronto: Clarkson W. James, 1923.
- "Physical Education in Canada." *Bulletin of the Canadian Physical Education Association* 1, no. 1 (1933): 3–9.
Landi, Dillon, Katie Fitzpatrick, and Hayley McGlashan. "Models Based Practices in Physical Education: A Sociocritical Reflection." *Journal of Teaching in Physical Education* 35, no. 4 (2016): 400–11.
Lathrop, Anna H. "Contested Terrain: Gender and 'Movement' in Ontario Elementary Physical Education: 1940–1970." *Ontario History* 94, no. 2 (2002): 165–82.
- "Elegance and Expression, Sweat and Strength: A Portrait of the Margaret Eaton Schools (1901–1941) through the Life History of Emma Scott Nasmith, Mary G. Hamilton, and Florence A. Somers." *Vitae Scholasticae* 16, no. 1 (1997): 69–92.
- "Elegance and Expression, Sweat and Strength: Body Training, Physical Culture and Female Embodiment in Women's Education at the Margaret Eaton Schools (1901–1941)." PhD diss., University of Toronto, 1997.
- "Portrait of 'A Physical': A Case Study of Elizabeth Pitt Barron (1904–98)." *Historical Studies in Education / Revue d'histoire de l'éducation* 11, no. 2 (1999): 131–46.
- "'Strap an Axe to Your Belt': Camp Counselor Training and the Socialization of Women at the Margaret Eaton School (1925–1941)." *Sport History Review* 32, no. 2 (2001): 110–25.
Lathrop, Anna H., and Valerie A. Drake. "'The Canadian Climber': Resurrection or Rejection of a Canadian Innovation?" *CAHPERD Journal de l'ACSEPLD* 64, no. 4 (1998): 14–19.
Lawther, John. *The Learning and Performance of Physical Skills*. Englewood Cliffs, NJ: Prentice Hall, 1977.
Leduc, Yvan, and André Girard. "Le statut professionnel des éducators physiques à la Commission des écoles catholiques de Montréal de 1938 à 1965." *Revue des sciences de l'éducation* 19, no. 2 (1993): 327–43.
Lenskyj, Helen. "Femininity First: Sport and Physical Education for Ontario Girls, 1890–1930." *Canadian Journal of the History of Sport* 13, no. (1982): 4–17.
- *Out of Bounds: Women, Sport and Sexuality*. Toronto: Women's Press, 1986.
Leslie, John. "The Bagot Commission: Developing a Corporate Memory for the Indian Department." *Historical Papers/Communications historiques* 17, no. 1 (1982): 31–52.
Living and Learning: The Report of the Provincial Committee on Aims and Objectives of Education in the Schools of Ontario. Toronto: Newton Publishing, 1968.
Lloyd, Rebecca, and Stephen Smith. "Physical Literacy." In *Teaching Physical Education Today Canadian Perspectives*, edited by Daniel B. Robinson and Lynn Randell, 226–42. Toronto: Thompson Educational Publishing, 2014.
Lorusso, Jenna R., Chris Markham, and Janice Forsyth. "Indigenous Youth in Ontario School-Based Health and Physical Education Programs: A Scoping Review." *Revue phénEPS/PHEnex Journal* 11, no. 3 (2021): 1–18.
Lorusso, Jenna R., and K. Andrew R. Richards. "Expert Perspectives on the Future of Physical Education in Higher Education." *Quest* 70, no.1 (2018): 114–36.
Lorusso, Jenna R., Kaitlyn Watson, Jocelyn Brewer, Madison Hubley, Reid Lenders, and Megan Pickett. "Learning to Infuse Indigenous Content in Physical Education: A Story of Growth towards Reconciliation." *Revue phénEPS/PHEnex Journal* 10, no. 2 (2019): 1–21.
Lu, Chunlei, Nancy Francis, and Ken Lodewyk. "Movement Domains." In *Teaching Physical Education Today: Canadian Perspectives*, edited by Daniel B. Robinson and Lynn Randell, 208–25. Toronto: Thompson Educational Publishing, 2014.

Lupton, Deborah. "Data Assemblages, Sentient Schools and Digitized Health and Physical Education (Response to Gard). *Sport, Education and Society* 20, no. 1 (2014): 122–32.

Macdonald, Charlotte. *Strong, Beautiful and Modern: National Fitness in Britain, New Zealand, Australia and Canada, 1935–1960.* Vancouver: UBC Press, 2011.

MacDonald, Robert H. *Sons of the Empire: The Frontier and the Boy Scout Movement, 1890–1918.* Toronto: University of Toronto Press, 1993.

Macintosh, Donald. "The Challenges Facing Physical Education." *CAHPER Journal* 39, no. 5 (1973): 3–8.

– "Glancing Back, Looking Forward: The R. Tait McKenzie Address 1992." *CAHPER Journal/Journal de L'ACSEPL* 58, no. 4 (1992): 9, 11, 13, 15, 17.

Macintosh, Donald, Tom Bedecki, and C.E.S. Franks. *Sport and Politics in Canada: Federal Government Involvement since 1961.* Montreal and Kingston: McGill-Queen's University Press, 1987.

Macintosh, Donald, and Michael Hawes. *Sport and Canadian Diplomacy.* Montreal and Kingston: McGill-Queen's University Press, 1994.

Macintosh, Donald, and Alan J.C. King. *The Role of Interscholastic Sports Programs in Ontario Secondary Schools – A Provincial Analysis.* Toronto: Ontario Ministry of Education, 1976.

Macintosh, Donald, and David Whitson. *The Game Planners: Transforming Canada's Sport System.* Montreal and Kingston: McGill-Queen's University Press, 1990.

Macleod, David. "A Live Vaccine: The YMCA and Male Adolescence in the United States and Canada 1870–1920." *Histoire sociale / Social History* 11, no. 21 (1978): 5–25.

MacNeill, Margaret, and Debra Kriger. "Bartering with Fate: Imagination, Health, and the Body." In *Body Studies in Canada: Critical Approaches to Embodies Experiences*, edited by Valerie Zawilski, 95–113. Toronto: Canadian Scholars, 2021.

Maletic, Vera. *Body-Space-Expression: The Development of Rudolf Laban's Movement and Dance Concepts.* Berlin: Mouton de Gruyter, 1987.

Marr, Lucille M. "Church Teen Clubs, Feminized Organizations? Tuxis Boys, Trail Rangers, and Canadian Girls in Training, 1919–1939." *Historical Studies in Education/Revue d'histoire de l'éducation* 3, no. 2 (1991): 249–67.

Martens, Fred L. "Daily Physical Education – A Boon to Canadian Elementary Schools." *Journal of Physical Education, Recreation & Dance* 53, no. 3 (1982): 55–8.

Mason, Fred. "R. Tait McKenzie's Medical Work and Early Exercise Therapies for People with Disabilities." *Sport History Review* 39, no. 1 (2008): 45–70.

Matthews, Jill Julius. "They Had Such a Lot of Fun: The Women's League of Health and Beauty between the Wars." *History Workshop: A Journal of Socialist and Feminist Historians* 30 (Autumn 1990): 22–54.

McCracken, Krista. "Archival Photographs in Perspective: Indian Residential School Images of Health." *British Journal of Canadian Studies* 30, no. 2 (2017): 163–82.

McDermott, Lisa. "'Thrash Yourself Thursday': The Production of the 'Healthy' Child through a Fitness-Based PE Practice." *Sport, Education and Society* 17, no. 3 (2012): 405–29.

McKee, Taylor, and Janice Forsyth. "Witnessing Painful Pasts: Understanding Images of Sports at Canadian Indian Residential Schools." *Journal of Sport History* 46, no. 2 (2019): 175–88.

McKenzie, R. Tait. *Exercise in Education and Medicine.* Philadelphia: W.B. Saunders, 1909.

– "Frederick S. Barnjum and His Work." *American Physical Education Review* 2, no. 2 (1897): 73–80.

McMurray, J. David. "The Organizational Growth and Development of the Ontario Student Leadership Centre 1948–1988." MHK thesis, University of Windsor, 1989.

McNeill, William H. *Keeping Together in Time: Dance and Drill in Human History.* Cambridge, MA: Harvard University Press, 1995.

McNutt, Steven. "Shifting Objectives: The Development of Male Physical Education in Nova Scotia from 1867 to 1913." *Canadian Journal of the History of Sport* 22, no. 1 (1991): 32–51.

Meagher, John W. "Professional Preparation." In *Physical Education in Canada*, edited by M.L. van Vliet, 64–81. Scarborough, ON: Prentice Hall 1967.

Metcalfe, Alan. *Canada Learns to Play: The Emergence of Organized Sport, 1807–1914*. Toronto: McClelland and Stewart, 1987.

Miller, J.R. *Compact, Contract, Covenant: Aboriginal Treaty-Making in Canada*. Toronto: University of Toronto Press, 2009.

– *Shingwauk's Vision: A History of Native Residential Schools*. Toronto: University of Toronto Press, 1996.

Milloy, John S. *A National Crime: The Canadian Government and the Residential School System, 1879 to 1986*. Winnipeg: University of Manitoba Press, 1999.

Ministry of Education. *Moving and Growing: Physical Education in the Primary School, Part One*. London: Her Majesty's Stationery Office, 1952.

– *Planning the Programme: Physical Education in Primary School, Part Two*. London: Her Majesty's Stationery Office, 1953.

Moody, Barry M. "GRAVES, MARY ELIZABETH." In *Dictionary of Canadian Biography*, vol. 13. University of Toronto/Université Laval, 2003–. Accessed 20 March 2021. http://www.biographi.ca/en/bio/graves_mary_elizabeth_13E.html.

– "SAWYER, ARTEMAS WYMAN." In *Dictionary of Canadian Biography*, vol. 13. University of Toronto/Université Laval, 2003–. Accessed 22 March 2021. http://www.biographi.ca/en/bio/sawyer_artemas_wyman_13E.html.

Morrow, L. Donald. "Selected Topics in the History of Physical Education in Ontario: From Dr. Egerton Ryerson to the Strathcona Trust, 1844–1939." PhD diss., University of Alberta, 1975.

– "The Strathcona Trust in Ontario, 1911–1939." *Canadian Journal of History of Sport and Physical Education* 8, no. 1 (1977): 72–90.

Mosby, Ian. "Administering Colonial Science: Nutrition Research and Human Biomedical Experimentation in Aboriginal Communities and Residential Schools, 1942–1952." *Histoire sociale / Social History* 46, no. 91 (2013): 145–72.

Mossman, Gary. *Lloyd Percival: Coach and Visionary*. Revised and Fully Referenced Edition. Gary Mossman, 2022.

Mott, Morris. "Confronting 'Modern' Problems through Play: The Beginning of Physical Education in Manitoba's Public Schools, 1900–1915." In *Schools in the West: Essays in Canadian Educational History*, edited by Nancy M. Sheehan, J. Donald Wilson, and David C. Jones, 57–71. Calgary: Detselig, 1986.

Munrow, A.D. *Pure and Applied Gymnastics*. London: Edward Arnold, 1955.

Murray, Heather. "Making the Modern: Twenty-Five Years of the Margaret Eaton School of Literature and Expression." *Essays in Theatre/Études* 10, no. 1 (1991): 39–57.

Murray, Kenneth Hemsley. "The Status of Physical Education in the Public and Elementary Schools in the Provinces of Canada." Thesis for the Higher Diploma of Physical Education, McGill University, 1935.

Nachman, Jessica, Janelle Joseph, and Caroline Fusco. "'What If What the Professor Knows Is Not Diverse Enough for Us?': Whiteness in Canadian Kinesiology Programs." *Sport, Education and Society* 27, no. 7 (2022): 789–802.

National Report on New Perspectives for Elementary School Physical Education Programs in Canada. School Activity Programs Committee of CAHPER, 1976.

Neatby, Hilda. *So Little for the Mind*. Toronto: Clark, Irwin, 1953.

Neil, Graham Ivan. "A History of Physical Education in the Protestant Schools of Quebec." MA thesis, McGill University, 1963.
Nesdoly, Autumn, Douglas Gleddie, and Tara-Leigh F. McHugh. "An Exploration of Indigenous Peoples' Perspectives of Physical Literacy." *Sport, Education and Society* 26, no. 3 (2021): 295–308.
Nicholas, Jane. *The Modern Girl: Feminine Modernities, the Body, and Commodities in the 1920s.* Toronto: University of Toronto Press, 2015.
Nicholas, Larraine. *Dancing in Utopia: Dartington Hall and Its Dancers.* Alton, UK: Dance Books, 2007.
Norman, Mark, Peter Donnelly, and Bruce Kidd. "Gender Inequality in Canadian Interuniversity Sport: Participation Opportunities and Leadership Positions from 2010–11 to 2016–17." *International Journal of Sport Policy and Politics* 13, no. 2 (2021): 207–23.
Ogrodnik, Lucie. "Sport Participation in Canada, 1998." *Focus on Culture* 12, no. 2 (2000): 3–6.
Ontario Department of Education. *Physical Education Junior Division Grades 4,5,6*, 1959.
– *Physical Education Primary Division Grades I II III*, 1956.
Orban, William A.R. "The Fitness Movement." In *Physical Education in Canada*, edited by M.L. van Vliet, 238–48. Scarborough, ON: Prentice-Hall, 1965.
Outdoor Play Canada. *Outdoor Play in Canada: 2021 State of the Sector Report.* July 2021. Accessed 25 January 2022. https://www.outdoorplaycanada.ca/wp-content/uploads/2021/09/OPC_SSR_english_FINAL.pdf.
Park, Roberta J. "A Long and Productive Career: Franklin M. Henry – Scientist, Mentor, Pioneer." *Research Quarterly for Exercise and Sport* 65, no. 4 (1994): 295–307.
– "The Second 100 Years: Or, Can Physical Education Become the Renaissance Field of the 21st Century?" *Quest* 41, no. 1 (1989): 1–27.
ParticipACTION. *The Future Is Physical: Moving to a Better Normal.* The 2021 ParticipACTION Report Card on Physical Activity for Adults. Toronto: ParticipACTION, 2021. Accessed 28 February 2022. https://www.participaction.com/en-ca/resources/adult-report-card.
– *Lost & Found: Pandemic Related Challenges and Opportunities for Pysical Activity.* The 2022 ParticipACTION Report Card on Physical Activity for Children and Youth. Toronto: ParticipACTION, 2022. Accessed 24 April 2023. https://www.participaction.com/the-science/children-and-youth-report-card/.
Pearl-Cartu, Lynda. "Social and Political Changes and the Development of Physical and Health Education within the Ontario Public Education System 1841–1918." MEd thesis, Brock University, 1980.
Pedersen, Diana. "'Building Today for the Womanhood of Tomorrow': Businessmen, Boosters, and the YWCA, 1890–1930." *Urban History Revue / Revue d'histoire urbaine* 15, no. 3 (1987): 225–42.
– "'Keeping Our Good Girls Good': The YWCA and the 'Girl Problem,' 1870–1930." *Canadian Woman Studies / Les cahiers de la femme* 7, no. 4 (1986): 20–4.
– "The Photographic Record of the Canadian YWCA, 1890–1930: A Visual Source for Women's History." *Archivaria* 24 (Summer 1987): 10–34.
– "'The Power of True Christian Women': The YWCA and Evangelical Womanhood in the Late Nineteenth Century." In *Changing Roles of Women within the Christian Church of Canada*, edited by Elizabeth Gillan Muir and Marilyn Färdig Whiteley, 321–37. Toronto: University of Toronto Press, 1995.
Peers, Danielle, Nancy Spencer-Cavaliere, and Lindsay Eales. "Say What You Mean: Rethinking Disability Language in *Adapted Physical Activity Quarterly*." *Adapted Physical Activity Quarterly* 31, no. 3 (2014): 265–82.
Pennington, Gary, Jack Stevens, Barbara Kallus, and Peter Moody. "Education through Challenge and Adventure." Report No. 3, Educational Research Institute of BC, 1971.

Pennington, Jo. *The Importance of Being Rhythmic*. New York and London: G.P. Putnam & Sons, 1925.
Percival, Lloyd. "Our Flabby Muscles Are a National Disgrace." *MacLean's Magazine*, 15 April 1953, 20–1, 71–2.
Petherick, LeAnne Dorothy. "Curriculum, Pedagogy and Embodied Experience: The (Re)production of Health Discourse in Grade 9 Health and Physical Education." PhD diss., University of Toronto, 2008.
– "Race and Culture in the Secondary School Health and Physical Education Curriculum in Ontario, Canada: A Critical Reading." *Health Education* 118, no. 2 (2018): 144–58.
Philpot, Rod. "Critical Pedagogies in PETE: An Antipodean Perspective." *Journal of Teaching in Physical Education* 34, no. 2 (2015): 316–32.
Philpot, Rod, Göran Gerdin, and Wayne Smith. "Socially Critical PE: The Influence of Critical Research on the Social Justice Agenda in PETE and PE Practice." In *Critical Research in Sport, Health and Physical Education*, edited by Richard Pringle, Håkan Larsson, and Göran Gerdin, 134–46. New York: Routledge, 2019.
Physical Work Capacity of Canadian Children. Canadian Association for Health, Physical Education and Recreation, 1968.
Plewes, Doris W. "Affiliated Organizations: V. The Canadian Physical Education Association." *Journal of Health and Physical Education* 17, no. 5 (1946): 273–4, 313–15.
– "Canadian News." *Journal of Health and Physical Education* 16, no. 4 (1945): 203–5.
– "Canadian News." *Journal of Health and Physical Education* 16, no. 6 (1945): 334–6.
– "Canadian News." *Journal of Health and Physical Education* 16, no. 7 (1945): 397–9.
– "Canadians: Rugged or Ragged?" *Journal of CAHPER* 23, no. 7 (1957): 21–3.
– "Physical Education in the Primary School." *Journal of CAHPER* 19, no. 5 (1953): 37–8.
– "Physical Fitness – Its Problems and Implications for Physical Education." *Report of the Second British Empire and Commonwealth Conference on Physical Education*. Glamorgan Training College, Barry Wales, 11–17 July 1958, 56–9.
Posse, Nils. *The Special Kinesiology of Educational Gymnastics*. Boston: Lee and Shephard, 1903.
Potts, Robert Earl Kent. "The Development of Physical Education in Nova Scotia Schools." MEd thesis, Acadia University, 1966.
Prang, Margaret. "'The Girl God Would Have Me Be': The Canadian Girls in Training, 1915–39." *Canadian Historical Review* 66, no. 2 (1985): 154–84.
Prentice, Alison L. *The School Promoters: Education and Social Class in Mid-Nineteenth Century Upper Canada*. Toronto: University of Toronto Press, 2004.
Preston-Dunlop, Valerie. *Rudolf Laban: An Extraordinary Life*. London: Dance Books, 1998.
Priest, Simon, and Morten Asfeldt. "The History of Outdoor Learning in Canada." *International Journal of the History of Sport* 39, no. 5 (2022): 489–509.
Proceedings of the American Association for the Advancement of Physical Education, Seventh Annual Meeting, Philadelphia, 1892. Springfield, MA: Springfield Printing and Binding, 1893.
Prochner, Larry. "Placing a School at the Tail of a Plough – The European Roots of Indian Industrial Schools in Canada." In *Knowing the Past, Facing the Future: Indigenous Education in Canada*, edited by Sheila Carr-Stewart, 53–84. Vancouver: University of British Columbia Press, 2019.
"Proposal for the Closure of the Bachelor of Physical and Health Education Programs, School of Kinesiology and Health Studies, Queen's University at Kingston, 2017."
Province of Manitoba. *Education and Recreation in the Province of Manitoba*. Winnipeg: Queen's Printer, 1958.

Proyer, Valerie A. "Formal and Educational Gymnastics – Why the Dichotomy?" *Journal of CAHPER* 40, no. 2 (1973): 13–19.

Purc-Stephenson, R.J., M. Rawleigh, H. Kemp, and Morten Asfeldt. "We Are Wilderness Explorers: A Review of Outdoor Education in Canada." *Journal of Experiential Education* 42, no. 4 (2019): 364–81.

Putnam, J.H., and G.M. Weir. *Survey of the School System*. Province of British Columbia. Victoria, B.C., 1925.

Reid, Eileen, and Ruth Duncan. "Anglo-American Course on Physical Education for Children under 12 Years of Age." *Journal of CAHPER* 23, no. 2 (1956): 12–15.

Reid, Greg. *From Bloomers to Body Mass Index: 100 Years of Kinesiology and Physical Education at McGill*. Montreal: McGill University, 2012.

–. "Moving Toward Inclusion." In *Adapted Physical Activity*, edited by Robert D. Steadward, Garry D. Wheeler, and Jane Watkinson, 131–47. Edmonton: University of Alberta Press, 2003.

Reid, Greg, and Ian F. Jobling. "R. Tait McKenzie: Inspirational Sculptor and Pioneer Advocate of Physical Activity for People with Disabilities." *International Journal of Disability, Development and Education* 59, no. 3 (2012): 231–42.

Reid, Greg, and Heidi Stanish. "Professional and Disciplinary Status of Adapted Physical Activity." *Adapted Physical Activity Quarterly* 20, no. 3 (2003): 213–29.

Report of the Royal Commission on Aboriginal Peoples: Gathering Strength. Volume 3. Ottawa: Canada Communications Group, 1996.

Report of the Royal Commission on Aboriginal Peoples: Perspectives and Realities. Volume 4. Ottawa: Canada Communications Group, 1996.

Report of the Royal Commission on the Status of Women in Canada. Ottawa: Information Canada, 1970.

Robinson, Daniel B., Lisa Lunney Borden, and Ingrid M. Robinson. "Charting a Course for Culturally Responsive Physical Education." *Alberta Journal of Educational Research* 58, no. 4 (2013): 526–46.

Robinson, Daniel B., and Lynn Randall. "Marking Physical Literacy or Missing the Mark on Physical Literacy? A Conceptual Critique of Canada's Physical Literacy Assessment Instruments." *Measurement in Physical Education and Exercise Science* 21, no. 1 (2017): 40–55.

–. "Smooth Sailing or Stormy Seas? Atlantic Canadian Physical Educators on the State and Future of Physical Education." *Canadian Journal of Education/Revue canadienne de l'éducation* 39, no. 1 (2016): 1–31.

–, eds. *Social Justice in Physical Education: Critical Reflections and Pedagogies for Change*. Toronto: Canadian Scholars' Press, 2016.

–, eds. *Teaching Physical Education Today: Canadian Perspectives*. Toronto: Thompson Educational Publishing, 2014.

Robinson, Daniel B., Lynn Randall, Doublas L. Geddie, Joe Barrett, and Stephen Berg. "Canada's 150-Minute 'Standard' in Physical Education: A Consideration of Research Evidence Related to Physical Education Instructional Time." *Curriculum Studies in Health and Physical Education* 10, no. 3 (2019): 226–46.

Rogers, Irene L. "MACKIESON, JOHN." In *Dictionary of Canadian Biography*, vol. 11. University of Toronto/Université Laval, 2003–. Accessed 20 March 2021. http://www.biographi.ca/en/bio/mackieson_john_11E.html.

Ross, Murray G. *The Y.M.C.A. in Canada: The Chronicle of a Century*. Toronto: Ryerson Press, 1951.

Roy, Arundhati. "The Pandemic Is a Portal." *Financial Times*, 3 April 2020. Accessed 25 January 2022. https://www.ft.com/content/10d8f5e8-74eb-11ea-95fe-fcd274e920ca.

Russell, Peter. *Canada's Odyssey: A Country Based on Incomplete Conquests*. Toronto: University of Toronto Press, 2017.
Ruyter, Nancy Lee Chalfa. "American Delsartism: Precursor of an American Dance Art." *International Journal of the History of Sport* 26, no. 13 (2009): 2015–30.
– *The Cultivation of Body and Mind in Nineteenth-Century American Delsartism*. Westport, CT: Greenwood Press, 1999.
Ryerson, Egerton. "Military Drill in Public Schools." *Journal of Education for Upper Canada* 15, no. 8 (1862): 113–14.
– "Papers on Military School Drill." *Journal of Education for Upper Canada* 19, no. 10 (1866): 145–52.
– "Physical Training in Schools, Gymnastic Exercises No. 1." *Journal of Education for Upper Canada* 5, no. 5 (1852): 65–7.
– "Report by Dr. Ryerson on Industrial Schools, 26 May 1847 [Appendix A]." *Statistics Respecting Indian Schools*. Ottawa: Government Printing Bureau, 1898.
– *Report on a System of Public Elementary Instruction for Upper Canada*. Montreal: Lovell and Gibson, 1847.
– *"The Story of My Life."* Edited by J. George Hodgins. Toronto: William Briggs, 1884.
Schrodt, Phyllis Barbara. "Federal Programmes of Physical Recreation and Fitness: The Contributions of Ian Eisenhardt and BC's Pro-Rec." *Canadian Journal of History of Sport* 15, no. 2 (1984): 45–61.
– "A History of Pro-Rec: The British Columbia Provincial Recreation Programme – 1934 to 1953." PhD diss., University of Alberta. 1979.
Schwartz, Hillel. "Torque: The New Kinaesthetic of the Twentieth Century." In *Incorporations*, edited by Jonathan Crary and Sanford Kwinter, 71–126. New York: Zone, 1992.
Sexton, Ella B. "Teacher Recruitment in Physical Education." *Journal of CAHPER* 22, no. 8 (1956): 21–2, 27–8 and *Journal of CAHPER* 22, no. 9 (1956): 13–17.
Shawn, Ted. *Every Little Movement: A Book about François Delsarte*. 2nd ed. New York: Dance Horizons, 1963.
Sheehan, Dwayne, Daniel Robinson, and Lynn Randall. "Physical Literacy in Canada." In *Physical Literacy across the World*, edited by Margaret Whitehead, 125–42. London: Routledge, 2019.
Shephard, Roy J. *Endurance Fitness*, 2nd ed. Toronto: University of Toronto Press, 1977.
Shephard, Roy J., and François Trudeau. "Quality Daily Physical Education for the Primary School Student: A Personal Account of the Trois-Rivières Regional Project." *Quest* 65, no. 1 (2013): 98–115.
Sheppard, Joanna, and Doug Gleddie. "Curriculum Models." In *Teaching Physical Education Today Canadian Perspectives*, edited by Daniel B. Robinson and Lynn Randell, 34–46. Toronto: Thompson Educational Publishing, 2014.
Siedentop, Daryl, ed. *Sport Education: Quality PE through Positive Sport Experience*. Champaign, IL: Human Kinetics, 1994.
Simons, Wm. M. "Educational Gymnastics – It's Meaning, Uses and Abuses," *Journal of CAHPER* 32, no. 5 (1966): 6, 26.
Singleton, Ellen, and Aniko Varpolotai, eds. *Pedagogy in Motion: A Community of Inquiry for Human Movement Studies*. London, ON: Althouse Press, 2012.
– *Stones in the Sneaker: Active Theory for Secondary School Physical and Health Educators*. London, ON: Althouse Press, 2006.
Slack, Zerada. "Development of Physical Education for Women at McGill University." Thesis for the Higher Diploma of Physical Education, McGill University, 1934.
Smith, Donald B. "Egerton Ryerson and the Mississauga, 1826 to 1856, an Appeal to Further Study." *Ontario History* 113, no. 2 (2021): 222–38.

- *Mississauga Portraits: Ojibwe Voices from Nineteenth-Century Canada*. Toronto: University of Toronto Press, 2013.
- *Seen but Not Seen: Influential Canadians and the First Nations from the 1840s to Today*. Toronto: University of Toronto Press, 2021.
Solmon, Melinda A. "Physical Education and Sport Pedagogy: The Application of the Academic Discipline of Kinesiology." *Kinesiology Review* 10, no.2 (2021): 331–8.
Somers, Florence A. "Ideals for Girls' Athletics." *Bulletin of the Canadian Physical Education Association* 3, no. 9 (1936): 9–10.
- *Principles of Women's Athletics*. New York: A.S. Barnes, 1930.
Spence, John C., Guy Faulkner, Christa Costas Bradstreet, Mary Duggan, and Mark S. Tremblay. "Active Canada 20/20: A Physical Activity Plan for Canada." *Canadian Journal of Public Health* 106, no. 8 (2015): 470–3.
Spencer-Cavaliere, Nancy, and E. Jane Watkinson. "Inclusion Understood from the Perspectives of Children with Disability." *Adapted Physical Activity Quarterly* 27, no. 4 (2010): 275–93.
Stack, Prunella. *Zest for Life: Mary Bagot Stack and the League of Health and Beauty*. London: Peter Owens, 1988.
Stanley, Sheila. *Physical Education: A Movement Orientation*. Toronto: McGraw-Hill, 1969.
Statistics Respecting Indian Schools with Dr. Ryerson's Report of 1847 Attached. Ottawa: Government Printing Bureau, 1898.
Statten, Taylor. "Canadian Standard Efficiency Training for Boys." In *Proceedings of the Fifty-Eighth Annual Convention of the Ontario Educational Association*, 180–90. Toronto: Ryerson Press, 1919.
Syllabus of Physical Exercises for Schools. Published by the Executive Council, Strathcona Trust. Toronto: Copp, Clark, 1911.
Syllabus of Physical Training for Schools 1919. London: Published by His Majesty's Stationary Office, 1922.
Syllabus of Physical Training for Schools 1933. London: Published by His Majesty's Stationary Office, 1935.
Tamtik, Merli, and Melissa Guenter. "Policy Analysis of Equity, Diversity and Inclusion Strategies in Canadian Universities – How Far Have We Come? *Canadian Journal of Higher Education* 49, no.3 (2019): 41–56.
Te Hiwi, Braden Paora. "Physical Culture as Citizenship Education at Pelican Lake Indian Residential School, 1926–1970." PhD diss., University of Western Ontario, 2015.
- "Unlike Their Playmates of Civilization, the Indian Children's Recreation Must Be Cultivated and Developed: The Administration of Physical Education at Pelican Lake Indian Residential School, 1926–1944." *Historical Studies in Education / Revue d'histoire de l'éducation* 29, no. 1 (2017): 99–118.
Te Hiwi, Braden, and Janice Forsyth. "'A Rink at This School Is Almost as Essential as a Classroom': Hockey and Discipline at Pelican Lake Indian Residential School, 1945–1951." *Canadian Journal of History* 52, no. 1 (2017): 80–108.
Third Congress of the Universities of the British Empire 1926. Report of Proceedings. London: G. Bell & Sons, 1926.
Thomson, Dianne C., and Lorayne Robertson. "Fit for What? Critical Analysis of Canadian Physical Education Curriculum." *Critical Education* 5, no. 19 (2014): 1–19.
Titley, Brian E. "Indian Residential Schools in Western Canada." In *Schools in the West: Essays in Canadian Educational History*, edited by Nancy M. Sheehan, J. Donald Wilson, and David C. Jones, 133–53. Calgary: Detselig, 1986.

Truth and Reconciliation Commission. *Canada's Residential Schools: Reconciliation.* Final Report of the Truth and Reconciliation Commission of Canada. Volume 6. Montreal and Kingston: McGill-Queen's University Press, 2015.
– *Canada's Residential Schools: The History, Part 1, Origins to 1939.* Final Report of the Truth and Reconciliation Commission of Canada, Volume 1. Montreal and Kingston: McGill-Queen's University Press, 2015.
– *Canada's Residential Schools: The History, Part 2, 1939 to 2000.* Final Report of the Truth and Reconciliation Commission of Canada, Volume 1. Montreal and Kingston: McGill-Queen's University Press, 2015.
– *Honouring the Truth, Reconciling the Future.* Final Report of the Truth and Reconciliation Commission of Canada. Volume One: Summary. Toronto: Lorimer, 2015.
Tyrrell, Joyce Plumptre. "Watch Britain." *Journal of CAHPER* 19, no. 2 (1953): 14–16.
UNESCO. *International Charter of Physical Education, Physical Activity and Sport,* 2015. Accessed 27 February 2022. https://en.unesco.org/themes/sport-and-anti-doping/sport-charter.
University of British Columbia, Faculty of Education. *Task Force on Race, Indigeneity and Social Justice Final Report,* 28 June 2021. Accessed 25 February 2022. https://educ.sites.olt.ubc.ca/files/2021/06/Final-Report-Task-Force-on-Race-Indigeneity-and-Social-Justice.pdf.
University of Manitoba, Faculty of Kinesiology and Recreation Management. *Strategic Plan 2015–2020.* Accessed 25 February 2022. https://umanitoba.ca/faculties/kinrec/media/fkrm_strategic_plan_2015_2022.pdf.
University of Toronto, Faculty of Kinesiology and Physical Education. *Equity Report 2019–2020.* Accessed 25 February 2022. https://kpe.utoronto.ca/sites/default/files/equity_report_2020_27_june_final_0.pdf.
– *Task Force on Race and Indigeneity Final Report,* 4 December 2018. Accessed 25 February 2022. https://kpe.utoronto.ca/sites/default/files/kpe_task_force_on_race_and_indigeneity_-_final_report.pdf.
– *Creating Capacity, Cultivating Change,* 2018–2022 Academic Plan Extension. Accessed 25 February 2022. https://kpe.utoronto.ca/sites/default/files/academic_plan_2019_web.pdf.
Varpalotai, Aniko, and Ellen Singleton. "So Little for the Body." In *Pedagogy in Motion: A Community of Inquiry for Human Movement Studies,* edited by Ellen Singleton and Aniko Varpolotai, 1–13. London, ON: Althouse Press, 2012.
Veder, Robin. "The Expressive Efficiencies of American Delsarte and Mensendieck Body Culture." *Modernism/Modernity* 17, no. 4 (2010): 819–38.
Verbrugge, Martha H. *Active Bodies: A History of Women's Physical Education in Twentieth-Century America.* New York: Oxford University Press, 2012.
Vertinsky, Patricia A. "'Building the Body Beautiful' in *The Women's League of Health and Beauty*: Yoga and Female Agency in 1930s Britain." *Rethinking History: Journal of Theory and Practice* 16, no. 4 (2012): 517–42.
– *The Eternally Wounded Woman: Women, Exercise and Doctors in the Late Nineteenth Century.* Manchester: Manchester University Press, 1990.
– "A Question of the Head and the Heart: From Physical Education to Kinesiology in the Gymnasium and the Laboratory." *Kinesiology Review* 6, no. 2 (2017): 140–52.
– "Reclaiming Space, Revisioning the Body: The Quest for Gender-Sensitive Physical Education." *Quest* 44, no. 3 (1992): 373–96.
– "Schooling the Dance: From Dance under the Swastika to Movement Education in the British School." *Journal of Sport History* 31, no. 3 (2004): 401–23.
– "Transatlantic Traffic in Expressive Movement: From Delsarte and Dalcroze to Margaret H'Doubler and Rudolf Laban." *International Journal of the History of Sport* 26, no. 13 (2009): 2031–51.

Vertinsky, Patricia, and Bieke Gils. "'Watch Britain': Movement Education, Transnational Exchanges, and the Contested Terrain of Physical Education in Mid-Twentieth-Century Canada." *Journal of Sport History* 44, no. 3 (2017): 456–75.

Waite, Peter B., ed. *The Confederation Debates in the Province of Canada, 1865: A Selection*. Montreal and Kingston: McGill-Queen's University Press, 2006.

Wall, A.E. (Ted). "The History of Adapted Physical Activity in Canada." In *Adapted Physical Activity*, edited by Robert D. Steadward, Garry D. Wheeler, and Jane Watkinson, 27–44. Edmonton: University of Alberta Press, 2003.

Wall, Jennifer, and Nancy Murray. *Children and Movement: Physical Education in the Elementary School*. Madison, WI: Brown & Benchmark, 1990.

Wall, Sharon. *The Nurture of Nature: Childhood, Antimodernism, and Ontario Summer Camps, 1920–55*. Vancouver: UBC Press, 2009.

Walsh, Shannon L. *Eugenics and Physical Culture Performance in the Progressive Era: Watch Whiteness Workout*. Cham, Switzerland: Palgrave Macmillan, 2020.

Walton, Yvette M. "The Life and Professional Contributions of Ethel Mary Cartwright, 1880–1955." MA thesis, University of Western Ontario, 1976.

Webb, Ida M. *The Challenge of Change in Physical Education: Chelsea College of Physical Education – Chelsea School, University of Brighton 1898–1998*. London: Falmer Press, 1999.

West, J. Thomas. "Physical Fitness, Sport and the Federal Government 1909 to 1954." *Canadian Journal of History of Sport and Physical Education* 4, no. 2 (1973), 24–42.

Whitehead, Margaret, ed. *Physical Literacy across the World*. London and New York: Routledge, 2019.

– *Physical Literacy throughout the Lifecourse*. London and New York: Routledge, 2010.

– "Under the Critical Eye. An Insider's Experience of the Female Tradition." In *The Female Tradition in Physical Education. Women First Reconsidered*, edited by David Kirk and Patricia Vertinsky, 62–74. London and New York: Routledge, 2016.

Whitson, David J., and Donald Macintosh. "The Scientization of Physical Education: Discourses of Performance." *Quest* 42, no. 1 (1990): 40–51.

Winther, Neil. "A Comprehensive Overview of Sports and Recreation Issues Relevant to Aboriginal Peoples of Canada." Paper prepared as part of the Research program of the Royal Commission on Aboriginal Peoples, 1994.

Wipper, Kirk A.W. *Retrospect and Prospect: A Record of the School of Physical and Health Education, University of Toronto, 1940–1965*. Toronto: University of Toronto, 1965.

Wright, Gordon A. "Youth Leadership through Camping and Athletics in Ontario." *Report on the Second British Empire and Commonwealth Conference on Physical Education*, Glamorgan Training College, Barry Wales, 11–17 July 1958, 14–17.

Zeigler, Earle F. *History of Physical Education and Sport*. Englewood Cliffs, NJ: Prentice Hall, 1976.

– "Jacks-of-All-Trades and Masters of None?" *CAHPER Journal* 59, no. 2 (1993): 36.

– "What Should the Field of Physical Activity Education Promote in the 21st Century?" *PHE America* 8 (September 2017).

Index

Page numbers with (f) refer to illustrations; pages with (t) refer to tables.

Aboriginal peoples. *See* Indigenous people
Acadia University, Nova Scotia, 31
Active for Life, 197
Active Living Alliance for Canadians with a Disability, 211, 263n73
adaptive physical activity, 209–12, 212(f)
adolescence, overview, 65–6. *See also* children and youth
Alberta: curriculum revisions (2000s), 192–3, 261n12; Depression-era recreation, 115–17; EDI issues, 202, 204; evaluation of school programs, 133; instructional time, 106, 190–1, 191(f); movement education, 144; neoliberalism, 193, 261n15; teacher education, 155; wellness education, 192–3, 261n12. *See also* University of Alberta
– Indigenous education: cadets, 56–7; Edmonton (St. Albert) School, 39, 153, 258–9n83; health, 52–3; reports on, 151; St. Paul's School, 46, 56–7; youth organizations, 66, 120–2
Algoma University, Ontario, 254n24
Alnwick Industrial School, Alderville, Ontario, 27, 46
Amateur Athletic Association of Canada, 33
Anglicans, 17, 25, 109, 154

approaches to teaching. *See* pedagogy
Armington, Helen Ward, 84
arts: arts culture (MES), 76, 84–6, 89, 96–7, 98–9; new kinesthetic of modernism, 78–82; voice culture, 83–4, 89. *See also* dance; Margaret Eaton School (MES), Toronto; movement education
Ashton, Robert, 42
associations and organizations. *See* children and youth organizations; professional organizations
Austin, Patricia, 210–11, 237
Australia, 14, 216

Baden-Powell, Robert and Lady, 71–2, 250n77
Bagot Commission, 25–6
Bailey, Donald, 167–8, 167(f), 239
Barker, Mary Ross, 87–8, 87(f), 102, 236
Barnes, Findlay, 153, 258–9n83
Barnjum, Frederick S., 12, 29–31, 30(f), 32(f), 34
Barnjum, Helen, 31
Bartlett, Fred, 102, 161, 237
baseball, 42–3, 44
basketball, 31, 33, 78, 212(f)
Battleford Industrial School, Saskatchewan, 39, 42–4, 43(f), 46

Beaton, Mary, 69(f)
Beers, George W., 8, 31, 33
Bélisle, René, 105, 253n13
Bergman-Österberg, Madame, 77
Birtle Residential School, Manitoba, 152(f)
Bishop, Emily, 80, 81
Black people, 5, 202, 204, 209, 218, 225
Boorman, Joyce, 144, 149(f), 240
Borden, Frederick, 49–50, 55–6
boys. *See* gender/sex
Boy Scouts, 66, 71–2, 120
Britain. *See* United Kingdom
British Columbia: cadets, 57–8; EDI issues, 202, 204; Indigenous education, 121, 151; instructional time, 106, 190–1, 191(f); movement education, 144–5; physical literacy, 197; Pro-Rec program, 112–17, 114(f), 115(f), 124, 128, 254n27; public education, 46; QDPE programs, 171–2; teacher education, 155; Vanves model (⅓ system), 13–14, 163–6, 164(f), 168. *See also* University of British Columbia
British North America Act (1867), 20, 28, 36, 38
Brock University, 265n23
Brown, G.A., 32(f)
Bryans, Helen, 95–6, 236, 253n53
Bryce, Peter, 52–3
Bukh, Niels, 104, 253n10
Byl, John, 251n3

CAAWS (Canadian Association for the Advancement of Women and Sport, *now* Canadian Women & Sport), 177, 177(f), 179
CAHPER (Canadian Association for Health, Physical Education and Recreation): fitness research, 132–3; francophones, 108; history committee, 11, 183; movement education equipment, 142; name changes, 174, 260n43; pan-Canadian curriculum, 160; publications, 130, 135, 183; QDPE recommendations, 171–3, 172(f), 190–1, 191(f), 214, 260n30; teaching resources, 142, 171. *See also* PHE Canada (Physical and Health Education Canada)
CAHPERD (Canadian Association for Health, Physical Education and Recreation and Dance), 174, 260n43

calisthenics: overview, 37–8, 41–2; facilities and equipment, 21, 41; girls, 23, 37–8, 46, 57, 59(f), 65(f); Indigenous education, 41–2, 54–5, 57, 59(f); music with, 41–2; teachers, 37–8; teaching resources, 37–8, 48, 51(f), 54–5. *See also* gymnastics
Cameron, W.A., 32(f)
camps. *See* outdoor education; summer camps
Camp Tanamakoon (MES), Ontario, 76, 90–2, 91(f), 92(f), 97, 98
Canada: British North America Act (1867), 20, 28, 36, 38; British ties, 47, 158; Confederation, 28, 47; Constitution Act (1982), 159; Depression, 100–1; federal/provincial jurisdiction, 28, 38–9, 128, 134, 215; imperialism, 47–8; militarism, 24, 47–8; multiculturalism, 158–9; national narratives, 3–5, 15–16; National Physical Fitness Act (1943), 118, 123–5, 127–8, 134, 153, 155; nationhood, 24, 46–7; neoliberalism, 193, 215–16, 261n15; pre-Confederation, 16–20, 246n2. *See also* federal–provincial–territorial relations; Indigenous and settler relations; national narratives
Canadian Association for Health, Physical Education and Recreation. *See* CAHPER (Canadian Association for Health, Physical Education and Recreation)
Canadian Association for the Advancement of Women and Sport, *now* Canadian Women & Sport (CAAWS), 177, 177(f), 179
Canadian Camping Association, 220–1
Canadian Council of University Physical Education and Kinesiology Administrators (CCUPEKA), 185–6, 198–202, 204–5, 227, 262nn, 43, 46, 262nn42, 43
Canadian Girls in Training (CGIT), 73, 120
Canadian Intercollegiate Athletic Union (*now* U SPORTS), 181
Canadian Journal of the History of Sport, 11
Canadian Kinesiology Alliance/Alliance Canadienne de Kinésiologie (CKA/ACK), 186, 201
Canadian League, 114
Canadian Parks and Recreation Association, 197

Canadian Physical Education Association (CPEA), 68, 74, 93, 98, 102–3, 126, 133
Canadian Physical Efficiency Tests, 129
Canadian Sport Policy (2012), 15, 161
Canadian Standard Efficiency Training (CSET), 71–2, 73
Canadian Women & Sport (CAAWS), 177, 177(f), 179
Canadian Youth Commission (CYC), 122–4, 255n53
Canadian Youth Congress, 120
Cartwright, Ethel Mary, 13, 50, 62–4, 63(f), 74, 88, 104, 105(f), 235
Caudwell, Margaret, 144
CCUPEKA (Canadian Council of University Physical Education and Kinesiology Administrators), 185–6, 198–202, 204–5, 227, 262nn, 43, 46, 262nn42, 43
CECM (Commission des écoles catholiques de Montréal), 104, 105, 107
Celia Jeffrey Residential School, Kenora, Ontario, 151(f)
certification of teachers. *See* teacher education; teacher education, institutions and certifications
CGIT (Canadian Girls in Training), 73, 120
character and citizenship, 66, 72–3, 127
Chatwin, Nora, 141–5, 237, 257nn45, 46, 49
child-centred learning: decline of militarism, 60; Hall-Dennis report (1968), 157; holistic approach, 227–9; meaningful physical education, 228–9; modern dance, 13, 82, 138–40, 174, 197, 228; movement education, 13, 138–41, 147–8, 228; optional vs. required courses, 162; Vanves model (⅓ system), 13–14, 163–6, 164(f), 168
children and youth: overview, 120–5; adaptive physical activity, 211–12, 212(f); adolescence as concept, 65–6; character and citizenship, 66, 72–3, 127; digital technologies, 221–3; fitness tests, 129–30, 132–3, 223–4; movement guidelines, 189; need for exercise, 167–8; optional approaches to education, 157, 162; pandemic's impacts, 188–9, 217–22; ParticipACTION, 214, 225; physical literacy, 193–4; reports on (CYC), 122–4, 255n53; statistics, 186, 189; vision of the future, 217–19. *See also* child-centred learning; education; outdoor education; physical literacy; school physical education; summer camps
children and youth organizations: overview, 65–74, 120–5; Boy Scouts, 66, 71–2, 120; CGIT (Canadian Girls in Training), 73, 120; CSET (Canadian Standard Efficiency Training), 71–2, 73; CYC (Canadian Youth Commission), 255n53; Girl Guides, 66, 72–3, 120, 121(f), 254n46; Indigenous youth, 66, 120–2; leadership training, 66–7; patriotism, 71; statistics, 120, 254n46; Woodcraft Indians, 69–71, 250n73, 250n77; YMCAs, 33–4, 60, 66–73, 67(f), 128, 129; YWCAs, 13, 68–9, 69(f), 72–3, 87(f), 88
Christianity: Anglicans, 17, 25, 109, 154; Catholics, 55; Methodists, 16–17, 24–5, 27, 84; missionaries, 24–5; moral education, 17, 20; muscular Christianity, 33; residential school operations, 27, 38–9, 111–12; Ryerson's influence, 16–17; YMCAs and YWCAs, 69, 71; youth organizations, 66, 72–3, 247n46
CKA/ACK (Canadian Kinesiology Alliance/Alliance Canadienne de Kinésiologie), 186, 201
Clark, Ruth, 64
class. *See* social class
colleges. *See* universities and colleges
Commission des écoles catholiques de Montréal (CECM), 104, 105, 107
Cosentino, Frank, 11
Couchiching, Lake, summer camps, 97, 116(f), 117, 136, 136(f), 137(f)
Council on Physical Fitness, National, 118–19, 119(f), 123–5, 127–9, 153
Coventry, Ivy, 88
COVID-19 pandemic, 188–9, 217–22
CPEA (Canadian Physical Education Association), 68, 74, 93, 98, 102–3, 126, 133
creative dance. *See* movement education
Credit Mississauga, 24–5
cricket, 42–4, 43(f)
critical pedagogy, 207–9, 227–8
Crocker, J. Howard, 11, 67–8, 67(f), 87, 235

CSET (Canadian Standard Efficiency Training), 71–2, 73
Cunningham, Jean, 142
curricula: overview, 189–93, 223–6; Alberta's revisions (2000–1, 2021), 192–3, 261n12; arts and physical culture (MES), 76, 84–6, 94–9; combined health and physical education, 190–3, 191(f); comprehensive school health (CSH), 192; consistency across provinces, 104; culturally relevant, 205–7; curricular models, 198, 224–5, 228–9, 262n33; EDI issues, 225–6; education *of* vs. *for* the physical, 225; health education, 190–1, 191(f), 196–7, 224; instructional time, 190–1, 191(f), 260n32; meaningful physical education, 228–9, 265n30; neoliberalism, 193, 215–16, 261n15; online access, 261n3; physical literacy, 196–7, 198; policy analysis framework, 224–5; political influence, 190, 192–3, 223; progression principle, 21, 37; provincial jurisdiction, 189–90, 191(f), 260n32, 261n3; *Syllabus*, 49–52, 51(f), 104; territorial adoption of provincial curricula, 190; vision of the future, 225–6; wellness education, 192, 261n12. *See also* Indigenous education; teaching and learning resources
Curry, Samuel Silas, 83
CYC (Canadian Youth Commission), 122–4, 255n53

Dalcroze, Émile Jaques-, 13, 79, 81–2, 90, 139
dance: overview, 80–1, 147–8, 173–4; child-centred approach, 13, 138, 140, 147–8, 174, 197, 228; costumes, 96–7; creative dance, 142, 144, 146, 149(f), 174; Delsartism, 13, 79–83, 193–4; eurythmics, 81–2, 90, 139; folk dance, 64, 80, 88, 96, 174; gendered preferences, 140, 146–8; Laban's approach, 13, 79, 81–2, 139–40, 139(f), 142, 144, 146, 197; modern dance, 79–82, 96–7, 138–40, 145–6, 174, 258n57; movement education, 78–82, 138–41, 144, 146–8, 149(f), 174, 258n57; physical literacy, 195(f), 196; rhythmic gymnastics, 107; *Syllabus* (1933), 174; teacher education, 145–6, 174; terminology, 146. *See also* movement education

Danish gymnastics, 104, 253n10
Davidson, Stewart, 11–12, 166, 235, 238
Davin, Nicholas Flood, 39
day schools, 24–8, 39, 46, 53–5, 112, 121, 148, 151–2, 159, 258n75. *See also* Indigenous education
Delsarte, François, 13, 79–83, 193–4
Dennis, Lloyd, 157
developmental physical activity. *See* kinesiology
Devenney, Hart, 256n32
Dewar, John, 11
Dewar, W. Alex, 68
digital technologies, 221–3
disability: overview, 209–12; ability groups, 211; adaptive physical activity, 209–12, 212(f); critical pedagogy, 207–9, 227–8; digital technologies, 223; early approaches, 31, 210; EDI issues, 202, 204, 209–12, 263n73; leaders with disabilities, 67; learning resources, 210, 263n73; legislation, lack of, 211–12; teacher education, 210–11, 212; terminology, 209–10
diversity, terminology, 230. *See also* equity, diversity, and inclusion (EDI)
drill. *See* military drill
Drover, Victoria, 259–60n26
Duncan, Isadora, 80
Duncan, Ruth, 140–1

Eaton, Margaret Wilson Beattie, 83(f), 84, 86, 97. *See also* Margaret Eaton School (MES), Toronto
Eaton Company, 84–5, 86, 93, 97
EDI. *See* equity, diversity, and inclusion (EDI)
Edmonton Residential School, St. Albert, Alberta, 39, 153, 258–9n83
Educating the Body (Hall, Kidd, and Vertinsky), 10–14
education: education *of* vs. *for* the physical, 225; holistic approach, 192, 199, 227–9; meaning in, 228–9; neoliberalism, 193, 215–16, 261n15; pandemic's impacts, 188–9, 217–22; professionalization, 94, 99; provincial jurisdiction, 36, 215; technologies, 221–3; universal education, 15–16, 19–21; vision of the future, 217–26, 232–3. *See also* physical education

- early history: overview, 19–24, 36–8, 37(t), 38(t), 45–7; educational psychology, 21, 23; historical context, 17–20, 24; moral education, 20, 23; Ontario system, 36–8, 37(t), 38(t); practical education, 26–7; private schools, 19–20; secondary schools, 45, 56; statistics, 36–8, 37(t); teachers, 36–8, 37(t); teaching resources, 21, 22(f), 23, 37–8; uniform curriculum, 19–20; universal education, 15–16, 19–21, 24, 26–7, 45. *See also* history of physical education, early history; history of physical education, 1900–1930s; Ryerson, Egerton

educational gymnastics. *See* movement education

educational psychology, 21, 23, 65–6

educators. *See* teachers

Eisenhardt, Ian (Jan), 112–13, 115–16, 118–19, 119(f), 127–8, 150–4, 150(f), 258nn71, 75, 78

elite sports. *See* sports and games, high-performance

Elkhorn Residential School, Manitoba, 56–7

Elliot, Digby, 262n41

Ellis, Margaret, 144

England. *See* United Kingdom

equipment. *See* facilities and equipment

equity, diversity, and inclusion (EDI): overview, 4–5, 202–12, 229–33; adaptive physical activity, 209–12, 212(f); CCUPEKA on anti-racism, 204–5; critical pedagogy, 207–9, 227–8; critical physical literacy, 224; critiques of ParticipACTION, 214–15; curricula, 225–6; digital technologies, 222–3; Indigenous education overview, 6–8, 202, 204–5, 226, 229–32; intersectionality, 207, 230; outdoor education, 219–21; physical literacy as inclusive, 195(f), 196; task forces on, 230–1; teaching resources, 263nn75, 76; terminology, 209–10, 230; university faculties and students, 202, 204–5; vision of the future, 217–19, 232–3. *See also* disability; gender/sex; Indigenous education; LGBTQ2S; racialized people; social justice

Europe: dance and movement, 138–40; influences on Ryerson, 21, 26; leaders in physical education, 31; movement education, 79–82, 137–8; Vanves model (⅓ system), 13–14, 163–6, 164(f), 168. *See also* Swedish gymnastics

eurythmics, 81–2, 90, 139

exercise sciences. *See* kinesiology

facilities and equipment: costs, 187; digital technologies, 221–3; gymnasiums, 134–5; for gymnastics, 21, 64; movement education, 138, 142, 143(f), 149(f); residential schools, 109–12, 110(f), 151–4; secondary schools, 134; universities, 64; YMCAs, 33–4

FAS (Fitness and Amateur Sport Directorate), 166–7, 183

federal jurisdiction for Indigenous education. *See* Indigenous education; Indigenous education, residential schools

federal-provincial-territorial relations: overview, 28, 129; cadets, 49, 56; *Canadian Sport Policy* (2012), 15; Fitness and Amateur Sport Act (1961), 132; fitness programs, 118–20, 119(f), 123–5, 126–8; funding for education, 46, 205; high-performance sports, 133, 178–9; Indigenous education, 38–9, 134; jurisdictional issues, 36, 38–9, 117, 128, 134, 171–2, 215; National Council on Physical Fitness, 118–20, 119(f), 123–5, 127–8; ParticipACTION overview, 168–70, 169(f), 214–15, 225; QDPE programs, 171–3; Sport Canada, 133; Strathcona Trust overview, 48–52; territories, 134, 190

Fellenberg, Philipp Emanuel von, 21, 26, 246n26

feminism. *See* women and girls

First Nations. *See* Indigenous people

First World War, 56–7, 88, 210. *See also* wartime

fitness: children's exercise needs, 167–8; critiques of tests, 223–4; curricula, 190–1, 191(f), 224–5; physical literacy, 128, 193–8, 195(f), 224–5, 262n22

- 1900–1945: overview, 73, 124–5; early history, 65; federal-provincial programs, 117–20, 119(f), 126–8; fitness exams, 65; national council, 118–20, 119(f), 123–5,

fitness (*continued*)
  127–8; National Physical Fitness Act (1943), 118, 123–5, 127–8, 134, 153, 155; Pro-Rec program, 112–17, 114(f), 115(f), 124, 128, 254n27; reports on youth (CYC), 122–4, 255n53; wartime shortage of fit recruits, 126; Women's League of Health and Beauty, 113–14; WWII fitness tests, 118
– 1945–1970s: critiques of, 146–8; federal-provincial programs, 126–8; Fitness and Amateur Sport Act (1961), 132; "heroic agenda," 126; media, 129–30; Prince Philip's recommendations, 130, 132, 134; public learning resources, 129; research institutes, 132; surveys and tests, 129–30, 132–3
– 1970s–2020s: overview, 13–14, 186–7, 223–5; curricula, 190–2, 223–5; digital technologies, 221–3; pandemic's impacts, 217–19; ParticipACTION overview, 168–70, 169(f), 214–15, 225, 259–60n26; QDPE programs, 171–3, 172(f), 190–1, 191(f), 214; research on children's exercise needs, 167–8; social barriers, 170; tests, 173, 223–4; Vanves model (⅓ system), 13–14, 163–6, 164(f), 168, 173
Fitness and Amateur Sport Act (Bill C-131) (1961), 132
Fitness and Amateur Sport Directorate (FAS), 166–7, 183
forest schools, 220, 264n10. *See also* outdoor education
Forster, Jean, 98
Forsyth, Janice, 244, 258n75
Foster, Ruth, 144
Fourestier, Max, 163–6

games. *See* sports and games
gender/sex: overview, 5, 176–9; biological determinism, 94–5, 96; character formation in youth, 66; competition vs. play for play's sake, 94–7; critique of ParticipACTION, 214–15; female teachers, 60, 64; high-performance sports, 178–9; human rights actions, 179; integration vs. segregation of students, 23, 36, 38, 163, 177; manliness and muscular Christianity, 33; militarism and masculinity, 35–6; school attendance rates, 45; sports culture, 175–80; sports vs. movement education preferences, 140, 146–8; universities, 179–82, 181(f); youth movements, 66. *See also* history of physical education, early history, girls; LGBTQ2S; women and girls
Germany, 31, 138–40
Gettas, Irene, 87–8
Girl Guides, 66, 72–3, 120, 121(f), 254n46
girls. *See* gender/sex; history of physical education, early history, girls; women and girls
Gjoa Haven, Nunavut, 208(f)
Godwin, Henry, 35
Goodwin, Helen, 144–5
Goodwin, Major H., 21
Graves, Mary Elizabeth, 31
Greer, Allan, 10
Grenier, Cécile, 104, 105, 107–8, 107(f), 236
gymnasia. *See* facilities and equipment
gymnastics: overview, 29–31, 36–8; Barnjum's leadership, 12, 29–31, 30(f), 32(f), 34; critiques of, 61; Danish gymnastics, 104, 253n10; early history, 21, 22(f), 36–8; eurythmics, 81–2, 90, 139; facilities and equipment, 21, 29, 31, 32(f), 37–8, 64, 138; girls and women, 23, 30–1, 32(f), 37–8, 64, 107; Indigenous education, 27; ladder pyramids, 29–30; mind–body relations, 30; movement education, 80–2; movement theory overview, 78–82; pan-Canadian curriculum, 12–13, 49–52, 52(t), 73, 104–5; Pro-Rec program, 128; rhythmic gymnastics, 107; Swedish gymnastics, 12–13, 49–50, 77–8, 107, 138, 251n7; *Syllabus,* 49–50, 51(f), 104, 138; teacher education, 64, 76; teaching resources, 21, 22(f), 23, 37–8, 51(f), 104, 251n7; uniforms and costumes, 49, 78, 113, 114. *See also* calisthenics; movement education

Hall, Emmett, 157
Hall, G. Stanley, 65–6, 70
Hall, Kathlyn, 121(f)
Hall, M. Ann, 10, 257n36
Hall-Dennis report *(Living and Learning)*, 157
Hamilton, Mary, 13, 76, 86–93, 89(f), 91(f), 92(f), 97–8, 102

Harris, Dorothy J., 239, 257n55
H'Doubler, Margaret, 145, 257n55
health: children's exercise needs, 167–8; EDI issues, 224–6; Indigenous students, 52–3, 54–5; kinesiology as health profession, 5, 186, 201–2, 226; lifestyle choices, 224; medical exams, 78; mental health, 123, 130; social determinants, 170, 224; vaccinations, 250n65
health education: overview, 224–6; Alberta's curriculum (2000s), 190–3, 191(f), 261n12; Boy Scouts and Girl Guides, 72; breathing exercises, 53, 54, 78, 80, 83; combined with physical education, 190–3, 191(f); curricula, 189–93, 191(f), 224–6; degree programs, 97–8; digital technologies, 221–3; early programs, 31; education *of* vs. *for* the physical, 225; Indigenous education, 205–7, 229–32; instructional time, 106, 190–1, 191(f); meaningful physical education, 228–9, 265n30; neoliberalism, 193, 261n15; physical literacy, 193–8, 195(f), 262n22; reports on youth (CYC), 122–4, 255n53; school curricula, 118, 190–3, 191(f); social marketing of fitness, 168–70, 169(f); teaching resources, 171–2; Vanves model (⅓ system), 13–14, 163–6, 164(f), 168, 173; wellness education, 192–3, 261n12. *See also* fitness; physical literacy
Henry, Franklin, 183–4
Higgins, Andy, 162–3
higher education. *See* universities and colleges
HIGH FIVE, 197–8
high-performance sports. *See* sports and games, high-performance
Hill, Martha, 145
Hill, Rose, 146, 174, 238, 257n45, 258n57
history of physical education: overview, 3–5, 12–14; archives, 11–12, 20, 99; author's backgrounds, 10–11; historical sources, 11–12; Indigenous peoples, 6–10, 9(f); interviews with leaders, 11–12, 235; R. Tait McKenzie Honour Award winners (1948–2023), 235–44; scholarly research, 11–12; state school programs, 3–5; terminology, 11, 14, 146, 156; universal education, 4, 15–16. *See also* Indigenous education; Indigenous education, residential schools

– early history: overview, 12, 16; Christian instruction, 26, 27; disability and activity, 210; facilities and equipment, 23–4; gymnastics and calisthenics, 21–3, 22(f), 36–8, 38(t), 41–2; historical context, 17–20, 24, 34–6; military drill, 23, 34–8, 38(t), 42; organizations, 33–4; Ryerson's influence, 16–24, 18(f), 22(f), 26–7; sports, 31–4; statistics, 36–8, 37(t), 38(t); teacher education, 23–4; teaching resources, 21, 22(f), 23, 37–8; transnational influences, 20–1, 23. *See also* education, early history; Indigenous education; Ryerson, Egerton

– early history, girls: overview, 23, 37–8; after-school sports, 33; gendered curricula, 37–8, 41; gymnastics and calisthenics, 23, 31, 36–8, 38(t), 57, 59(f); Indigenous education, 41, 59(f); military drill, 37–8, 38(t); school attendance, 45; sex segregation, 23, 36, 37–8, 41; summer camps, 116(f); teachers, 36, 60, 64; teaching resources for, 37–8. *See also* Margaret Eaton School (MES), Toronto

– 1900-1930s: overview, 12–13, 45–7, 73–4; cadets, 49, 55–8, 58(f); calisthenics, 46, 54–5; historical context, 45–7; military drill, 48, 55–62, 73; pan-Canadian curriculum, 12–13, 49–52, 52(t), 73, 104–5; professional organizations, 74; statistics, 47, 52(t); Strathcona Trust overview, 48–52, 52(t), 73; teachers, 46, 74; teaching resources, 46; wartime, 57–8, 210; youth movements, 65–73. *See also* education, early history; Indigenous education; Margaret Eaton School (MES), Toronto; Strathcona Trust

– 1930s–1945: overview, 13, 100–1, 124–5; fitness, 126–7; historical context, 67–8, 100–1; pan-Canadian curriculum, 104–5; professional organizations, 101–3; *Syllabus* as curriculum, 104; wartime, 101, 124–5. *See also* fitness; Indigenous education

– 1945–1970s: overview, 13, 126; child-centred approaches, 13, 138, 140, 148, 228; disability and activity, 210–11; "heroic agenda," 126; movement education, 13, 137–48, 149(f); school physical education, 133–7; teacher education, 135, 137–48, 155; teacher shortages, 135, 137, 141;

history of physical education (*continued*)
universities, 155. *See also* fitness; Indigenous education
- 1970s–1990s: overview, 13–14, 157–60, 186–7; child-centred approaches, 157; compulsory vs. optional courses, 157, 162, 176, 187; funding, 159, 205; Hall-Dennis report (1968), 157; high-performance sports, 178–9; kinesiology, 14, 156, 182–7; ParticipACTION, 168–70, 169(f), 197, 214–15, 218, 224–5, 259–60n26; private recreation, 158, 173; QDPE programs, 171–3, 172(f), 190–1, 191(f), 214, 260n30; sports and games, 174–82; university programs, 179–82; Vanves model (⅓ system), 13–14, 163–6, 164(f), 168; women's activism, 179–82, 181(f). *See also* fitness; Indigenous education
- 2000s–2020s: overview, 14, 188–9, 213–16; curricula, 188–93, 191(f), 223–6; curricula (2014), 190–1, 191(f); digital technologies, 221–3; EDI issues, 202–12, 225–6, 230; federal funding, 205, 213; fitness, 223–5; health and well-being, 224–6; high-performance sports, 213; Indigenous reconciliation, 205–7, 229–32; kinesiology, 226–8; marginalization of physical education, 191; meaningful physical education, 228–9; outdoor education, 219–21; ParticipACTION, 214–15, 225; Physical Activity and Sport Act (2003), 205; physical literacy, 15, 193–8, 195(f), 224–5, 262n22; research needed, 215–16; statistics, 190–1, 191(f), 201; teacher education, 198–200, 226–8; TRC calls to action, 6–8, 205, 230–1; universal physical education, 15–16. *See also* fitness

Hobday, Marion, 96
hockey, ice: federal support, 133; films, 129, 256n12; Indigenous players, 44, 55, 110, 153–5, 155(f), 208(f)
Holmstrom, Vendla M., 77–8
Houghton, E.B., 12, 37–8
Howell, Maxwell, 11, 237
Hughes, James L., 48, 56, 248n11
Hughes, Sam, 56
human kinetics. *See* kinesiology
Hutton, Maurice, 48

ice hockey. *See* hockey, ice
IEP (Institut d'éducation physique), Montreal, 107
illiteracy. *See* physical literacy
immigrants, non-British: EDI issues, 225–6; multiculturalism, 158–9; national pride, 5; settlement houses, 251n2; sports, 175; vision of the future, 217–19
inclusion terminology, 230. *See also* equity, diversity, and inclusion (EDI)
Indigenous and settler relations: abuse and hardships, 46, 101, 154–5, 159; assimilation, 7–9, 25, 39–41, 42–4, 43(f), 53–5, 92, 110–12, 148, 150, 159; Bagot Commission, 25–6; colonialism, 7–10, 28–9; cultural appropriation, 31, 33, 70–1, 90–2, 252n41; forced adoptions, 159; Indian Act, 10, 28, 153; Indigenous activism, 159; land titles, 18–19, 28; photos, analysis of, 154–5, 155(f); racial distinctions, 19; reconciliation, 6–7, 229–32; reserves, 9–10, 25, 28, 205–6; rights under Constitution Act (1982), 159; Royal Commission on Aboriginal Peoples (RCAP), 6, 111, 159–60; treaties and agreements, 10, 18–19, 28; Truth and Reconciliation Commission (TRC), 6–8, 205, 230–1; Two-Eyed seeing, 231; wartime, 57
Indigenous education: overview, 6–10, 38–41, 40(f), 46, 52–5, 148, 150–5, 159–60, 229–32; abuse and hardships, 46, 101, 154–5, 159; assimilation, 7, 25, 39–41, 42–4, 43(f), 53–5, 110–11, 148, 150, 159; attendance, 46, 54; Bagot Commission, 25–6; boarding schools, 39, 44, 46, 52–5; boys, 39–41, 40(f), 55, 110–11, 154–5, 155(f); cadets, 56–8, 58(f); calisthenics, 41–2, 53, 54–5, 59(f); Christian education, 27, 38–41, 40(f); critique of ParticipACTION, 214–15; culturally relevant curricula, 205–7; curricula, 39–41, 40(f), 53–5, 153, 190, 205–7, 225–6; day schools, 24–8, 39, 46, 53–5, 112, 121, 148, 151–2, 159, 258n75; early history, 24–5; EDI issues, 202, 204–5, 225–6, 229–32; Eisenhardt's role, 152–3; everyday life, 8–10; facilities and equipment, lack of, 13, 151–4; federal jurisdiction, 38–9, 46, 101, 134, 148, 150–3, 205; funding, 53, 101, 205; girls, 27,

41, 42, 44, 53–5, 59(f), 150, 154–5; health and wellness, 46, 52–5, 111–12, 152, 192, 205–7, 206(f), 208(f), 229–32; Indigenous authority, 152–3, 159, 206; Indspire, 231, 265n41; industrial schools, 26–8, 39–41, 40(f), 44, 46; lacrosse *(tewaarathon)*, 8–9, 9(f), 31, 33, 206(f), 245n12; military drill, 42, 54, 55, 56–8, 58(f); music, 41–2, 59(f); on-reserve schools, 205–6; physical education, 13, 27, 205; recreation and games, 42–4, 43(f), 53–5, 151(f), 152–5, 152(f), 155(f), 159–60, 206(f); statistics, 27, 39, 46, 53–5, 108, 109, 121, 151, 159, 205; teacher education, 202, 204–5; terminology for schools, 53–4; territorial adoption of provincial curricula, 190; traditional culture, 160; traditional games, 8–9, 9(f), 31–2, 44, 206(f); universities, 202, 204–5, 265n41; vision of the future, 217–19, 229–32; youth groups, 66, 120–2. *See also* Indigenous education, residential schools

– residential schools: overview, 9–10, 25–8, 39–41, 40(f), 46, 52–5, 108–12, 121, 148–55, 159; abuse and hardships, 46, 101, 110–12, 154–5, 159; assimilation, 7, 26, 39–41, 42–4, 43(f), 53–5, 110–12, 148, 150; Bagot Commission, 25–6; boarding schools, 39, 43, 44, 46, 52–5; boys, 39–41, 40(f), 55, 110–11, 154–5, 155(f); calisthenics, 41, 53, 54, 57, 59(f), 111(f), 112; church-state relations, 26–7, 38–9, 111–12; closures, 154, 159; curricula, 26–8, 39–41, 53–5, 108, 110–12; day schools, 24–8, 39, 121, 151, 159, 258n75; Eisenhardt's role, 150–1, 150(f); facilities and equipment, 109–12, 110(f), 151–4; first residential school (1831), 25; funding, 111, 152; girls, 25, 27, 41, 53, 55, 111, 111(f), 154; health failures, 46; industrial schools, 12, 26–8, 39–41, 40(f), 44, 46, 52–8, 58(f), 109–12; military drill, 42, 53–5, 56–8, 58(f); photos, analysis of, 154–5, 155(f), 259n86; physical education and recreation, 42–4, 43(f), 110–12, 150–4, 151(f), 152(f), 155(f); Ryerson's role, 24–8; statistics, 27, 39, 46, 53–5, 108, 109, 121, 151, 154, 249n26; teachers, 46, 53–4, 112, 152; terminology, 53–5; TRC calls to action, 6–8, 205, 230–1; youth groups, 66, 120–2

Indigenous people: overview, 6–10, 229–32; collective ownership, 10; health, 41, 46, 52–3, 54–5; languages, 24–5; traditional culture, 8–9, 160; women and girls, 151. *See also* Indigenous and settler relations; Indigenous education; Indigenous education, residential schools

industrial schools, 12, 26–8, 44, 46. *See also* Indigenous education, residential schools

Institut d'education physique (IEP), Montreal, 107

instructional resources. *See* teaching and learning resources

International Charter of Physical Education, Physical Activity and Sport (UNESCO), 233

International Physical Literacy Association, 194, 196, 262n22

intersectionality, 207, 230. *See also* equity, diversity, and inclusion (EDI)

interviews with leaders in physical education, 11–12, 235

Inuit, 190, 208(f)

Irwin, Marion, 144

Jackson, Dorothy, 98
Jahn, Frederick Ludwig, 21, 31
Janzen, Henry, 172
Jaques-Dalcroze, Émile, 13, 79, 81–2, 90, 139
Jarman, Robert, 126, 235, 255n1
Jones, Peter, 24–5
Journal of Education for Upper Canada, 21, 22(f), 23, 35

Kelm, Mary-Ellen, 112
Kennedy, Frank, 133
Kenora Boarding School, Lake of the Woods, Ontario, 39, 55
Kidd, Bruce, 10–11, 255n9
kinesiology: overview, 5, 156, 182–7, 198–202, 226–8; EDI issues, 202, 204–5, 230–3; health profession, 5, 186, 201–2, 226; Indigenous education, 229–32, 265n41; interdisciplinary field, 5, 183–5, 201–2, 226–7; organizations, 201–2, 227; research focus, 183–5, 226–7; shift from physical education, 5, 156, 182–7, 200–1, 226–8; statistics, 186, 201, 227; teacher education, 186, 198–9, 226–8;

kinesiology (*continued*)
  terminology, 11, 156, 184, 185; university degrees and accreditation, 156, 185–6, 198–9, 200–2, 204–5, 226–7; visions of future, 226–8
kinesthetic of modernism, 13, 78–82. *See also* movement education
King, Alan, 175–6, 178, 179
Kirchner, Glenn, 142, 257n50
Kirk, David, 14
Kraus-Weber fitness test, 129–30
Kretchmar, Scott, 228–9

Laban, Rudolf, 13, 79, 81–2, 138–40, 139(f), 142, 144, 146, 197
lacrosse (*tewaarathon*), 8–9, 9(f), 31, 33, 206(f), 245n12
Lac Seul First Nation, Ontario, 109
Lakehead University, 212, 257n52
Lamb, Arthur S., 12–13, 60–3, 61(f), 72, 74, 101–3, 117–19, 235, 250n60, 254n41
LAMPE (Learning About Meaningful Physical Education), 228–9, 265n30
Lang, Jack G., 105, 235
Lasserre, Madeleine Boss, 90
Lathrop, Anna, 75, 251n3, 257n42
Laurentian University, 11
Laval University, 31, 155
learning resources. *See* teaching and learning resources
Lee, Ernest, 128
leisure. *See* recreation and leisure
Leonidoff, Leon, 90
LGBTQ2S: critical studies, 5; heterosexual norms, 92–3, 96; lesbianism, 92–3; vision of the future, 217–19. *See also* equity, diversity, and inclusion (EDI); gender/sex
L'Heureux, Bill, 129, 256n12
Liddell, Mary, 142, 257n45
Ling, Per Henrik, 12–13, 31, 77, 78, 107, 138
literacy, physical. *See* physical literacy
Littlechild, Wilton, 6–7
London, England. *See* United Kingdom

Macintosh, Donald, 160, 161–2, 161(f), 175–6, 178, 179
Mackenzie, Jack, 165

Manitoba: combined health and physical education, 190; Depression-era recreation, 117; early history of physical education, 47; evaluation of school programs, 133; fitness of teachers, 166; instructional time, 106, 190–1, 191(f). *See also* University of Manitoba
– Indigenous education: Birtle School, 152(f); calisthenics and drill, 41–2, 57–8, 59(f); EDI initiatives, 231, 265n38; Elkhorn School, 56–7; health, 52–3; Rupert's Land (St. Paul's) School, 41, 44, 46, 57, 58(f); St. Boniface School, 41–2, 46
Manual of Drill and Calisthenics (Hughes), 48
manuals. *See* teaching and learning resources
marching drills. *See* military drill
Margaret Eaton School (MES), Toronto: overview, 13, 75–7, 85(f), 98–9; arts culture, 76, 84–6, 89, 96–7, 98–9; Camp Tanamakoon, 76, 90–2, 91(f), 92(f), 97, 98; competition vs. play for play's sake, 94–7; curriculum, 76, 84–6, 94–9; Delsartism, 82–6; Eaton Co., 84–5, 86, 93, 97; femininity, 91, 94–5; fitness, 88–93; gender/sex ideologies, 76–7, 92–6, 98–9; health, 84–5, 97–8; marriage preparation, 75, 76–7, 83, 85, 92–3, 96; M. Eaton as sponsor, 84, 85(f); Modern Girls, 76–7; movement theorists, 13, 78–82; outdoor education, 76, 90–2, 91(f), 92(f), 97, 98; physical culture, 75, 79–84; school building, 84, 85(f), 86; social class, 75, 76–7, 84, 99; sports and games, 94–5; statistics, 76, 86, 89, 93, 96, 99; teacher education, 69, 75–6, 88, 93, 97–8, 106, 117; teaching staff, 76, 89–90, 95–8; transnational influences, 82–6; University of Toronto relations, 76, 82, 88, 93, 96–9; vocational preparation, 13, 75–6, 85–6, 88, 90, 92–3, 96, 99, 117, 251n2; whiteness, 77
– principals, 13, 76. *See also* Hamilton, Mary; Nasmith, Emma Scott Raff; Somers, Florence
Martens, Fred, 172
Martin, Paul, 128
Martineau, Harriet, 23
McGill University, Montreal: degrees, 74, 155–6; facilities and equipment, 29, 78; fitness exams, 56, 65, 78; gymnastics, 29–30, 77–8; leaders, 31, 32(f), 77–8; MSPE

(McGill School of Physical Education), 62–4, 88, 102, 103–4, 249–50n53; required courses, 56, 62; Royal Victoria College, 48–9, 62, 78; sports, 180–1; teacher education, 29, 62–4, 77–8, 106, 155, 212; Wickstead Medals, 32(f); women students, 56, 62, 65, 78

McKaye, Steele, 79

McKenzie, R. Tait, 11, 31, 32(f), 64, 78, 80, 210, 235. *See also* R. Tait McKenzie Honour Award winners (1948–2023)

McMaster University, 145, 155, 185

McNeill, William, 57–8

meaningful physical education, 228–9, 265n30

men and boys. *See* gender/sex

mental health, 123, 130

MES. *See* Margaret Eaton School (MES), Toronto

Metcalfe, Alan, 11

Methodists, 16–17, 24–5, 27, 84

Métis, 6, 192, 206, 220, 226, 232

militarism: overview, 24, 34–6, 55–8, 106; Boys' Brigade, 247n46; cadets, 35, 49, 55–8, 58(f), 247n46; critiques of, 58–61, 103, 106; federal role, 49, 56, 103, 106; historical context, 24, 34–6, 49; Indigenous education, 42, 56–8, 58(f); militias, 24, 34–6; moral discipline, 49; post-WWII, 120; Strathcona Trust's support, 49, 55–6, 62, 73; university training, 56; wartime, 56–7

military drill: overview, 23–4, 34–8, 55–62, 73; as collective ritual, 57–8; critiques of, 58–61, 103, 106; girls, 23, 37–8; historical context, 24, 34–6; Indigenous education, 42, 54, 55, 56–8, 58(f); as marching in unison, 12–13, 21, 23–4, 37; masculinity, 35–6; music with, 42, 57, 59(f); Ryerson's advocacy for, 12, 21, 23–4, 35–6; Strathcona Trust, 45, 48–9, 73; teachers, 21, 24, 35, 36–8, 57, 61–3, 106; teaching resources, 23, 37–8, 106

Miller, J.R., 112

Milloy, John S., 111

missionaries, 24–5. *See also* Ryerson, Egerton

modernism, 76–82

Mohawk Institute Residential School, Brantford, Ontario, 25, 41, 56, 57, 246n28

Montreal, Quebec: CECM (Commission des écoles catholiques de Montréal), 104, 105, 107; facilities and equipment, 34; gymnastics, 29–31, 32(f), 34; IEP (Institut d'éducation physique), 107; Indigenous students, 206(f); teacher education, 106, 107–8; YMCAs and YWCAs, 34, 68. *See also* McGill University, Montreal

Mount Allison University, New Brunswick, 65(f)

Mount Elgin (Muncey) Industrial Institute, London, Ontario, 27, 46, 246n28

movement education: overview, 13, 78–82, 137–48, 143(f); child-centred approach, 138, 140, 148, 197, 228; creative dance, 142, 144–6, 148, 149(f), 174; critiques of, 146–8; Dalcroze, 13, 79, 81–2, 90, 139; Delsartism, 13, 79–83, 193–4; eurythmics, 81–2, 90, 139; expressive forms, 79–83; facilities and equipment, 138, 142, 143(f), 149(f); gendered preferences, 140, 146–8; Laban's approach, 13, 79, 81–2, 139–40, 139(f), 142, 144, 146, 197; meaningful approach, 228–9, 265n30; modern dance, 80, 82, 96–7, 138–40, 144–6, 174; modernist theory, 78–82; rhythmic gymnastics, 107; social class, 79–80; statue posing compositions, 80, 81(f); teacher education, 137–48; teaching resources, 50, 80, 138, 139–42; terminology, 11, 146; transnational influences, 13, 79–82, 137–48, 257n54. *See also* dance

MSPE (McGill School of Physical Education), 62–4, 88, 102, 249–50n53

Muncey (Mount Elgin) Institute, London, Ontario, 27, 246n28

Munro, Iveagh, 249–50n53

Munrow, A.D. (Dave), 145, 147

music: eurythmics and movement, 81–2, 90, 139; Indigenous education, 41–2, 57, 59(f). *See also* dance

Naismith, James, 31, 32(f)

Nasmith, Emma Scott Raff, 13, 76, 82–6, 83(f), 252n25, 252n26, 252n32

Nasmith, George G., 85, 252n32

National Academy of Health and Physical Literacy, 196

national associations. *See* professional organizations

National Council on Physical Fitness, 118–20, 119(f), 123–5, 127–8, 153

national narratives: overview, 3–5, 15–16, 28–9; fitness and nationalism, 170; multiculturalism, 158–9; nation-building vision, 4–5, 15–16, 21, 24, 28–9; order and discipline, 20, 22–3; universal education, 15–16, 19–21, 24

National Physical Fitness Act (1943), 118, 123–5, 127–8, 134, 153, 155

National Physical Fitness League, 117

nature. See outdoor education; recreation and leisure; summer camps

Neatby, Hilda, 147–8, 156

neoliberalism, 193, 215–16, 261n15

New Brunswick: early history, 23, 45–6; Indigenous youth, 121; instructional time, 106, 190–1, 191(f); teacher education, 155

New England Company (NEC), 25

Newfoundland and Labrador: instructional time, 106, 190–1, 191(f)

New York School of Expression, 81(f)

Nishnawbe-Aski Nation, 109

Nissen, Hartwig, 77

Noble, Hugh, 134, 144, 237, 256n31

North American Indigenous Games, 7

Northwest Territories, 134, 190

Nova Scotia: early history of physical education, 47, 64; facilities, 31; fitness, 134; instructional time, 106, 190–1, 191(f); movement education, 144; recreation centres (NFB film), 256n31; school physical education, 134, 144; Strathcona Trust, 49, 134; summer camps, 34; teacher education, 77–8, 134; women students, 64, 77; YWCAs, 68

Nunavut, 190, 208(f)

OAC (Ontario Athletic Commission), 97, 116(f), 117

OALC (Ontario Athletic Leadership Camp), 136, 136(f), 137(f), 257n36

OCE (Ontario College of Education), Toronto, 88, 95–6

Olympics: overview, 213–14; 1976 (Montreal), 178; 2010 (Vancouver-Whistler), 213; 2020 (Tokyo), 213; conduct and ethics, 214; first team, 67; gender issues, 178; media coverage, 178; Own the Podium (OTP), 213, 263–4n79; Paralympics, 213, 263–4n79; professionalization of sports, 178–9; women athletes, 178–9, 213

⅓ system (Vanves model), 13–14, 163–6, 164(f), 168, 173

online learning, 221–3

Ontario: early history, 12, 36–8; EDI issues, 202, 204; facilities and equipment, 134, 142; health and physical education, 190, 196–7; instructional time, 106, 190–1, 191(f); kinesiology, 201–2, 226; Lake Couchiching camps, 97, 116(f), 117, 136, 136(f), 137(f); leadership camps (OALC), 136, 136(f), 137(f), 257n36; movement education, 140–6; outdoor education, 220–1; pan-Canadian curriculum, 12–13, 50–1, 73; pandemic's impacts, 217, 220; physical literacy, 196–7; professional organizations, 74, 102; rural schools, 134; school physical education, 134, 179; Scouting movement, 71–2; statistics, 36–8, 37(t), 38(t), 47, 50–1, 52(t); Strathcona Trust, 48–52, 52(t); summer camps, 90–2, 91(f), 116(f), 136, 136(f), 220–1, 257n36; teacher certifications, 96, 106; teacher education, 23–4, 50–1, 109(f), 155–6; Vanves model (⅓ system), 13–14. See also Margaret Eaton School (MES), Toronto; Ryerson, Egerton

– Indigenous education: overview, 39; Alnwick School, 27, 46; Celia Jeffrey School, 151(f); Kenora School, 39, 55; military drill, 56, 57; Mohawk Institute, 25, 41, 56, 57, 246n28; Mount Elgin (Muncey) School, 27, 46, 246n28; Pelican Lake (Sioux Lookout) School, 109–12, 110(f), 111(f), 153–5, 155(f); reports on, 151; Shingwauk School, 39–41, 40(f), 112, 254n24; youth groups, 66, 121

Ontario Athletic Commission (OAC), 97, 116(f)

Ontario College of Education (OCE), Toronto, 88, 95–6, 253n53

Ontario Physical and Health Education Association (OPHEA), 74, 102

OPC (Outdoor Play Canada), 219–20

organizations, child and youth. See children and youth organizations

organizations, professional. *See* professional organizations
Osborne, Robert, 11, 237
Österberg, Madame, 77
outdoor education: overview, 219–21, 264n12; EDI issues, 219–20; forest schools, 220, 264n10; pandemic's impacts, 219–21; play-based learning, 70–1, 104; recommendations, 120; school programs, 162; summer camps, 97; Vanves model (⅓ system), 13–14, 163–6, 164(f), 168, 173; vision of the future, 219–21; Woodcraft Indians, 69–71, 250n73, 250n77. *See also* summer camps
Outdoor Play Canada (OPC), 219–20
Own the Podium (OTP), 213, 263–4n79

pandemic, COVID-19, 188–9, 217–22
Paralympics, 263–4n79
Parent Commission, 165
ParticipACTION, 168–70, 169(f), 197, 214–15, 218, 224–5, 259–60n26
pedagogy: overview, 5, 156, 226–8; ability groups, 162–3; adaptive physical education, 209–12, 212(f); child-centred approach, 13, 60, 138, 140, 148, 157, 197, 228–9; critical pedagogy, 207–9, 227–8; critical studies, 5, 10; culturally relevant, 205–7; kinesiology, 5, 156, 226–8; meaningful approach, 228–9, 265n30; PETE/PESP terminology, 199–200; play-based learning, 70–1, 104; teacher education, 199–200; Vanves model (⅓ system), 13–14, 163–6, 164(f), 168, 173. *See also* curricula
Pedagogy in Motion (Singleton and Varpalotai, eds.), 189
Pedersen, Diana, 250n70
Pelican Lake Residential School (also Sioux Lookout School), Ontario, 13, 109–12, 110(f), 111(f), 153–5, 155(f)
Penney, Marian Henderson, 237, 253n53
Percival, Lloyd, 129–30, 131(f), 256n18
Pestalozzi, Johann Heinrich, 21
PETE/PESP, terminology, 199–200. *See also* teacher education
PHE Canada (Physical and Health Education Canada): instructional time, 106, 190–1, 191(f); McKenzie award winners (1948–2023), 236–44; name changes, 174, 260n43; pandemic's impacts, 217–22; physical literacy, 195(f), 196, 197; vision of the future, 219–21
Philip, Prince, Duke of Edinburgh, 130, 132, 134, 256n20
Physical Activity and Sport Act (2003), 205
physical culture, 52(t), 60–1, 75, 79–84, 224
Physical Culture (Houghton), 37–8
physical education: overview, 3–5, 228–33; adaptive physical activity, 209–12, 212(f); combined with health education, 190–3, 191(f); culturally relevant programs, 205–7; curricula, 189–93, 191(f), 224–6; digital technologies, 221–3; EDI issues, 202–12; education *of* vs. *for* the physical, 225; as "fundamental right," 233; goals, 4, 60–1, 160–1; Indigenous education, 6–7; neoliberalism, 193, 215–16, 261n15; pandemic's impacts, 188–9, 217–22; requirements by province, 190–1, 191(f); schooling the body, 14; shift to kinesiology, 5, 156, 182–7, 200–2, 226–8; state schools, 3–5; terminology, 11, 60–1, 146, 156; universal education, 15–16, 19–21; vision of the future, 217–19, 232–3; wellness education, 192, 261n12. *See also* curricula; education; fitness; health education; history of physical education; Indigenous education; kinesiology; school physical education
physical fitness. *See* fitness
physical literacy: overview, 193–8, 195(f); critical physical literacy, 224; curricula, 196–7, 198, 224; inclusivity, 196; Indigenous culture, 207; mind–body relation, 194; PHE model, 195(f), 196; teacher education, 198; terminology, 193–4, 196, 197, 262n22
Plewes, Doris W., 128–32, 131(f), 134–5, 137, 138, 194, 235, 255n9, 256n32
Plumptre, Joyce, 87, 140, 250n60
policy analysis framework, 224–5. *See also* curricula
Posse, Nils, 77, 251n7
post-secondary education. *See* universities and colleges

power relations: critical pedagogy, 207–9, 227–8; curricular models, 224–6; schooling the body, 14
Prendergast, Winnifred, 134
Prince Edward Island: generalist vs. specialist teachers, 166; instructional time, 106, 190–1, 191(f)
private schools, 19–20, 21, 33, 187. *See also* Margaret Eaton School (MES), Toronto
private sports and recreation, 158, 173, 178
professional organizations: overview, 33, 74, 101–3, 160; CCUPEKA, 185–6, 198–202, 227, 262n43; CPEA, 68, 74, 93, 98, 102–3, 126, 133; early history, 33–4, 74, 101–2; membership difficulties, 102–3; recent new organizations, 215. *See also* CAHPER (Canadian Association for Health, Physical Education and Recreation); PHE Canada (Physical and Health Education Canada)
Pro-Rec program, 112–17, 114(f), 115(f), 124, 128, 254n27
provincial governments: curricula, 189–91, 191(f), 260n32; education requirements by province, 190–1, 191(f); instructional time, 106; jurisdiction over education, 45, 134, 215, 260n32; kinesiology as profession, 226; optional physical education (K–12), 187; recreation programs, 112–19, 114(f), 115(f); school board relations, 45–6; Strathcona Trust, 49; teaching certificates, 106. *See also* curricula; federal–provincial–territorial relations
Proyer, Valerie, 144, 257n52
Putnam, J.H., 58–9, 73
Pye, Lois, 144

QDPE (quality daily physical education), 171–3, 172(f), 190–1, 191(f), 214, 260n30
Qu'Appelle Industrial School, Saskatchewan, 39, 41, 46
Quebec: combined health and physical education, 190; Depression-era recreation, 115; EDI issues, 202, 204; educators, 106–8; generalist vs. specialist teachers, 166; Indigenous education, 151; instructional time, 106, 190–1, 191(f); lacrosse *(tewaarathon)*, 8–9, 9(f); nationalism, 4, 13, 158; professional organizations, 74; public education, 45; Quiet Revolution, 164–5; Royal Commission on Education (Parent), 165; *Syllabus,* 50, 104; teacher education, 88, 155; Vanves model (⅓ system), 13–14, 163–6, 164(f), 168, 173; YMCAs and YWCAs, 34, 68. *See also* McGill University, Montreal; Montreal, Quebec
Quebec Physical Education Association (QPEA), 74, 101–2
Queen's University, Kingston, Ontario, 56, 64, 155, 160, 161–2, 200

racialized people: overview, 4–5, 229–33; Black people, 5, 202, 204, 209, 218, 225; CCUPEKA on anti-racism, 204; critical pedagogy, 207–9, 227–8; critique of ParticipACTION, 214–15; curricula, 225–6; EDI in universities, 202, 204–5, 224–5, 230–3; multiculturalism, 158–9; vision of the future, 217–19; whiteness, 77, 209, 225–6. *See also* equity, diversity, and inclusion (EDI); immigrants, non-British; Indigenous people
Raff, Emma Scott (later Nasmith), 13, 76, 82–6, 83(f), 252nn25, 26, 252n32
Randall, Lynn, 189, 207–9
recreation and leisure: Depression-era programs, 112–19, 114(f), 115(f); facilities and equipment, 113, 115; Indigenous education, 229–32; learning resources, 129; pandemic's impacts, 217–22; ParticipACTION, 168–70, 169(f), 197, 214–15, 218, 224–5, 259–60n26; physical literacy, 195(f), 197; Pro-Rec program, 112–17, 114(f), 115(f), 124, 128, 254n27; reports on youth (CYC), 122–4, 255n53; training of instructors, 198, 231–2; Vanves model (⅓ system), 13–14, 163–6, 164(f), 168, 173; vision of the future, 219–21. *See also* children and youth organizations; fitness; outdoor education; sports and games; summer camps
religion. *See* Christianity
research insights: Vanves model (⅓ system), 13–14, 163–6, 164(f), 168, 173
residential schools. *See* Indigenous education, residential schools

resource materials. *See* teaching and learning resources
Rice Lake mission, 25, 27
Robbins, Dorothy Walker, 134, 144, 238, 245n17, 256n31
Robbins, Stuart, 171
Robinson, Daniel, 188, 189, 207–9
Ross, Marion, 249–50n53
Ross, Murray G., 255n53
Royal Commission of Inquiry on Education in Quebec (Parent Commission), 165
Royal Commission on Aboriginal Peoples, 6, 111, 159–60
Royal Commission on the Status of Women (1970), 160
Royal Victoria College. *See* McGill University, Montreal
R. Tait McKenzie Honour Award winners (1948–2023), 235–44
Rupert's Land (St. Paul's) Industrial School, Manitoba, 41, 44, 46, 57, 58(f)
Ryerson, Egerton: overview, 12, 16–25, 18(f), 233; girls' education, 23, 36; historical context, 16–21, 23–4, 28, 35–6, 246n2; Indigenous education, 16, 24–8, 246n22; Methodist missionary, 16–17, 24–5; military drill, 21, 23–4, 35–6; moral education, 20, 23; nation-building vision, 15–16, 24, 26–7; physical education, 20–4, 22(f), 27–8; *Report* (1847), 19, 26–7; superintendent of education, 16, 18, 24; teaching resources, 21, 22(f), 23–4; transnational influences on, 16, 20–1, 26, 35; universal education, 15–16, 18–21, 26–8, 233
Ryerson, E. Stanley, 97–8

Sargent, Dudley A., 80, 84–5
Sargent, Franklin H., 80
Sargent School, 86, 88, 90, 93, 94, 96
Saskatchewan: Depression-era recreation, 117; instructional time, 106, 190–1, 191(f); physical education curricula, 104, 106; teacher education, 155; Vanves model (⅓ system), 13–14, 163–6, 164(f), 168. *See also* University of Saskatchewan
– Indigenous education: Battleford Industrial School, 39, 42–4, 43(f), 46; health and education, 52–3, 151; Qu'Appelle Industrial School, 39, 41, 46
schooling the body, 14
school physical education: overview, 3–5, 15–16, 103–8, 133–7; ability groups, 162–3, 211; adaptive physical education, 209–12, 212(f); after-school recreation, 123, 187; compulsory vs. optional, 157, 162, 176, 184, 187, 189; critiques of, 102–3; curricula (2014), 190–1, 191(f); decline in physical activity, 186–7; EDI issues overview, 202–12; evaluation of programs, 133–5; facilities and equipment, 134–5, 142; funding, 46, 187, 205; gender inequalities, 175–7; goals of universal education, 15–16, 19–21; instructional time, 190–1, 191(f); outdoor education, 219–21; pan-Canadian curriculum, 104–5; pandemic's impacts, 188–9, 217–22; physical literacy, 193–8, 195(f); provincial jurisdiction, 134–5, 190, 215; QDPE programs, 171–3, 172(f), 190–1, 191(f), 214; rural schools, 133, 134, 187; secondary schools, 45, 56, 134–6, 162–3, 176, 187, 190, 191; sports, 174–9; teacher shortages, 135, 137, 141; vision of the future, 219–21. *See also* curricula; equity, diversity, and inclusion (EDI); health education; Indigenous education, residential schools; movement education; pedagogy; Strathcona Trust; teacher education; teaching and learning resources
Scott, Duncan Campbell, 53–4, 248n24
Scott, Henri-Thomas, 56
Scott Raff, Emma (later Nasmith), 13, 82–6, 83(f), 252n25, 252n26, 252n32
Scouting movement, 66, 71–2, 120
Second World War: overview, 118, 124–5; disability and activity, 210; fitness of youth, 118, 124–6; National Physical Fitness Act (1943), 118, 123–5, 127–8, 134, 155; women's army corps (CWAC), 87; youth, 120, 124–5. *See also* wartime
Seton, Ernest Thompson, 69–71, 250n73, 250n77
settings. *See* facilities and equipment
Sexton, Ella, 135

sexuality: critical pedagogy, 207–9, 227–8. *See also* gender/sex
Shawn, Ted, 80, 193–4
Shephard, Roy J., 168–9
Shingwauk Indian Residential School, Ontario, 39–41, 40(f), 112, 254n24
Siedentop, Daryl, 198
Simon Fraser University, 200–1
Sinclair, Murray, 6–7
Singleton, Ellen, 189
Sioux Lookout (Pelican Lake) Residential School, Ontario, 13, 109–12, 110(f), 111(f), 153–5, 155(f)
Six Nations Reserve, Brantford, Ontario, 25
skating, ice, 55, 110, 151(f), 153–5, 155(f)
skiing, 164(f)
Slack, Zerada, 249–50n53
Smith, Donald. *See* Strathcona, Lord (Donald Smith)
social class: overview, 4–5; access to technologies, 222; critical pedagogy, 207–9, 227–8; critique of ParticipACTION, 214–15; fear of "others," 23; high-performance sports, 179; MES students, 75, 76–7, 84, 99; movement gymnastics, 79–80; private schools, 19–20; sports organizations, 33; universal education, 19–21, 46
social Darwinism, 248n10
social justice: overview, 207–9; CCUPEKA statement on, 204–5; critical pedagogy, 207–9, 227–8; curricular models, 224–6; EDI initiatives, 230–3; vision of the future, 230–3. *See also* equity, diversity, and inclusion (EDI)
Social Justice in Physical Education (Robinson and Randall, eds.), 207–9
Somers, Florence, 13, 76, 87, 93, 94–8, 95(f)
Sport Canada, 133, 178–9, 215, 263–4n79
Sport for Life Society, 197–8, 215
sports and games: overview, 174–82, 224–5; after-school sports, 33, 174–5; competition vs. play for play's sake, 94–7; curricula, 224–5; early history, 31, 33–4, 174–5; as fundamental right, 233; gendered activities, 94–5, 175–7; girls, 33, 44, 94–5, 175–6; Indigenous education, 7–8, 9(f), 41, 42–4, 43(f), 54–5, 229–32; optional vs. required courses, 162, 176; organizations, 33; physical literacy, 195(f), 197; public learning resources, 129; secondary education, 176; statistics, 186; summer camps, 97; teachers' gendered preferences, 140, 146–8; universities, 179–82; vision of the future, 217–19
- high-performance: overview, 178–9, 213; critiques of, 213; eligibility of student athletes, 182; federal funding, 158, 214; federal–provincial–territorial relations, 132–3, 178–9; gender equity, 178–82; international games, 7, 178; Own the Podium (OTP), 213, 263–4n79; physical literacy, 194; professionalization of system, 178–9; Sport Canada, 133, 178–9; university programs, 182. *See also* Olympics
Stack, Mary Bagot and Prunella, 113–14
St. Albert (Edmonton) Residential School, 39, 153, 258–9n83
Stanley, Sheila, 142, 257nn45, 49
Statten, Taylor, 71–2
St. Boniface Industrial School, Manitoba, 41–2, 46
St. Denis, Ruth, 80
Stebbins, Genevieve, 79–80, 81(f)
St. Francis Xavier University, Nova Scotia, 64
Stones in the Sneaker (Singleton and Varpalotai, eds.), 189
St. Paul's Industrial School, Alberta, 46, 56–7
St. Paul's (Rupert's Land) Industrial School, Manitoba, 41, 46, 56–8, 58(f), 59(f)
Strathcona, Lord (Donald Smith), 48–9, 48(f), 55–6, 62, 71, 248n13
Strathcona Trust: overview, 12–13, 48–52, 233; cadets, 49, 55–6; critiques of, 58, 60–2, 103; federal–provincial relations, 49–52; film on, 248n13; girls, 51(f), 62; health education, 50; historical context, 46–8; militarism, 12–13, 45, 49, 55–6, 106; pan-Canadian curriculum, 12, 49–52, 73, 104–5; Swedish gymnastics, 12–13, 49, 77; *Syllabus*, 49–52, 51(f), 58, 61, 104, 138, 174; teacher education, 49–50, 62, 106
student-centred learning. *See* child-centred learning

summer camps: overview, 66, 136–7, 221; Camp Tanamakoon (MES), 76, 90–1, 91(f), 92(f), 97, 98; CGIT camps, 73; early history, 34, 66, 73; girls, 73, 137(f); Indigenous cultural appropriation, 70–1, 90–2, 252n41; Lake Couchiching camps, 97, 116(f), 117, 136, 136(f), 137(f); leadership camps (OALC), 136, 136(f), 137(f), 257n36; pandemic's impacts, 220–1; staff, 13, 90; statistics, 73; woodcraft, 66, 71, 250n73, 250n77. *See also* outdoor education

Swedish gymnastics, 12–13, 49–50, 77–8, 107, 138, 251n7

swimming, 31, 65, 66, 69(f)

Syllabus of Physical Exercises, 49–52, 51(f), 58, 61, 104, 138, 174

Tanamakoon, Camp (MES), Ontario, 76, 90–2, 91(f), 92(f), 97, 98

teacher education: overview, 5, 74, 155–6, 182–7, 198–200, 226–8; critical pedagogy, 207–9, 227–8; critical studies, 5, 10; critiques of, 62–3, 146–8, 156; early history, 19, 23–4; EDI issues, 202, 204–5, 212, 225–6; facilities and equipment, 64, 142; federal funding, 158, 182; fitness of teachers, 166; generalists vs. specialists, 36, 105–6, 109(f), 166, 198; holistic approach, 227–9; Indigenous reconciliation, 6–7, 205, 229–32; in-service training, 134, 141, 144, 146, 166; kinesiology overview, 156, 182–7, 198–9, 226–8; meaningful physical education, 228–9, 265n30; militarism, 60–3, 106; movement education, 137–48; national legislation, 155; PETE/PESP terminology, 199–200; physical literacy, 198; secondary school teachers, 106–7; social justice issues, 207–9, 231, 233; statistics, 198, 227; Strathcona Trust, 49–52, 62, 106; summer schools, 62, 64, 106, 117, 134, 141, 144, 252n37; Vanves model (⅓ system), 13–14, 163–6, 164(f), 168; vision of the future, 189, 217–19, 226–8; women instructors in, 60. *See also* kinesiology; Margaret Eaton School (MES), Toronto; teaching and learning resources
– institutions and certifications: overview, 106, 155, 198–9; accreditation, 185–6, 198–9, 200, 201–2, 204, 227; adaptive physical education, 212; degree and after-degree programs, 95–8, 134, 155–6, 179–80, 182–3, 198–9; EDI requirements, 204–5; Indigenous education, 205, 229–32; institutions for, 106, 262n43; MES program, 88, 93, 97–8; normal schools, 21, 23–4, 60, 106; qualifications of instructors, 60–3, 106; recommendations (CYC), 122–4, 255n53; statistics, 135, 201, 227; Strathcona certificates, 49, 50, 52, 106; university programs, 60–4, 155, 179–80, 198–9

teachers: EDI issues, 225–6; fitness of, 166; gendered preferences for activities, 140, 146–8; gender of, 35, 36, 135; generalists vs. specialists, 36, 105–6, 109(f), 135, 166, 198; military drill, 21, 24, 35, 57, 61–3, 106; QDPE programs, 171–3, 172(f), 190–1, 191(f); reduced demand for, 184, 201; shortages, 135, 137, 141; social justice issues, 207–9, 231, 233; sports coaches, 176–7, 178–9, 187; statistics, 36, 37(t), 38(t), 135, 198; Vanves model (⅓ system), 13–14, 163–6, 164(f), 168. *See also* teacher education; teaching and learning resources

teaching and learning resources: calisthenics, 37–8, 48, 54–5, 189; disability and activity, 210; films, 129, 142, 256n12; first Canadian textbook, 48; first manual, 21, 22(f), 23; for girls, 37–8; gymnastics, 21, 22(f), 23, 37–8; *Manual of Drill and Calisthenics,* 48; meaningful approach, 265n30; military drill, 37–8; movement education, 80, 138, 139–42; *Physical Culture,* 37–8; public learning resources, 129; QDPE resources, 171–3, 172(f); recent trends, 189; *Syllabus of Physical Exercises* (1911, 1919, 1933 eds.), 49–52, 51(f), 58, 61, 104, 138, 174

Teaching Physical Education Today (Robinson and Randall, eds.), 189

technologies, digital, 221–3

teens. *See* children and youth

terminology: adaptive physical activity, 209; equity, diversity, and inclusion, 230; kinesiology, 11, 156, 184; movement, 11; movement education, 146; outdoor education, 220; persons experiencing

terminology (*continued*)
　　disability, 209–10; physical education, 156; physical literacy, 193–4, 196, 197, 262n22; schooling the body, 14; wellness, 192
territories: adoption of provincial curricula, 190; federal jurisdiction, 134
tewaarathon (lacrosse), 8–9, 9(f), 31, 33, 206(f), 245n12
Tilley, Anne, 145, 257n54
time for instruction, 106, 190–1, 191(f)
tobogganing, 152(f)
Toronto. *See* Ontario
track and field, 66, 97, 131(f), 165
Trail Rangers, 72, 120
training teachers. *See* teacher education
Trudeau, Pierre, 159
Truth and Reconciliation Commission (TRC), 6–8, 205, 230–1
Tudor-Hart, Edith, 257n40
Tuxis Boys, 72, 120
Tyrrell, Joyce Plumptre, 87, 140, 250n60

Ullmann, Lisa, 139
Unemployment and Agricultural Assistance Act (1937), 114–15
UNESCO, 11, 251n14, 258n71
United Kingdom: Boys' Brigade, 247n46; Boy Scouts, 71–2; Chelsea College, 64, 141; child-centred approach, 137–8; elite schools, 19–20, 21; girls' physical education, 23, 77; movement education, 137–47; Prince Philip's recommendations for Canada, 130, 132, 134; Swedish gymnastics, 49–50, 77; *Syllabus,* 51(f); teacher education, 64, 77, 89, 137–46; Women's League of Health and Beauty, 113–14
United States: curricular models, 198, 262n33; Delsartism, 13, 79–83, 81(f), 193–4; fitness, 129, 146; Indigenous education, 39; meaningful education, 228–9; modern dance, 80, 96–7, 145–6; movement education, 79–80, 145–6, 148; physical literacy, 196; summer camps, 90; teacher education, 94, 145, 252n37; Woodcraft Indians, 69–71, 250n73, 250n77; YMCA leadership training, 66, 67
Université de Montréal, 132

universities and colleges: overview, 5, 155–6, 226–8; activism, 179–81, 181(f); critical pedagogy, 207–9, 227–8; dance studies, 145, 146, 174; degree programs, 74, 97–8, 155–6, 179–80, 182–3, 258n57; EDI issues, 202, 204–5, 225–6, 229–32; Indigenous education, 202, 204–5, 229–32; integration of women's and men's departments, 179, 180, 182; kinesiology overview, 182–7, 198–202, 226–8; pay-for-play, 180; physical education, 62–5, 179–82; racialized people, 202, 204–5; research focus, 132, 183–5, 199; shift from physical education to kinesiology, 5, 156, 182–7, 200–2, 226–8; sports and games, 33, 179–82; statistics, 101, 201, 258n57; teacher education, 60–4, 155, 179–80, 198–201, 226–8; women students, 64, 179–82. *See also* kinesiology; Margaret Eaton School (MES), Toronto; teacher education; teacher education, institutions and certifications
University of Alberta: disability studies, 210–11, 212; evaluation of school programs, 133; fitness research institute, 132; Indigenous education, 231–2; kinesiology, 186(f), 201, 226–7, 231–2; military training, 56; movement education, 144; physical drill, 56; sports, 11, 180–1; teacher education, 155, 210–11, 212, 231–2
University of British Columbia: archives, 11; EDI task force, 231; movement education, 144–5; Pro-Rec, 115(f); sports, 180–1; teacher education, 155, 253n53
University of Manitoba, 133, 231, 265n38
University of Montreal, 155
University of New Brunswick, 155
University of Ottawa, 155
University of Saskatchewan, 63, 74, 104, 106, 132, 155, 167, 167(f)
University of Toronto: degrees, 74, 155–6; EDI task force, 230–1; fitness, 65, 132; kinesiology, 201; MES relations, 82, 88, 93, 96–9; statistics, 108; teacher education, 88, 106, 108, 109(f), 155; team sports, 180–1
University of Waterloo, 156, 200
University of Western Ontario (UWO) (*now* Western University), 11, 67–8, 87, 130, 155, 184, 203

University of Windsor, 11
U SPORTS (*was* Canadian Intercollegiate Athletic Union), 181

Vanves model (⅓ system), 13–14, 163–6, 164(f), 168, 173
Varpalotai, Aniko, 189
Vertinsky, Patricia, 10–11

Walker, Dorothy (later Robbins), 134, 144, 238, 245n17, 256n31
Wall, Ted, 211
Warrell, Eileen, 142
wartime: disability and activity, 210; First World War, 56–7, 88, 210; Indigenous soldiers, 57. *See also* militarism; Second World War
Waterloo, University of, 156, 200
Watkinson, Jane, 211
Watt, Tom, 162–3
Weir, George M., 60, 73, 113, 115–16
wellness education, 192–3, 261n12. *See also* health education
Western University (*was* University of Western Ontario), 11, 67–8, 87, 130, 155, 184, 203
Whitehead, Margaret, 194
whiteness, 77, 202, 204–5, 209, 225–6
Whitton, Charlotte, 152
wilderness. *See* outdoor education; summer camps
Wilson, Marie, 6
Wiseman, Evelyn, 145
women and girls: activism, 179–82, 181(f); biological determinism, 94–5, 96; competition vs. play for play's sake, 94–7; critical studies, 5; domestic training, 23; early history, 19, 28–9, 30–1, 32(f); EDI issues, 202, 204; femininity, 91, 94–5; feminism, 160, 175; high-performance sports, 178–9; Indigenous cultural appropriation, 90–2; inequalities, 175–7; Modern Girls, 76–7; sex segregation, 23, 36, 179; sports culture, 175–9; sports organizations, 33; university students, 64; YWCAs, 13, 68–9, 69(f), 72–3, 87(f), 88. *See also* gender/sex; history of physical education, early history, girls; Margaret Eaton School (MES), Toronto
Women's League of Health and Beauty, 113–14
woodcraft youth groups, 69–71, 250n73, 250n77
Workers' Sports Association, 4–5
Wreyford, Constance, 84
Wright, Gordon, 141, 142, 237

YMCA (Young Men's Christian Association), 33–4, 60, 66–73, 67(f), 128, 129
youth. *See* children and youth; children and youth organizations
Youth Training Act (1939), 115
Yukon Territory, 134, 190
YWCA (Young Women's Christian Association), 13, 68–9, 69(f), 72–3, 87(f), 88

Zeigler, Earle F., 130, 148, 184, 203–4, 203(f), 204(f), 238

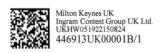

Milton Keynes UK
Ingram Content Group UK Ltd.
UKHW051922150824
446913UK00001B/1